CARDIOTONIC DRUGS

BASIC AND CLINICAL CARDIOLOGY

Series Editors

Henri Denolin, M.D.

Director of Cardiological Research Center
Hôpital Universitaire Saint-Pierre
Brussels, Belgium

H. J. C. Swan, M.D., Ph.D.

Director, Department of Cardiology
Cedars-Sinai Medical Center
Los Angeles, California

Other Volumes in Preparation

CARDIOTONIC DRUGS
A Clinical Survey

Edited by

CARL V. LEIER

OHIO STATE UNIVERSITY
COLLEGE OF MEDICINE
COLUMBUS, OHIO

MARCEL DEKKER, INC.   New York • Basel

LIBRARY OF CONGRESS CATALOGING-IN-PUBLICATION DATA

Cardiotonic drugs.

   (Basic and clinical cardiology; v. 7)
   Includes index.
   1. Cardiotonic agents. I. Leier, Carl V., [date]
II. Series. [DNLM: 1. Cardiotonic Agents—therapeutic
use. 2. Heart Failure, Congestive—drug therapy.
W1 BA813St v. 7 / QV 150 C2655]
RM349.C38 1986 615'711 86-8983
ISBN 0-8247-7611-9

MARCEL DEKKER, INC.
270 Madison Avenue, New York, New York 10016

Current printing (last digit):
10 9 8 7 6 5 4 3 2 1

PRINTED IN THE UNITED STATES OF AMERICA

To the families of the contributing authors and my own, my wife, Jolene, and my children, Rachel, Andrew, and Joseph, who, in their special way, have contributed greatly to medical research and to the betterment of humankind

Introduction

Inotropic drugs are used extensively for the support of the cardiovascular system, acutely or chronically compromised by ventricular dysfunction. In the past two decades, the availability first of the catecholemines and other sympathomimetic agents, followed by drugs with completely different forms of action (e.g., phosphodiesterase inhibitors) have given the treating physician a great many options in place of, or in addition to, management with the digitalis-like glycosides.

Dr. Leier and his collaborators have provided a comprehensive review of the extensive literature on each of these several classes of positive inotropic drugs. The authors, with their extensive investigative background in clinical pharmacology and bedside investigation, bring together a wealth of experience in a concise presentation. The complex interaction of each of these agents, dosage and dose scheduling, and application in specific subgroups of patients with heart failure is summarized. This should materially assist the cardiology consultant and clinical teacher alike. The role of digitalis is importantly reevaluated and these compounds remain useful. The constraints and precautions identified for this agent, now 200 years with us, apply also to a greater or lesser extent to other cardiotonic drugs.

Great current interest in cardiotonic drugs is their possible role in the earlier (subclinical) phases of ventricular dysfunction. Information to this point is eagerly awaited, since the long-term outcome in Class IV patients remains unsatisfactory.

Cardiotonic Drugs fulfills the broad objective of the "Basic and Clinical Cardiology" series in the provision of a succinct account of a clinically relevant, yet complex, topic.

H. J. C. SWAN

v

Preface

It is the intent of this book to provide to basic and clinical scientists and practicing physicians a comprehensive current treatise on the group of cardioactive drugs generally referred to as "positive inotropes." The emphasis is placed on clinical studies and the application of the findings of these clinical investigations to the management of patients with cardiac failure. Basic laboratory investigations are utilized to present data on mechanisms of action, metabolism, drug disposition, and other information not available or not well defined in humans.

The contributing authors were selected by the editor on the basis of their long-standing interest in a particular inotropic agent (e.g., "Digitalis" by Richard P. Lewis) or because of the author's investigative experience with an inotrope (e.g., phosphodiesterase inhibitors by Barry F. Uretsky). Expertise as a clinical investigator, integrity as a scientist, and honesty as a reporter were additional mandatory requirements. Each author is an active and excellent clinician.

The editor is most grateful for the contributions made by these authors, not only for their splendid chapters, but also for their contributions to the clinical investigation of cardiac-myocardial failure and the treatment thereof. The contributing authors and editor thank H.J.C. Swan, M.D., Ph.D., Series Editor, and Marcel Dekker, Inc. for the privilege of writing and assembling this treatise.

CARL V. LEIER

Contributors

Philip F. Binkley, M.D. Assistant Professor of Medicine and Radiology, Division of Cardiology, Ohio State University College of Medicine, Columbus, Ohio

Harisios Boudoulas, M.D. Professor of Medicine, Division of Cardiology, Ohio State University College of Medicine, Columbus, Ohio

Robert DiBianco, M.D. Associate Clinical Professor of Medicine, Georgetown University, Cardiology Staff, and Director, Cardiology Research Clinics, Veterans Administration Medical Center, Washington, D.C., and Washington Adventist Hospital, Takoma Park, Maryland

Philip C. Kirlin, M.D. Assistant Professor of Medicine, Cardiology Section, Michigan State University, East Lansing, Michigan

Carl V. Leier, M.D. James W. Overstreet Professor of Medicine and Pharmacology, Division of Cardiology, Ohio State University College of Medicine, Columbus, Ohio

Richard P. Lewis, M.D. Professor of Medicine, Division of Cardiology, Ohio State University College of Medicine, Columbus, Ohio

Donald V. Unverferth, M.D. Associate Professor of Medicine, Division of Cardiology, Director, Cardiology Research, Ohio State University College of Medicine, Columbus, Ohio

Barry F. Uretsky, M.D. Associate Professor of Medicine, Department of Medicine, University of Pittsburgh School of Medicine, Co-Director, Cardiac Catheterization Laboratories, Presbyterian-University Hospitals, Pittsburgh, Pennsylvania

Contents

CARDIOTONIC DRUGS

1

The "Cardiotonic" Agents
An Introduction

CARL V. LEIER
Ohio State University College of Medicine, Columbus, Ohio

"Cardiotonic drugs" is a rather broad term used to denote those agents which change cardiac contractility. It is generally assumed that the change is in a "positive" direction, that is, an increase in contractility. "Negative" cardiotonic drugs or agents which decrease contractility (for example, beta blockade, certain calcium channel blockers) will not be addressed. In this work, "positive inotropic" will be used in place of "cardiotonic" because the former term is somewhat more specific and more current.

The common denominator for virtually all forms of low-output congestive heart failure is depression of myocardial contractility. The loss of contractility results in a reduction in stroke volume, cardiac output and organ perfusion. The human organism responds to this threatening situation by activating the sympathetic nervous system and the renin-angiotensin-aldosterone axis. Although these responses may improve some aspects of cardiovascular function (for example, contractility, ↑ preload to augment ventricular function), if the responses are excessive they result in further deterioration of cardiovascular function through vasoconstriction (↑ afterload) and excess fluid retention (↑ preload). Therapeutic interventions may, therefore, be directed at curbing the body's responses to low output or at treating the underlying culprit, depression of myocardial contractility. The former intervention is accomplished by afterload reduction (vasodilators) and preload reduction (diuretics and venodilators) and the latter by positive inotropic agents ("cardiotonics").

Positive inotropic agents or positive inotropes are compounds that improve myocardial contractility through a direct action on the myocardial cell. These agents are not to be confused with drugs that indirectly improve contractility; for example, afterload-reducing agents may improve ventricular contraction by reducing systemic vascular resistance and aortic impedance without directly

1

stimulating the myocardium. The common cellular mechanism of action for the positive inotropes involves the release, utilization, and/or sequestration of intracellular calcium; these events are regulated by calcium channels, various sarcolemmal and intracellular proteins and enzymes, and cyclic AMP. Positive inotropes may augment contractility by altering Na-Ca kinetics through inhibition of Na-K ATPase (for example, digitalis), by increasing cyclic AMP through activation of adenylate cyclase (for example, beta-adrenergic agonists, glucagon), or inhibition of phosphodiesterase (for example, milrinone, MDL 17043), and by other, yet undescribed, mechanisms (for example, myocardial alpha-adrenoceptor agonist effect). The cellular and biochemical mechanisms of inotropy, as they relate to various drug groups, will be discussed further by each contributing author.

Positive inotropic therapy is directed at augmenting contractility in states of depressed cardiac contraction and function. The investigative and clinical methodology used to establish and quantitate the level of depressed cardiac contractility and to assess improvement in the inotropic state with therapy is critical to the study and presentation of cardiotonic drugs; the methods and major issues involved in analyzing inotropy of the myocardium in human subjects are discussed in Chap. 2.

The clinical role of acute inotropic intervention (Chap. 3) is fairly well delineated. This form of therapy is indicated for short-term support of severe and/or acute cardiac-ventricular dysfunction; by "short-term" is meant until the problem resolves spontaneously or the patient undergoes a definitive procedure (such as cardiac surgery). The role of chronic positive inotropic therapy in the management of chronic heart failure is less well defined. Positive inotropic therapy is often regarded as the approach that "whips a tired horse," an expression which in my view is comparable in validity and wisdom to the saying "If men were meant to fly, they would have been born with wings." Unfortunately, the "time-tested" use (200-year life span) of digitalis does not directly address this issue; many of the beneficial clinical effects of digitalis in heart failure are probably mediated via noncardiac and noninotropic properties (such as modulation of the autonomic nervous system, resetting of baroreceptors, and renal effects). Nevertheless, investigation into improving chronic inotropic therapy should continue with the assumption that a positive inotrope can be developed to improve cardiac function well above any harmful effects or that an inotrope can be formulated to deliver other beneficial effects (for example, selective vasodilation of coronary or renal vascular beds, myocardial cellular repair, and peripheral conditioning response) in addition to improving contractility. Of course, the ultimate therapy for myocardial failure must be designed to prevent or eradicate the underlying cause(s) prior to the development of cardiac-ventricular dysfunction.

A substantial number of endogenous substances (such as hormones, calcium) are capable of augmenting cardiac contractility. Although the primary role of these substances is to maintain overall homeostasis of the organism, they may be released in excess in certain disease states (for example, hyperthyroidism) and are occasionally administered as positive inotropic intervention (such as calcium, glucagon). Chapter 8 provides a unique discussion of endogenous positive inotropic substances whose role in normal health and in the pathophysiology and therapy of heart failure is beginning to unfold.

2

Measurement of Myocardial Inotropy

PHILIP F. BINKLEY AND HARISIOS BOUDOULAS
Ohio State University College of Medicine, Columbus, Ohio

At the most fundamental level, the inotropic state of the ventricle is determined by the characteristics of individual sarcomeres. The collective effects of such individual characteristics are studied in the laboratory by examination of isolated muscle strips. Under such conditions, the many factors that influence inotropy may be individually controlled so that the effect of a single variable may be determined. Extrapolations of these fundamental laboratory techniques comprise the basis for inotropic parameters employed in the clinical setting. However, clinical scientists are limited in that they are not afforded total control of the complex interaction of variables that may alter inotropy. Consequently, they are forced to rely on inotropic indices that are not pure in their measurement of the intrinsic inotropic state of the ventricle. Much like the ancient alchemists who futilely attempted to arrive at the formula for gold, clinicians have for many years attempted to find the ideal inotropic index that is independent of extrinsic factors. Although clinical techniques for the measurement of inotropy have become increasingly refined, there probably will never be an ideal inotropic formula.

I. FUNDAMENTAL PRINCIPLES

Indices of inotropy used in the clinical setting may be likened to measurements obtained from isolated strips of myocardium (Fig. 1) (1-4). In such preparations, the muscle strip is connected to a gauge that measures force. At rest the force measured by the gauge is termed *preload*. The magnitude of the preload will be determined by the initial length of the muscle strip (Fig. 1A) (5).

If the muscle strip is then stimulated to contract, but is held at a constant length, a force greater than that measured at rest will result. This is termed an *isometric*

5

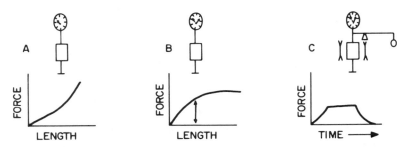

FIGURE 1   Contraction of an isolated muscle strip. A. Resting tension of the
muscle prior to contraction is termed the preload and is determined by length of
the muscle strip. B. The muscle strip contracts without a change in length in an
isometric contraction. C. Muscle contracts and shortens against a constant load in
an isotonic contraction.

contraction, and the magnitude of force generated is related to the initial length
of the muscle strip (Fig. 1B) (1,3,4). On a cellular level, this contraction is related
to the overlap of actin and myosin filaments within the individual sarcomeres. As
the length of the muscle strip increases, each sarcomere is stretched, resulting in
an increase in the number of overlapping actin and myosin filaments. This results
in a greater generation of force at the time of contraction (6). As the muscle is progressively stretched, the optimal degree of filament overlap is attained, and no increase in contractile force results from further increases in length (1,5).

In part C of Figure 1, a weighted lever is attached to the muscle strip, which is
then stimulated to contract and allowed to shorten. A brief period of time is required before the muscle generates sufficient force to overcome the weight (isometric contraction). As the force generated by the muscle becomes equal to that
exerted by the weight, muscle shortening occurs. The muscle will shorten to a
length at which the force generated is equal to the weight. The force exerted by
the weight and against which the contracting muscle must work is termed the *afterload*. Because the force generated by the muscle during shortening is constant, this
phase of contraction is referred to as isotonic (3-5).

In the above discussion and in Figure 1, the force generated by or the degree of
shortening of the muscle strip were used as indices of performance. Another important characteristic of myocardial function involves not only the absolute force
generated or the degree of muscle shortening, but the time over which force generation and muscle shortening occurs (2). As shown in Figure 2, in an isolated muscle
strip the velocity of muscle shortening reflects the additional dimension of time.
Figure 2 illustrates changes in the velocity of isotonic muscle shortening with increasing levels of preload and afterload. It is noted that as preload increases, the
velocity of shortening increases. In contrast, as afterload increases, the velocity of

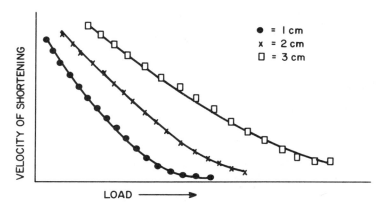

FIGURE 2   Velocity of fiber shortening in isotonically contracting isolated muscle strips with varying initial length (preload) and afterload (see text).

shortening decreases until a level of afterload is attained at which no shortening occurs and an isometric contraction results. It is important to note that the inotropic state of the muscle strip is the same in the three lines demonstrated in Figure 2. Thus, initial muscle length will influence an index of myocardial performance, such as rate of muscle shortening, without a change in inotropy. Similarly, the rate of muscle shortening varies with preload and afterload even though inotropy is constant (3-5).

Nakamura and Wiegner (7) studied the factors that control the duration of the phases of systole in an isolated rat papillary muscle preparation. They found that the duration of the sequential phases of the cardiac cycle in the isolated muscle strip responds consistently to alterations in preload and total load. Thus, increased preload causes an abbreviation in the preshortening (pre-ejection) period and an increase in the duration of the isotonic (ejection) phase with minor lengthening of total electromechanical systole. The ratio of the preshortening period to the isotonic phase thus decreases with increased preload. Increases in total load induce opposite changes with little influence on the duration of electromechanical systole (7).

Figure 3 demonstrates the situation in which initial muscle length and levels of afterload remain constant, but inotropy is changed. The initial curve indicates the velocity of muscle shortening in an isolated muscle strip at increasing levels of afterload. After an increase in inotropy, as may be provided by addition of an agent such as norepinephrine, the entire curve is shifted to the right. This indicates that with identical initial muscle lengths and equal levels of afterload, a greater velocity of muscle shortening results. Therefore, a measure of myocardial performance, such as velocity of shortening, may vary due to changes in initial length, afterload, or inotropic state (1-5).

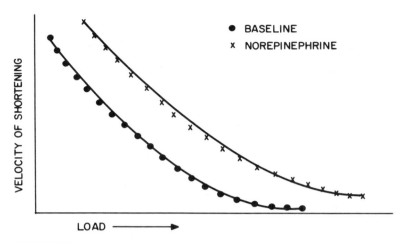

FIGURE 3 Velocity of fiber shortening in an isolated muscle strip with increasing afterload at baseline and after norepinephrine infusion. With increased inotropy, shortening velocity is increased for a given level of afterload and the entire curve is displaced above baseline.

Figure 4 demonstrates conditions in the intact ventricle analogous to those described for isolated muscle strips. In part A of Figure 4 the preload of the ventricle is determined by the volume of blood entering the ventricle during diastole. As filling occurs, ventricular volume increases as does intraventricular pressure. This is depicted in the bottom graph and is analogous to augmenting preload in the isolated muscle strip (Fig. 1A) (3-5). At the onset of ventricular contraction (Fig. 4B) both the mitral and aortic valves close. The ventricle now contracts with essentially unchanged volume, but it generates an increased pressure (this is depicted in the bottom graph by a vertical arrow). The situation resembles the isometric contraction of the isolated muscle strip (Fig. 1B) and in the intact ventricle it is termed an *isovolumic contraction* (1,3-5,8). Finally, as the pressure generated by the ventricle equals that exerted by the blood in the systemic circulation, the aortic valve opens and blood is ejected with a decrease in ventricular volume (Fig. 4C, arrow pointing from right to left). Ventricular volume continues to decrease until the left ventricular pressure equals the pressure in the systemic circulation. This phase of ventricular contraction is equivalent to isotonic shortening in the isolated muscle strip (Fig. 1C) (8).

The composition of the pressure/volume relations in the three phases of ventricular contraction describes the pressure/volume loop of the ventricle during a cardiac cycle (Fig. 5) (4,8-10). In diastole, pressure increases as volume in the ventricle increases with diastolic filling. As isovolumic contraction occurs, there is further increase in pressure without change in volume. As the pressure becomes

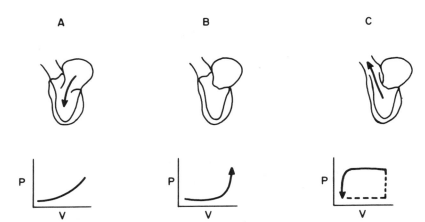

FIGURE 4   Phases of contraction in the intact ventricle (top panel) and corresponding changes in pressure and volume (bottom panel). A. Diastolic filling and determination of preload. B. Isovolumic contraction prior to opening of aortic valve. C. Opening of aortic valve and isotonic contraction (see text for details).

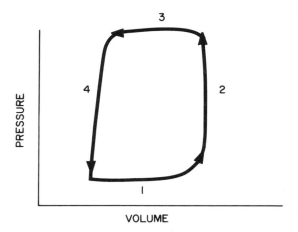

FIGURE 5   Ventricular pressure/volume curve. 1. Diastolic filling with increase in diastolic pressure. 2. Isovolumic contraction increase in pressure without volume change. 3. Ventricular ejection—decrease in volume equals the stroke volume. 4. Isovolumic relaxation decrease in ventricular pressure without change in volume during isovolumic relaxation.

equal to afterload, ejection occurs and ventricular volume decreases. The volume ejected during this period is the stroke volume of the contraction. At the completion of ejection, the ventricle relaxes without change in volume (downward-pointing arrow) indicating a period of isovolumic relaxation which precedes diastolic filling (8).

The effects of preload, afterload, and inotropy on contraction of the intact ventricle are shown in Figure 6. The influence of preload is illustrated in part A. It can be seen that increasing preload increases the rate of shortening of the ventricular wall during the isometric contraction and accelerates the rate of pressure development (3,4,5). In addition, the maximum pressure is increased. Thus, the effect of preload in the intact ventricle is similar to that observed in the isolated

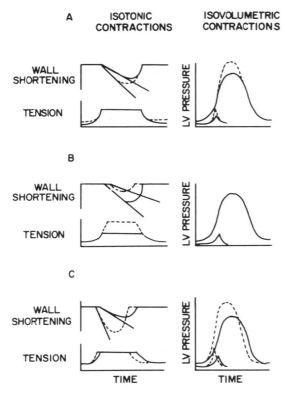

FIGURE 6   Effects of preload (A), afterload (B), and inotropic state (C) on rate of wall shortening, tension development, ventricular pressure, and rate of pressure development in intact ventricle (see text). (From E. Braunwald, ed., *Heart Disease*, 2nd ed., Philadelphia, Saunders, 1984, used with permission.)

muscle strip. Increasing afterload is accompanied by a decline in the rate of wall shortening as illustrated in part B of Figure 6 (2,4). This occurs despite a constant preload between contractions and with an unchanged inotropic state. The response of the intact ventricle to variations in afterload parallels that of the isolated muscle strip illustrated in Figure 2. Increasing the inotropic state of the ventricle results in an acceleration of muscle shortening and in an increase in the rate and amplitude of pressure development (Fig. 6C) (2,4,8). These events occur without changes in preload or afterload and resemble the enhanced rate of muscle shortening illustrated in Figure 3. Therefore, in a fashion similar to that of the isolated muscle strip, the measures of ventricular performance fall under the influence of preload, afterload, and inotropic state. Any one of these factors may independently alter measurements of ventricular performance (4,8).

Unlike bench laboratory conditions, in which individual factors affecting ventricular function may be selectively controlled, the clinical setting is complicated by the inability to completely control these individual influences. It is difficult to ascribe a change in ventricular performance purely to loading conditions or to an alteration in inotropic state. Clinical measures of inotropy have attempted to isolate these factors. As will be seen, many such indices have been proposed. Each in its proper place provides an insight into inotropy, yet none purely reflects this elusive entity.

II. LEFT VENTRICULAR PERFORMANCE

As stated earlier, left ventricular function is related not only to the intrinsic contractile state of the myocardial cells but also to the loading conditions. In addition, neural (autonomic) and endocrine factors, through their actions on loading and myocardial function, play a dominant role in modulating cardiac performance in an intact cardiovascular system (1,9,11,12).

An understanding of the determinants of the release of contractile energy in terms of the force, length, and rate of cardiac muscle contraction is essential to an interpretation of commonly employed hemodynamic parameters such as stroke volume, stroke work, ejection fraction, systolic time intervals, and the time derivatives of pressure, flow, and volume. As knowledge of such variables increases, our ability to reliably employ appropriate methodologies assessing myocardial contractility will also improve.

Abnormalities of the contractile function of the heart may result in diminished force generated by the myocardium, diminished degree of myocardial wall shortening, diminished volume of blood delivered to the circulation, and abnormal temporal relationships of the phases of contraction.

Indices used to assess ventricular performance are thus based on (1) the capacity of the heart to pump blood, (2) its ability to generate force, (3) the degree of shortening with each contraction, (4) the temporal relationships of contraction, and (5) combinations of these parameters.

A. Determination of Left Ventricular Function Based on Cardiac Output and Indices Primarily Dependent on Cardiac Output: The Frank-Starling Mechanism

1. Cardiac Output

Cardiac output is defined as the amount of blood ejected per unit of time, usually expressed in liters per minute. Output is calculated as the product of heart rate and stroke volume (8,9,13). Stroke volume is the difference between end-diastolic volume and end-systolic volume. Customarily, cardiac index (cardiac output per square meter of body surface area) and stroke index (stroke volume per square meter of body surface area) are used because the cardiac output and the stroke volume are generally proportional to the body surface area (4,9,13).

Of the various methods available, the direct Fick, the indicator dilution, and the thermodilution methods have established themselves as the standard techniques for the measurement of the cardiac output because of their accuracy, safety, reproducibility, and relative simplicity (13-17).

Cardiac output can also be measured indirectly using Doppler ultrasound techniques (18-20). It must be stressed that Doppler methods measure blood velocity and not blood flow, although the two may be closely related. In order to calculate flow, it is necessary to know the cross-sectional area of the vessel in which flow occurs, and the flow velocity profile (19,20). Although estimates of these factors may be made in conjunction with Doppler studies, this technique requires further refinement and validation (19).

Although cardiac output is commonly used as an index of ventricular function, it is a relatively insensitive parameter (13). In addition to the state of myocardial contractility, it is modified by many other factors, such as systemic oxygen requirements, circulating blood volume, mechanical loads (valvular disease, shunts), blood hemoglobin content and oxygen saturation, hormonal milieu, and other factors (8,9,11-13).

2. The Frank-Starling Mechanism

It is generally accepted that the relation of the end-diastolic volume to the stroke volume is governed by the Frank-Starling mechanism, which states that the mechanical energy expended depends on the length of the muscle fiber at end-diastole (preload) (8,21-27). For any given preload, the end-systolic volume is affected by the myocardial contractility and the afterload (5,8,24,25).

Simultaneous measurements of cardiac output and ventricular filling pressure provide more information regarding left ventricular function than measurement of cardiac output or pressure alone. With alterations in afterload and/or preload, serial determinations of cardiac output and ventricular filling pressures may be used to construct ventricular function curves (Fig. 7) (2,28). In normal subjects, small decreases in left ventricular filling pressure result in marked diminution of

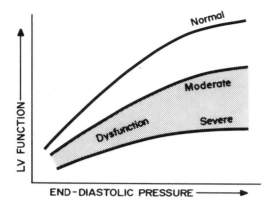

FIGURE 7 Effect of preload on left ventricular function. Ventricular function curves in normal subject and in patients with moderate and severe left ventricular (LV) dysfunction.

stroke volume. In contrast, in patients with severe left ventricular dysfunction, a large decrease in an elevated end-diastolic pressure may result in little or no change of stroke volume, indicating a plateau position on a depressed ventricular function curve (2,3,5,9).

The response to an increase in afterload produced by infusions of angiotensin or methoxamine or by isometric exercise provides further information regarding the ventricular function curve. Despite the increased resistance to left ventricular ejection, stroke volume increases or remains unchanged in normal subjects. In contrast, in patients with left ventricular dysfunction, a significant decrease in stroke volume results (Fig. 8) (4,28).

Because of the limitations of cardiac output as an index of myocardial contractility, several other indices based on cardiac output have been derived. These indices take into consideration time (mean systolic ejection rate), afterload (left ventricular work), preload and afterload (contractility index), and afterload and time (ventricular power).

Mean Systolic Ejection Rate. The mean systolic ejection rate (MER) represents the amount of blood ejected per second of systolic ejection (9,29). It is calculated using the following formula:

$$\text{MER} = \frac{\text{cardiac output or cardiac index}}{\text{left ventricular ejection time}} \quad (\text{ml/sec})$$

$$\text{MER per beat} = \frac{\text{stroke volume or stroke index}}{\text{left ventricular ejection time}} \quad (\text{ml/sec/beat})$$

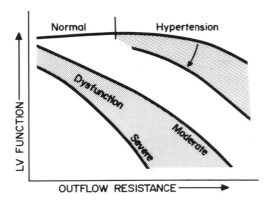

FIGURE 8 Effect of afterload on left ventricular function. Ventricular function curves in normal subject and in patients with moderate and severe left ventricular (LV) dysfunction.

Mean systolic ejection rate is greatly affected by preload, afterload, and myocardial contractility. It is increased by augmented preload and contractility and is decreased in left ventricular failure and in conditions associated with increased afterload (29). Thus, cardiac output (or stroke volume) corrected for ejection time is not a sensitive index of left ventricular function or inotropy.

Left Ventricular Work. Work is the product of force and distance moved from the point of application of the force. Assuming constant pressure during blood flow, work = pressure × volume of blood moved. An approximation of left ventricular stroke work could be obtained by the following formula which assumes a constant rate of ejection:

Stroke work (G–ml) = stroke index × mean left ventricular
    systolic pressure (9,10,30,31)

Left ventricular work per minute is obtained by this formula:

Work (kg/min) = stroke work × heart rate/1000 where
    1000 = conversion factor from g to kg

In evaluating left ventricular function utilizing left ventricular work, it is important to know the left ventricular volume at which a given amount of work is performed. For instance, left ventricular work in the curves shown in Figure 9 are from a normal subject (A) and a patient with primary cardiomyopathy (B), respectively. They show similar stroke volumes, systolic pressures, and systolic work; however, in primary cardiomyopathy this work is performed at a much larger ventricular volume. According to the law of Laplace, more wall tension is required to

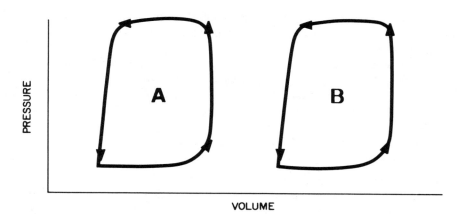

FIGURE 9 Pressure/volume curves obtained in a normal ventricle (A) and a dilated ventricle (B). Equal amounts of work are performed, but the dilated ventricle achieves this at the expense of greater tension.

generate a given pressure and perform a given level of work with a dilated ventricle (9,30,31). Therefore, any amount of work performed by a dilated ventricle is performed at the expense of higher levels of tension when compared to the normal ventricle. It should also be recognized that the magnitude of stroke work depends on all the fundamental factors capable of affecting stroke volume and cardiac output (afterload, preload, and myocardial contractility). Thus, stroke work alone is not a sensitive index of myocardial contractility (4,9,10,28).

Contractility Index.   To obviate the influence of end-diastolic volume on stroke work, the contractility index has been proposed as a parameter that corrects for the end-diastolic size of the left ventricle:

$$\text{Contractility index} = \frac{\text{stroke work}}{\text{end diastolic volume}}$$

The correction of stroke work for end-diastolic volume or end-diastolic pressure produces only a limited improvement in the diagnostic value of stroke work (9,32).

Ventricular Power.   Ventricular power represents the rate at which pressure-volume work is performed and is calculated by the formula:

Ventricular power = pressure × dV/dt where dV and dt are increments
of volume and time, respectively (9,33).

The commonly used approximation of stroke power is derived using the following formula.

$$\text{Stroke power} = \frac{\text{stroke work}}{\text{left ventricular ejection time}}$$

Although power takes into consideration time, it is not a sensitive index of myocardial contractility because it is influenced by a number of physiological variables (9,28).

First Derivative of the Aortic Flow (dQ/dt). The first derivative of aortic flow (dQ/dt) can be calculated using Doppler techniques; this parameter has been suggested as a good index of myocardial contractility. The validity of this index, however, has not been studied extensively (34).

B. Determination of Left Ventricular Function Based on Force and Indices Primarily Related to Force

Force is, in general, measured as a function of developed ventricular pressure. The first derivative of ventricular pressure development is defined as the rate of change of pressure and is usually expressed as dP/dt (9,35-44). Its maximum value, generally attained during early systole, is designated as peak dP/dt (Fig. 10) (36,39,40). Peak dP/dt cannot be reliably measured with the fluid-filled catheters used during routine cardiac catheterizations. To eliminate artifacts introduced by fluid-filled systems, high-fidelity catheter-tip micromanometers must be employed (2,9,41,42). Peak dP/dt has been found to increase with positive inotropic interventions. It decreases in conditions associated with depressed myocardial contractility (35-38). Augmented preload increases the peak dP/dt; tachycardia is also associated with an increase in this index due to rate enhancement of contractility (39,42,44). Therefore, these variables must be taken into consideration in evaluating the peak

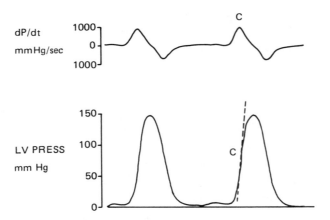

FIGURE 10   Time derivative (dP/dt) of the ventricular pressure curve (top panel) and simultaneous ventricular pressure (bottom). Maximum rate of rise in ventricular pressure (point C) equals peak dP/dt. (From Ref. 2, used with permission.)

dP/dt under different hemodynamic conditions in a given subject. Moreover, because of large individual variability, peak dP/dt has little value as an absolute index of contractility in a single subject or for comparison between different subjects under similar conditions (2,35-37).

The recognition that peak dP/dt is influenced by alterations in preload and afterload has led to other indices that take into consideration *time* (time to peak dP/dt); *preload* as determined by left ventricular end-diastolic pressure (LVEDP) or left ventricle end-diastolic volume (LVEDV) (peak dP/dt/LVEDP, peak dP/dt/LVEDV); and *afterload* (peak dP/dt/isovolumic developed pressure [IP] and peak dP/dt at common isovolumic pressure).

The time to peak dP/dt is defined as the time interval from the beginning of the left ventricular contraction to the peak dP/dt (9). When preload, afterload, and heart rate are held constant, an increased peak dP/dt and a shortened time to peak dP/dt are the hallmarks of a primary increase in myocardial contractility. In general, a change of time to peak dP/dt in a direction different from that of peak dP/dt itself indicates altered myocardial contractility. Parallel changes in these parameters suggest unchanged inotropic state (41,42).

The peak dP/dt/LVEDP is an index introduced to correct dP/dt for preload. In ventricular hypertrophy, this index may correct the peak dP/dt for the reduced ventricular compliance; however, poor correlation between ventricular diastolic volume and pressure in states of hypertrophy limits the value of this index to correct for preload (9,45).

The peak dP/dt/LVEDV is a second method introduced to correct peak dP/dt for preload. In ventricular hypertrophy, however, ventricular volume may be normal or low, and the increased muscle mass tends to raise peak dP/dt, even though peak dP/dt per unit of muscle is low. Thus the value of this index to correct peak dP/dt for preload is also limited (9,45).

The peak dP/dt/IP has been found to be independent of preload in experimental animals. However, changes in heart rate, myocardial contractility, and afterload may simultaneously influence this parameter, thus complicating the interpretation (9,46).

The peak dP/dt at the isovolumic pressure of 50 mmHg common to each of different ventricles or within the same ventricle (dP/dt/P50) is an accurate measure of the contractile state of the intact ventricle, assuming that no significant changes occur in preload. Because preload may vary widely within the same or between different ventricles, dP/dt at common isovolumic pressure could be further corrected by relating this ratio to left ventricular end-diastolic volume or left ventricular end-diastolic pressure (2,4).

Mean $\Delta P/\Delta t$ is an adaptation of more sophisticated measures of instantaneous dP/dt and can be calculated at the bedside using data derived from balloon-tipped, flow-directed catheters (47). Isovolumic pressure is equal to aortic diastolic pressure minus left ventricular diastolic pressure and is derived from the simultaneous recordings of the systemic arterial pressure and pulmonary capillary wedge pressure, respectively. Isovolumic time is equal to the pre-ejection period (PEP) minus the electromechanical delay. Electromechanical delay can be calculated from simultaneous recordings of the electrocardiogram and the apexcardiogram (Fig. 11).

$$\text{Mean } \triangle P/\triangle t = \frac{\text{isovolumic pressure}}{\text{isovolumic time}}$$

Because the electromechanical delay is relatively fixed over a wide range of pressure and contractility, the PEP instead of isovolumic time can be employed in the formula (47).

Maximum Velocity of Contractile Element Shortening (V_{max}). The velocity of shortening of the contractile element of the myocardial muscle is inversely proportional to the load with which it is confronted (2,9,47). It is possible in the intact heart to determine in a quantitative manner the level of myocardial contractility by extrapolating V_{max} from the instantaneous relation between dP/dt and its corresponding pressure in the left ventricle during isovolumic systole (Fig. 12) (2). Good approximation of contractile element velocity (VCE) can be obtained using this formula:

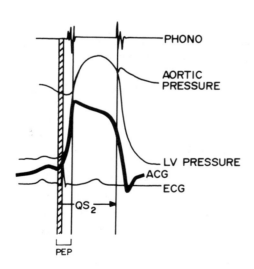

FIGURE 11   Schematic presentation of calculation of $\triangle P/\triangle t$. Phono = phonocardiogram, LV = left ventricle, ACG = apexcardiogram, ECG = electrocardiogram, QS2 = total electromechanical systole, PEP = pre-ejection period. The cross-hatched area represents the electromechanical delay. $\triangle P/\triangle t$ = isovolumic pressure/isovolumic time. Isovolumic time = P- electromechanical delay. See text for details.

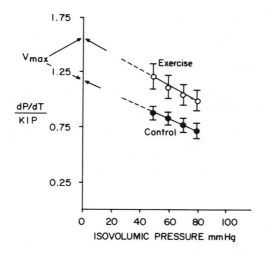

FIGURE 12   Velocity of shortening (approximated by dP/dt/KIP) versus simultaneous isovolumic ventricular pressure. The V_{max} is obtained by extrapolating the time to zero pressure. The V_{max} is increased over baseline with exercise. (From Ref. 2, used with permission.)

$$VcE = \frac{dP/dt}{KIP}$$

where IP is instantaneous isovolumic pressure and K is a constant (2,48). Extrapolation of this function to zero isovolumic pressure yields an accurate estimate of maximal contractile element velocity or V_{max}. This index theoretically provides a measure of myocardial contractility independent of preload and afterload (47). Unfortunately, the calculation of V_{max} in the intact heart is based on many assumptions and recent investigations show significant length dependence of V_{max} which declines with decreasing initial muscle length (2,4,9,48).

C. Determination of Left Ventricular Function Based on Indices Dependent Primarily on Distance of Length of Contraction

Indices dependent on distance or length of contraction are based on measurements of ventricular volumes or dimensions and their changes during contraction. The ejection fraction (EF) and the percentage of fractional shortening of the left ventricular internal diameter are clinically the most commonly employed indices of this type.

The ejection fraction has proved useful for detecting depressed ventricular performance. It is limited because it does not accurately reflect diminished ventricular function when the afterload is low (for example, in mitral regurgitation) (4,28). The ejection fraction can be calculated invasively from ventriculography (direct contrast or digital subtraction) or noninvasively from radionuclide angiography or two-dimensional echocardiography. In clinical cardiology, contrast ventriculography is still considered the standard for determining ejection fraction. Although contrast material can be injected into the pulmonary artery and left atrium, the left ventricle is outlined more clearly by direct injection into the left ventricular cavity (9,49-51). Biplane angiographic methods are superior to single-plane methods for the calculation of left ventricular volume; however, an approximation can also be obtained utilizing the single right anterior oblique projection (assuming that the short diameters of the two projections of the left ventricle are equal) (Fig. 13) (50). The prolate ellipsoid formula provides a reasonable mathematical model approximating left ventricular shape and volumes. The following formula is used to derive volume estimates:

$$\text{Volume} = \left(\frac{4\pi}{3}\right)\left(\frac{L}{2}\right)\left(\frac{D1}{2}\right)\left(\frac{D2}{2}\right)$$

where L = long ventricular and D1 and D2 = short ventricular diameters in right anterior oblique and left anterior oblique projections, respectively (52). The left ventricular EF is calculated from the end-diastolic volumes (EDV and ESV, respectively) using the following formula:

$$\text{EF} = \frac{\text{EDV}-\text{ESV}}{\text{EDV}} \times 100 \ (9,49\text{-}50)$$

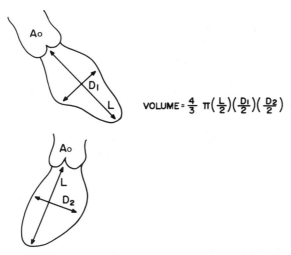

$$\text{VOLUME} = \frac{4}{3}\ \pi\left(\frac{L}{2}\right)\left(\frac{D1}{2}\right)\left(\frac{D2}{2}\right)$$

FIGURE 13   Calculation of left ventricular volumes from biplane ventriculography. L = long axis. D1 and D2-short diameters in the right anterior and left anterior oblique projections, respectively. Ao = aorta.

The normal left ventricular EF is $> 55\%$ (9). Injection of the contrast agent does not begin to produce hemodynamic changes until approximately the sixth beat after injection (49-52). The contrast agent can transiently increase blood volume, which may be followed by a diuretic effect. Thus, although direct contrast ventriculography is satisfactory for a single determination of ejection fraction it is not satisfactory for serial measurements of ventricular performance.

Radionuclide angiography can be used to measure the left ventricular ejection fraction and to assess regional ventricular performance (53,54). This information may be obtained by two different scintigraphic approaches—the first-pass technique and the equilibrium method. In the first-pass technique the initial passage of the radioactive bolus through the central circulation is studied. Sequential images follow the passage of the tracer through the central circulation. The right and left ventricular images are separated in time, and thus any desired view of the ventricle(s) can be obtained without the problem of overlap of the two images. The change in precordial count rate reflects the cyclical volume changes in the heart. The EF is calculated as

$$\frac{EDC - ESC}{EDC} \times 100$$

where EDC and ESC are the end-diastolic and end-systolic counts, respectively (53).

The equilibrium technique is also referred to as gated cardiac blood pool imaging, or more recently as multigated acquisition (MUGA) imaging (53,54). It relies on complete mixing of the radioactive tracer throughout the circulating blood volume and therefore requires a marker that remains intravascular. For this purpose, ^{99}Tc-labeled red blood cells are most commonly used. Because the marker has equilibrated with the blood volume at the time of imaging, all four cardiac chambers are seen simultaneously and various degrees of superimposition of the chambers occurs. In general, maximal separation of the right and left ventricles is achieved in the left anterior oblique view (Fig. 14). Again, the count rate is proportional to ventricular volume; thus, the EF can be determined by using end-diastolic and end-systolic counts as described for the first-pass technique.

Measuring the percentage of fractional shortening of the internal ventricular diameter ($\% \triangle D$) has proven useful for detecting decreased left ventricular performance (55,56). This technique has the same general limitations as the ejection fraction. In addition, because it is generally derived from the M-mode echocardiogram, it may neglect segmental contraction abnormalities. Thus left ventricular function may not be accurately reflected in patients with coronary artery disease. Using the M-mode echocardiogram, the transverse cavity dimension at end-diastole and end-systole can be measured (Fig. 15). The shortening fraction ($\% \triangle D$) is derived as

$$\frac{LVDd - LVDs}{LVDd} \times 100$$

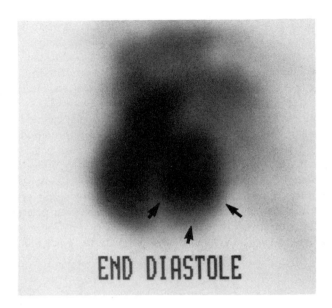

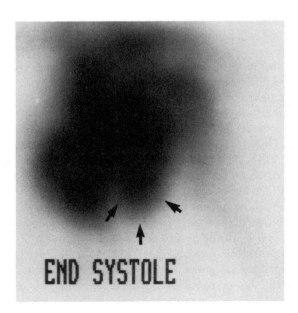

FIGURE 14   Multigated acquisition (MUGA) image of right and left ventricle obtained in left anterior oblique view. Images at end-diastole (top) and end-systole (bottom) may be used to calculate ejection fraction. The outline of the left ventricular cavity is depicted by arrows.

where LVDd and LVDs are left ventricular end-diastolic and end-systolic dimensions, respectively. The normal % △ D is > 30% (55). The cube of the transverse dimension of a normal-shaped left ventricle (ellipsoid model) approximates ventricular volumes from which the left ventricular EF can be estimated (56). However, left ventricular volumes derived from M-mode echocardiography in patients with dilated ventricles (for example, in congestive cardiomyopathy, regurgitant lesions)

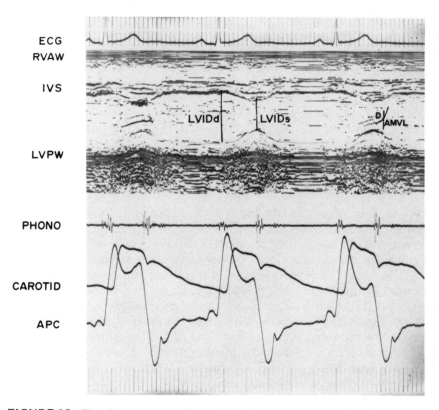

FIGURE 15 Simultaneous recordings of the electrocardiogram (ECG), echocardiogram, phonocardiogram (phone), carotid arterial pulse tracing (carotid), and apexcardiogram. RVAW = right ventricular anterior wall, IVS = intraventricular septum, LVPW = left ventricular posterior wall, LVIDd = left ventricular internal diameter of diastole, LIVIDs = left ventricular internal diameter at end systole. The percentage of shortening of the echocardiographic internal diameter (% △ D) can be calculated from the left ventricular diastolic and systolic diameters. The mean circumferential shortening of the left ventricle (VCF) is the ratio of fractional shortening to the left ventricular ejection time.

are subject to major error (57). Under such conditions, calculations should be treated as no more than semiquantitative estimations. Two-dimensional echocardiography allows assessment of regional wall abnormalities as well as measurement of ventricular size in the long axis and the short axis. Ventricular volumes may be approximated using these dimensions in models that resemble those used in contrast ventriculography (56). In this manner, a two-dimensionally derived echocardiographic ejection fraction may be calculated.

Calculation of the Circumferential Shortening of the Left Ventricle (VCF). Because EF can be altered by acute changes in afterload, the velocity of shortening of the circumferential fibers (VCF or fractional shortening rate), which takes into consideration the dimension of time, has been used to assess basal contractility (28,55). Mean VCF can be calculated using the contrast ventriculogram or the echocardiogram; it is the ratio of fractional shortening to left ventricular ejection time (Fig. 15). The magnitude of VCF is dependent on the duration of ejection, and thus could vary significantly with the heart rate even if the ejection fraction or the left ventricular fractional shortening remained unchanged (57). For this reason, it has been proposed that the rate-corrected left ventricular ejection time should be used to calculate the VCF. The normal mean VCF is > 1.1 cm/sec (55).

D. Determination of Left Ventricular Function Based on Indices Dependent on Temporal Relationship of Contraction: Systolic Time Intervals

Most tests of ventricular performance deal with force and/or distance. The systolic time intervals are unique because time is the only parameter measured. The three components of the systolic time intervals are the pre-ejection period (PEP), the left ventricular ejection time (LVET), and total electromechanical systole (QS2) (58-59) (Fig. 16). The measurements are obtained from simultaneous high-speed recordings (100 mm/sec) of an electrocardiographic lead best displaying the earliest onset of left ventricular depolarization, a carotid pulse tracing, and a phonocardiogram best displaying the initial high-frequency vibrations of the aortic closure sound. The patient is instructed to breathe quietly and at least ten cardiac cycles are averaged to obtain the systolic time intervals. The QS2 interval is measured from the onset of ventricular depolarization (as delineated by a sharp Q wave) to the first high-frequency vibration of the aortic component of the second heart sound. The LVET is calculated from the onset of the carotid upstroke to the incisural notch (carotid arterial pulse tracing). Because there is a transmission delay (average 18.5 msec) in the carotid pulse tracing, the PEP must be calculated by subtracting the LVET from the QS2. It has long been appreciated that all the components of the systolic time intervals vary inversely with heart rate. Thus, in order to interpret changes in the systolic time intervals, correction must be made for variations in resting heart rate; the normal values for the resultant indices (PEPI, LVETI, QS2I) are shown in Table 1 (58,59). The factors known to influence the PEPI and LVETI are shown in Figure 17.

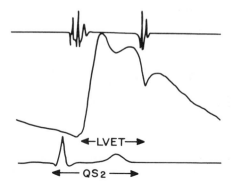

FIGURE 16 The measurement of systolic time intervals from simultaneous recordings of the electrocardiogram, phonocardiogram, and carotid arterial pulse tracing.

Several studies have been performed that relate systolic time intervals to other measurements of left ventricular performance. When left ventricular failure occurs, regardless of cause, the PEPI lengthens and the LVETI shortens (Fig. 18) (58-61). The prolongation of the PEPI can be attributed almost entirely to a diminished rate of left ventricular pressure rise during isovolumic contraction (62,63). However, the PEPI may fail to reflect a depression in dP/dt, especially if the pressure developed during isovolumic contraction is small. This may occur in patients with a high left ventricular end-diastolic pressure and low systemic diastolic pressure (64). Complete left bundle branch block usually delays activation of the left ventricle and therefore prolongs the PEPI (65-68). The PEPI may also be prolonged if preload is inadequate (for example, overdiuresis). A similar phenomenon occurs with the diminished preload induced by upright tilt or prolonged upright ambulatory activity (68,69).

TABLE 1 Calculation of Systolic Time Interval Index (1) Values from Resting Regression Equations

Sex	Equation	Mean normal values	
		(msec) + 1 SD	Range
Male	QS2I = 2.1 HR + QS2	546+14	518-574
Female	QS2I = 2.0 HR + QS2	459+14	521-577
Male	LVETI = 1.7 HR + LVET	413+10	393-433
Female	LVETI = 1.6 HR + LVET	418+10	398-438
Male	PEPI = 0.4 HR + PEP	131+10	111-151
Female	PEPI = 0.4 HR + PEP	133+10	113-153

Note: HR = heart rate.

	PEP	LVET	PEP/LVET	QS₂
INCREASED PRELOAD	↓	↑	↓	↓
INCREASED AFTERLOAD	↑	↓	↑	↓
POSITIVE INOTROPY	↓	↑,↓ =	↓	↓

FIGURE 17 Interventions that influence the systolic time intervals. Open arrows = small effect, solid arrows = strong effect.

The shortening of the LVETI with heart failure is more complex. A primary factor must be the relative lengthening of the PEP, which induces a delayed onset of ejection. During ejection, the velocity of fiber shortening is diminished when left ventricular failure is present, a condition that theoretically should prolong the LVETI. However, the extent of fiber shortening is also reduced and this would tend to shorten the LVETI. In patients with primary myocardial disease and left ventricular dysfunction, shortening of LVETI occurs when the left ventricular end-diastolic volume is increased, the ejection fraction is reduced, and the stroke volume and cardiac output are normal (59).

Unlike the PEPI, which responds in an opposite manner to positive and negative inotropic agents, the LVETI is generally shortened by both (70-75). With negative inotropic drugs, the mechanism is similar to that which occurs with left ventricular failure (76-78). Positive inotropic agents increase both the velocity and extent of fiber shortening. These two changes have opposite effects on the duration of the LVETI. Generally, the increased rate of shortening is the predominant effect so that the LVETI shortens or is unchanged. However, lengthening can occur when a marked hemodynamic change occurs (that is, a large increase in the stroke volume

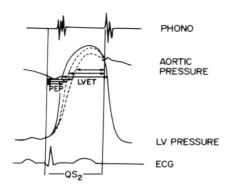

FIGURE 18 Relationship of the measured systolic time intervals to the normal cardiac cycle (solid line). The dotted lines illustrate the changes induced in left ventricular dysfunction. Pre-ejection periods (PEP) and left ventricular ejection times are also shown.

TABLE 2 Factors Influencing the Systolic Time Intervals

Intervals	Increase	Decrease
1. PEP	LV muscle failure Left bundle branch block preload Negative inotropic agents	Aortic valve disease LV isovolumic pressure Positive inotropic agents
2. LVET	Aortic valve disease	LV muscle failure preload Positive inotropic agents Negative inotropic agents
3. QS2	Left bundle branch block Aortic valve disease	Positive inotropic agents

after administration of vasodilators). Finally, diminished preload reduces the stroke volume and shortens the LVETI.

The duration of systole (QS2I) is one of the relative constants in the circulatory system (58,59). Although most types of heart disease may produce profound alterations in cardiac performance, manifested by directionally opposite changes in the PEPI and LVETI, the QS2I remains unchanged from normal unless high catecholamine levels or drug effects are present. Factors which may alter the septolic time intervals are summarized in Table 2. Alterations in preload and afterload influence QS2I only minimally, whereas positive and negative inotropic agents exert major reductions and increases (respectively) in the QS2I (79,80). Because of these characteristics of the QS2I, one can make inferences as to the inotropic state of the left ventricle. The finding of a QS2I less than 518 msec in the male or 521 msec in the female suggests a positive inotropic influence (59). Because positive inotropic agents generally shorten both the LVETI and PEPI, the QS2I is the most useful of the systolic time intervals in judging the presence of positive inotropic stimulation (59,72). The facts that the responses in the systolic time intervals are easily discernible and that the intervals can be measured repetitively without invasion of the vascular system allows sequential testing of the influence of pharmacologic agents and other therapeutic maneuvers in normal individuals as well as in patients with left ventricular dysfunction.

The diagnostic value of the systolic time intervals for identification of left ventricular dysfunction can be enhanced by determination of the ratio of PEP to LVET (58-61). At less than 110 beats/min, this ratio is unaffected by changes in heart rate because the PEP and LVET shorten proportionally as the heart rate increases. The PEP/LVET ratio may identify left ventricular dysfunction when either (or both) the PEPI and LVETI are still within the normal range. Consequently, the PEP/LVET ratio has become the single most useful measurement of left ventricular performance derived from the systolic time intervals. The normal PEP/LVET ratio is < 0.42. Other factors besides inotropy may alter systolic time intervals (Fig. 17). All these factors must be taken into consideration when left ventricular inotropy is determined using systolic time intervals.

E. Determination of Left Ventricular Function Based on Combinations of Distance, Force, and Time: End-Systolic Pressure/End-Systolic Volume Line

As noted earlier, the classic assessment of left ventricular function is found in the Frank-Starling relationship of end-diastolic pressure to left ventricular work (Fig. 7) (22,25,27). This model emphasizes that the myocardial fiber length at end-diastole is a major determinant of contractility in the subsequent systole. Recently, the slope of the end-systolic pressure/end-systolic volume line has been proposed as a measure of inotropy which, in contrast to the classic Frank-Starling relationship, uses changes in afterload in its assessment of contractility and is, in theory, independent of changes in preload (81-89). This measurement may represent the state of inotropy better than any of the previously proposed indices. In this method of analysis, the ventricle is considered to be a structure with a characteristic elastance (roughly defined as the ratio of pressure to volume). As with any structure, there is a limit to ventricular elastance, and thus there is a maximal value of the pressure/volume ratio (81,84,87,89). The maximal value of elastance determines the ventricular volume at end-systole for a given level of afterload (24,90). Because mechanical properties of the ventricle do not change over short intervals of time, elastance will remain constant for a given inotropic state, and the maximal ratio of pressure to volume is unchanged. Therefore, as afterload is increased, end-systolic volumes must increase as well. This may be demonstrated by plotting ventricular end-systolic volumes with varying afterload. As is shown in Figure 19, the relationship of end-systolic pressure to end-systolic volume is linear, having a slope that is directly related to maximal elastance (E_{max}) of that ventricle (81-87). If inotropy increases, the ventricle may then contract to a smaller volume for a given level of afterload. This reflects an increase in the maximal elastance of the

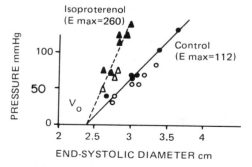

FIGURE 19 Linear relationship of end-systolic pressure and end-systolic dimension. Positive inotropic intervention (isoproterenol infusion) results in an increase in the slope of the line. E_{max} = maximal elastance (see text). (From Ref. 87, used with permission.)

ventricle and is indicated by an increase in the slope of the line relating end-systolic pressure and volume (81-88,91).

Catheterization studies utilizing angiographic volumes plotted against varying end-systolic pressures have confirmed the linearity of this relationship in humans. As would be predicted from the above models, the slope of the end-systolic pressure/volume relationship is greater for normal ventricles than for those with diminished function (as judged by ejection fraction) (82,83). Additionally, plotting end-systolic volume and end-systolic pressure for postextrasystolic beats generates a line with a slope increased above that of the baseline state, reflecting postextrasystolic potentiation of inotropy (82). Thus, within a range of physiologic pressures, in vivo end-systolic pressure/volume relations appear to be linear and to vary directly with the inotropic state of the ventricle.

To expand the application of the end-systolic pressure/end-systolic volume ratio to a wider range of clinical settings, techniques have been devised to obtain pressure and volume data by noninvasive means (92-96). Most commonly, the M-mode echocardiogram is utilized to determine left ventricular chamber size. A simultaneous phonocardiogram is recorded and the aortic component of the second heart sound is used to determine end-systole (Fig. 20). End-systolic left ventricular diameter is measured at this point. Systolic and diastolic blood pressure are determined indirectly by cuff-auscultation, or automated methods may be used to estimate central aortic systolic and diastolic pressures (95). From simultaneously recorded carotid pulse measurements, end-systolic pressure is interpolated at the dicrotic notch with systolic pressure assigned to the peak and diastolic pressure assigned to the nadir of the pressure tracing (96). In this manner, end-systolic pressure and end-systolic left ventricular diameter are derived (96,96). Such points must be obtained under varying levels of afterload in order to obtain a set of end-systolic pressure/volume values from which a line of best fit may be determined by least squares regression. The slope of the resultant line is then taken as a measure of inotropy (81,91,92,94). Preliminary studies in normal ventricles utilizing the noninvasive techniques described here have indicated that the slope of the end-systolic pressure/dimension line does increase over that obtained at baseline after the infusion of an inotropic agent such as dobutamine (95). Further refinements of this technique may add to its accuracy in clinical studies.

It has been noted that, in the setting of ventricular hypertrophy, the ratio of end-systolic pressure to end-systolic volume alone may not accurately reflect inotropic state. Hypertrophy may compensate for reduced inotropy and may result in end-systolic pressure to end-systolic volume ratios similar to those in normal ventricles (97-101). In such a case, the relationship of end-systolic stress to end-systolic dimension may provide a more reliable index of inotropy which corrects for ventricular wall thickness (Fig. 21) (97). A further modification takes into account the VCF. The relationship of end-systolic stress to VCF has been noted to be linear, to vary with inotropic state, and to be independent of loading conditions

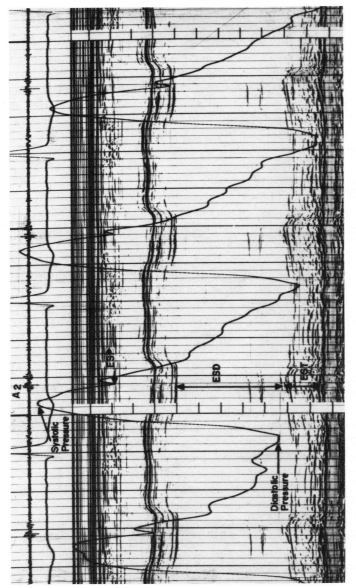

FIGURE 20 Simultaneous phonocardiogram (top channel), electrocardiogram (second channel), carotid pulse tracing, and echocardiogram through left ventricular chamber. End-systolic dimension (ESD) is measured at the time of the aortic component of the second heart sound (A2). Measured arterial diastolic pressure is assigned to the nadir and systolic pressure to the peak of the carotid pulse tracing. End-systolic pressure (ESP) is interpolated at the dicrotic notch.

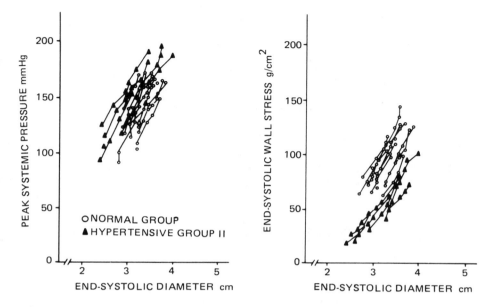

FIGURE 21 Peak systolic pressure (left panel) and end-systolic stress (right panel) plotted against end-systolic diameters in normals and patients with hypertension and ventricular hypertrophy. Measurement of stress/dimension relationship suggests decrease in inotropy in hypertrophy which is not indicated by pressure/ dimension relationship alone. (From Ref. 97, by permission of the American Heart Association, Inc.)

(Fig. 22) (102). It may be obtained by the noninvasive techniques noted above, and thus may provide an alternative load-independent index of inotropy to be utilized in clinical settings.

It has been suggested that the x-intercept of the pressure volume line may provide further information regarding inotropy (82). This remains controversial. In theory, the extrapolated volume at zero pressure (Vo) should be smaller under conditions of enhanced inotropy (81,82). However, clinical assessments of end-systolic pressure/volume ratios have not consistently demonstrated such a relationship (81,83). This variation from the theoretical prediction may in part result from reflex changes in inotropy which occur during the alterations in afterload required to obtain the pressure/volume line (103-105).

In hopes of simplifying this technique for clinical use, single pressure/volume points or stress/volume points have been utilized as estimates of the slope of the pressure or stress/volume line (106-110). However, estimates of the slope derived from a single pressure/volume point may not be accurate. The degree of error will relate to the magnitude of Vo compared to the measured volume (109). For this reason, error is magnified in small ventricles, and estimates of inotropy derived

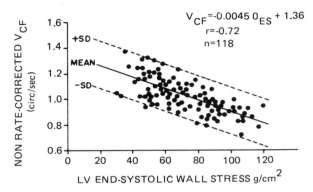

FIGURE 22 Velocity of circumferential fiber shortening (VCF) versus end-systolic wall stress. Mean + 1 SD in a group of normal patients. [From Ref. 102. Reprinted with permission from the *Journal of the American College of Cardiology*, 4: 715 (1984).]

from such single point determinations must be regarded with caution. Nevertheless, some success in clinical settings has been noted utilizing this adaptation. It has been possible to segregate patients with mitral regurgitation and poor surgical results due to left ventricular dysfunction from those with a good operative results by using a single measurement of the ratio of end-systolic stress to volume (106). Despite the limitations described above, potential exists for this simplification of the stress/volume ratio. Further investigation is warranted, particularly in patients with dilated ventricles.

The theoretical basis for the end-systolic pressure/volume line derives from animal models used to investigate the relationship of ventricular pressure and volume (that is, elastance) over time throughout the cardiac cycle (81,84,89,111). Suga and others (89) have demonstrated, in canine studies, that the ratio of instantaneous pressure (P) to volume (V) throughout systole forms a characteristic curve defined by the formula, $E(t) = P(t)/(V(t)-Vo)$, where t is any point in time following onset of systole and Vo is the volume of the ventricle at zero pressure. Originally, Vo was defined as the "dead space volume" of the ventricle at which no further volume could be ejected. It has since been determined that the dead space volume in fact occurs at subatmospheric pressures. Dead space volume is now labeled Vd to distinguish it from Vo (81). In the formula, E(t) is termed the "time-varying elastance" of the ventricle and the maximum value of E(t), E_{max}, occurs shortly before the end of systole and remains constant despite variations in preload and afterload. If the above equation is rearranged as $P(t) = E(t) \times (V(t)-Vo)$, the relationship of pressure to volume at a given time under various loading conditions describes a line with x-intercept (Vo) and a slope having the value of the elastance at that particular time. Under varying loading conditions but under constant inotropic state, the E_{max} points will form a line with a slope equal to E_{max}

(Fig. 23) (84,89). If, however, inotropy of the ventricle is increased, as through the infusion of epinephrine, E_{max} will be shifted to a higher value for a given pressure/volume curve, and the E_{max} line will become steeper (Fig. 23) (81,84,89). Hence, E_{max} appears to represent a quantity that expresses and is solely determined by contractility.

Several fundamental problems must be resolved to allow accurate interpretation of clinical estimates of E_{max}. In our experience it is necessary to obtain a minimum range of 30 mmHg in systolic blood pressure for the noninvasive determination of the end-systolic pressure/volume line, as this method may not be sensitive to blood pressure variations of less than 10 mmHg. Alterations in afterload necessary to obtain the multiple points used to construct an E_{max} line may be accompanied by reflex changes in inotropy. Under such conditions, end-systolic points are taken at varying inotropic states and the resultant line cannot truly represent E_{max} (104, 105). Autonomic blockade at the time measurements are acquired may minimize this effect (83). In addition, alpha-agonists are frequently used to vary afterload with the assumption that they are devoid of direct inotropic effects. However, recent evidence suggests that stimulation of myocardial alpha-receptors directly results in increased contractility (193). Other problems arise in the setting of regional wall motion abnormalities which may render inaccurate the estimates of left ventricular volume obtained by echocardiographic means or by angiographic models (109). In the case of valvular heart disease, (for example, aortic stenosis) aortic dicrotic notch pressure may not accurately reflect left ventricular end-systolic pressure (95). In the case of mitral regurgitation, left ventricular volume may continue to decrease after aortic valve closure, thus compromising the noninvasive determination of the end-systolic volume and pressure (95,109). Further-

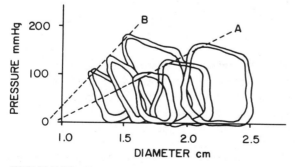

FIGURE 23   Pressure dimension curves for a single ventricle with varying afterload and inotropy. At baseline (A) connecting the points representing the maximum ratio of pressure to dimension (E_{max}) forms a line. After positive inotropic intervention (B) E_{max} increases as does the slope of the line connection the E_{max} points. (From Ref. 87, used with permission.)

more, careful examinations of the range of estimated values of E_{max} and changes observed after administration of inotropic agents in congestive heart failure have not been performed.

Thus, as with all proposed inotropic parameters, there are limitations to this method and it may not be devoid of the influence of loading conditions (81). Perhaps its most intriguing and useful potential lies in the evaluation of the failing ventricle, a situation for which relatively little information exists. As noted above, the normal ventricle is relatively sensitive to preload and independent of afterload (Figs. 7 and 8). Sugawa et al. have noted that the end-systolic pressure/volume relationship in normal ventricles may not be completely independent of preload (81). In contrast, the failing ventricle is minimally influenced by preload alterations as it has attained the plateau portion of its Frank-Starling curve (2,28). Alterations in afterload, however, may have a profound influence on depressed ventricular function. In such a setting, a parameter that is relatively insensitive to preload and that takes into account afterload may represent the ideal measure of ventricular function. Further investigation of this possibility and of clinical use of the end-systolic pressure/volume relationship will clarify its role in the assessment of inotropy.

III. RIGHT VENTRICULAR PERFORMANCE

The importance of right ventricular function in many disease states has been recently appreciated (112,113). Routine functional analysis of the right ventricle is limited because the complex shape of this chamber renders many of the geometric models used to determine left ventricular volume invalid (112). However, techniques which are relatively independent of geometric considerations have been successfully applied to the assessment of right ventricular function. Noninvasive methods including radionuclide angiography, M-mode echocardiography, two-dimensional and Doppler echocardiography, and systolic time intervals (obtained by M-mode echocardiography) have shed new light on the neglected right ventricle (113).

Radionuclide techniques (Fig. 24) now permit assessment of the right ventricular ejection fraction at rest and during exercise (53). At rest, the lower normal limit of the right ventricular ejection fraction is less than that of the left ventricle (normal value > 40%) using either first-pass or gated techniques. Two-dimensional echocardiography provides important, although semiquantitative, information of right ventricular performance (56). Systolic time intervals obtained from the pulmonary artery pressure pulse waves or noninvasively from the M-mode echocardiogram have been used to evaluate right ventricular function, particularly in children (112). Finally, the end-systolic pressure/volume relationship of the right ventricle is being defined in animal models and humans (83).

Some limited studies deal with the effect of inotropic drugs on right ventricular performance (112). Present and future technology will allow better definition of right ventricular performance at rest and during therapeutic interventions.

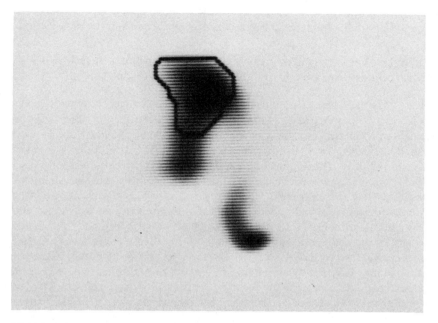

FIGURE 24 First-pass radionuclide angiogram of right ventricle (circled). Right and left ventricular images may be clearly separated allowing calculation of ejection fraction of each ventricle (see text). (Reproduced with permission from T. M. Bashore, and P. B. Shaffer. Nuclear cardiology, in J. V. Warren and R. P. Lewis, *Diagnostic Procedures in Cardiology: A Clinician's Guide*, Chicago, Year Book Medical Publishers, ©1985, used with permission.)

IV. DETERMINATION OF DIRECTIONAL CHANGES IN CONTRACTILITY

The assessment of directional changes in ventricular contractility is confounded by two major factors. First, as noted earlier, if loading conditions are varied between measurements, it is difficult to ascribe a change in a given parameter solely to an increase or decrease in inotropy. Second, the commonly used measures of loading conditions may themselves be inaccurate. Left ventricular filling pressure is only a rough estimate of preload; arterial pressure and mean systemic vascular resistance are incomplete approximations of afterload (4,5,9). Thus, even if filling pressures and peripheral resistance remain unchanged, we cannot with complete confidence assume that changes in ventricular performance are due only to changes in myocardial contractility.

The selection of an appropriate inotropic index must take these factors into consideration. Perhaps the most reliable data may be obtained by applying the inotropic parameter that is least sensitive to the conditions that are most variable in the given clinical setting. Recognition of these principles allows a reasonable interpretation of directional changes in inotropy as discussed in the next section.

A. Directional Changes of Left Ventricular Function Based on Indices Primarily Dependent on Cardiac Output

Cardiac output is an insensitive index of left ventricular inotropy because it is regulated by many other factors in addition to myocardial contractility. Similarly, indices derived from cardiac output, such as mean systolic ejection rate, stroke work, and left ventricular power, are altered by changes in preload, afterload, and myocardial contractility. These indices do not solely reflect left ventricular inotropy.

The determination of ventricular function curves (simultaneous measurements of cardiac output and ventricular filling pressures) allows qualitative assessment of ventricular performance and directional response to interventions which may alter loading conditions, contractility, or both. When afterload is held constant, the displacement of the entire curve upward or downward reflects a positive or negative inotropic effect, respectively (2,4,5,28). However, as previously noted, alterations in afterload may have significant effects on ventricular performance despite constant inotropic state, especially in the failing ventricle (28). An increase in afterload may result in a downward displacement of the function curve; a decrease in afterload will have the opposite effect. Therefore, interpretation of directional changes in the classic Frank-Starling ventricular function curve is not possible without knowledge of afterload conditions during the time of curve generation.

Related to cardiac output is the first derivative of aortic flow (dQ/dt), which has been suggested as an index reflecting changes in myocardial contractility. However, at present data are insufficient regarding the effects of inotropic interventions on dQ/dt (34).

B. Directional Changes of Left Ventricular Function Based on Indices Primarily Dependent on Force

As noted previously, peak dP/dt is dependent on loading conditions and thus is not useful for assessing directional changes in left ventricular contractility when alterations in preload or afterload also occur (34-42). Time to peak dP/dt, peak dP/dt/ LVEDP, peak dP/dt/LVEDV, peak dP/dt/IP, and peak dP/dt at common isovolumic pressure are less dependent on loading conditions and can be used to assess directional changes (9,45,46). Moreover, dP/dt/P50 is highly responsive to changes in the inotropic state and relatively insensitive to changes in preload and afterload (2,9). Because high-fidelity catheter-tip micromanometers must be employed for accurate measurement of this index, measurement of peak dP/dt/P50 is not practical when the long-term effects of a drug must be studied. The use of V_{max} does not seem to offer an advantage over the use of dP/dt/P50 (2,4,8).

Mean $\triangle P/\triangle t$ is a useful index to study directional changes of left ventricular performance, assuming that there are no major changes in loading conditions. In addition, mean $\triangle P/\triangle t$ can be used to study the time course (over several days) of inotropic effect of pharmacologic agents as the data required to derive this parameter may be obtained using balloon-tipped floating catheters (47).

C. Directional Changes of Left Ventricular Function Based on Indices Primarily Dependent on Length of Contraction

Changes in the extent of myocardial wall shortening may reflect acute changes in contractility if preload and afterload remain relatively constant. Acute elevations of afterload cause an inverse change in ejection fraction (2,4). However, as previously noted, ejection fraction is less sensitive to changes in preload. Left ventricular ejection fraction obtained from ventriculography with contrast injection is not useful in studying directional changes of left ventricular performance because the effect of hypersomolar contrast material on ventricular loading conditions will be present for several hours.

Ejection fractions obtained from radionuclide angiography are useful in evaluating directional changes of left ventricular performance, as EF can be calculated repetitively for approximately three hours with the same radioactive dose (53,54). The percentage of fractional shortening ($\% \triangle D$) obtained from M-mode echocardiography and the $\% \triangle D$ and the EF obtained from two-dimensional echocardiography are useful in studying directional changes of left ventricular contractility if the loading conditions are relatively constant (55,56). In addition, echocardiography is totally noninvasive and can be performed repeatedly over long periods of time.

D. Directional Changes of Left Ventricular Function Based on Indices Primarily Dependent on the Temporal Relationship of Contraction

The fact that changes in the systolic time intervals are easily discernible and that the intervals can be measured noninvasively and repetitively with no discomfort to the patient recommend them for use in serial studies of ventricular performance. The rate and extent of the cardiac response to loading conditions or inotropic agents can be evaluated by the serial observation of systolic time intervals (72-75, 79,80). The systolic time intervals are well suited for studying effects of pharmacologic agents upon the heart. Most studies have dealt with parameters of pharmacologic action such as the onset, magnitude, and duration of drug effect; establishment of dose response relationships; and studies of the interplay of agonists and antagonists. The clinical pharmacology of the various digitalis glycosides has been evaluated with the systolic time intervals (114-117). These studies have shown that the QS2I is the most sensitive of the systolic time intervals in assessing the presence of positive inotropic stimulation, whereas the hemodynamic response to the agent is reflected by the ratio of PEP to LVET (59,116,117).

The adrenergic subset of positive inotropic agents has also been studied with systolic time intervals. This class of drugs usually elicits a more striking change in the intervals than that found with digitalis (72-75). The effect of negative inotropic agents upon the systolic time intervals has been less extensively studied (76-78). In general, it appears that such agents induce the typical pattern of prolongation of the PEPI and shortening of the LVETI. Caution must be exercised to ensure that pharmacologic effects on the peripheral circulation do not cloud the interpretation of the systolic time intervals. This is particularly important when marked changes in afterload and preload occur (118).

E.   Directional Changes of Left Ventricular Function Based on Indices Combining Distance, Force, and Time

The end-systolic pressure/volume relationship and its related indices are relatively independent of preload and incorporate afterload as a factor in their determination; thus directional changes will more likely be governed purely by alterations in inotropy rather than loading conditions (81-89). Two types of changes have been described with increasing inotropy. First, the ventricle at a given level of afterload will be able to contract to a smaller dimension, indicating an increase in maximal elastance (E_{max}); hence, the slope of the end-systolic pressure/volume line increases with enhanced inotropic state (81,91,92,95). Although less thoroughly studied, by similar reasoning negative inotropic influences should lead to a decrease in slope. Second, rather than a change in slope, the entire line may be shifted up or down parallel to the baseline (8,82,87). Enhanced inotropy will result in a shift of the line above baseline, and diminished inotropy will cause the line to fall below baseline. These shifts are associated with changes in the x-intercept (Vo) which becomes smaller with increased inotropy and larger as inotropy decreases. Among the sources of error inherent in this method are variations in wall thickness which may result in alterations in the pressure/volume relationship. Therefore, correction for differences in wall thickness by use of stress rather than pressure may improve accuracy. Directional changes for wall stress/dimension relationships have been similar to those for pressure/dimension lines (94,97). Finally, the relationship of VCF to end-systolic stress has been similarly shown to shift above the baseline with enhanced inotropy and to fall below baseline with a decrease in inotropy (102). It has been proposed that VCF/stress relations may provide accurate clinical information using a single determination without alterations in afterload (102). This theory awaits further verification.

These indices have the advantages that they can be derived by noninvasive means, do not require the use of contrast media which may alter left ventricular volumes, and are suitable for long-term studies. Limitations arise in the necessity to alter blood pressure (which may be poorly tolerated in some patients), in the possible changes in inotropy which result either directly from a pressor agent or secondary to reflex mechanisms, and in that these indices may not be completely preload independent (81,84,103-105).

V. CLINICAL PITFALLS

Awareness of the complex interaction of factors influencing each of the inotropic indices is integral to the accurate interpretation of such parameters. The assessment of response to pharmacologic agents, such as cardiotonic drugs, is perhaps most prone to the pitfalls of these methodologies. In drugs with strong inotropic effects, it is likely that positive inotropy will be demonstrated with all or most of the indices used to measure ventricular performance. It is more difficult, however, to evaluate a less potent drug or one that has several physiologic effects (for example, with influences on afterload, preload, or both).

Such difficulties are illustrated in the recent evaluation of amrinone as a potential cardiotonic agent (119-129). Original reports suggested an improvement in the ventricular function curve after administration of this drug, and the initial interpretation of these data was that amrinone is a positive inotropic agent (119-121). Subsequent investigations, using several different inotropic parameters, have failed to show any change in inotropic state and have indicated that amrinone acts predominantly as a vasodilator (128,129). Again, one must take into account the limitations of the various methods used in assessment of inotropy.

Cumulatively, the pitfalls of the techniques used to measure inotropy are many. Each method has its limitations and the perfect inotropic parameter has not yet been found. In the clinical setting, we can only be aware of the shortcomings of each technique and select the methods that are least sensitive to the factors that are most altered in a given setting. The methods used must also be tailored to the type of clinical investigation; for example, in a chronic study a parameter requiring indwelling catheters is generally not feasible. Rhythm disturbances will also dictate which method is preferable. For example, in the setting of atrial fibrillation, an otherwise appropriate index may be inaccurate (130). It is also important to not lose sight of the fact that what is being measured is more important than the technique of measurement (Fig. 25). Much attention is often directed toward evaluation of the methodology when it is the inotropic state of the ventricle and its subsequent changes that are of ultimate importance. As was suggested in the introduction to this chapter, we remain much like the ancient alchemists in our persistent search for the elusive inotropic formula.

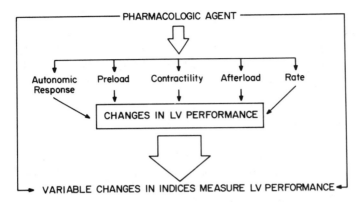

FIGURE 25 Multiple factors influence left ventricular (LV) performance. These changes may be detected by parameters of inotropy given adequate sensitivity of the method. Of central importance is the performance of the ventricle rather than the performance of the method.

REFERENCES

1. A. M. Katz. Energetics of muscle: Energy Utilization (Work and Heat). In *Physiology of the Heart*. Raven Press, New York, 1977, p. 73.
2. D. T. Mason, J. F. Spann, Jr., R. Zelis, and E. A. Amsterdam. Alterations of hemodynamics and myocardial mechanics in patients with congestive heart failure: Pathophysiologic mechanisms and assessment of cardiac function and ventricular contractility. *Prog. Cardiovasc. Dis. 12*: 507-557, (1970).
3. R. F. Rushmer. Functional anatomy of cardiac contraction. In *Organ Physiology: Structure and Function of the Cardiovascular System*. Saunders, Boston, 1972, p. 33.
4. E. Braunwald, E. H. Sonnenblick, and J. Ross, Jr. Contraction of the normal heart. In *Heart Disease: A Textbook of Cardiovascular Medicine*. E. Braunwald (ed.). Saunders, Boston, 1984, 1: 409.
5. R. C. Schland, E. H. Sonnenblick, and R. Gorlin. Normal physiology of the cardiovascular system. In *The Heart*. J. Willis Hurst, R. Bruce Logue, C. E. Rackley, R. C. Schland, E. H. Sonnenblick, A. G. Wallace, N. K. Wenter (eds.). McGraw-Hill, New York, 1982, p. 75.
6. A. M. Katz. Contractile proteins. In *Physiology of the Heart*. Raven Press, New York, 1977, p. 89.
7. Y. Nakamura, and A. W. Wiegner. Systolic time intervals: Assessment by isolated cardiac muscle studies. *J. Am. Coll. Cardiol. 2*: 973 (1983).
8. J. Ross, Jr. Cardiac function and myocardial contractility: A perspective. *J. Am. Coll. Cardiol. 1*: 52 (1983).
9. S. S. Yang, L. G. Bentivoglio, V. Maranhao, and H. Goldberg. *Assessment of Ventricular Function, from Cardiac Catheterization Data to Hemodynamic Parameters*. F. A. Davis Co., Philadelphia, 1972, p. 157.

10. I. L. Bunnell, C. Grant, and D. G. Green. Left ventricular function derived from the pressure-volume diagram. *Am. J. Med. 39*: 881 (1965).
11. S. R. Kjellberg, U. Rudhe, and T. Sjostrand. The influence of the autonomic nervous system on the contraction of the human heart under normal circulatory conditions. *Acta Physiol. Scand. 24*: 350 (1959).
12. A. F. Kelso, and W. C. Randall. Ventricular changes associated with sympathetic augmentation of cardiovascular pressure pulses. *Am. J. Physiol. 196*: 731 (1959).
13. R. F. Rushmer. The cardiac output. In *Organ Physiology: Structure and Function of the Cardiovascular System*. Sanders, Boston, 1972, p. 70.
14. A. Cournand, R. L. Riley, E. S. Breed, D. E. F. Baldwin, and D. W. Richard. Measurement of cardiac output in man using technique of catheterization of right auricle or ventricle. *J. Clin. Invest. 24*: 106 (1945).
15. J. V. Warren. Determination of cardiac output in man by right heart catheterization. *Methods Med. Res. 1*: 224 (1948).
16. P. S. Hetzel, H. J. C. Swan, A. A. Ramirez de Arellano, and E. H. Wood. Estimation of cardiac output from first part of arterial dye-dilution curves. *J. Appl. Physiol. 23*: 92 1958.
17. M. B. Visscher, and J. A. Johnson. The Fick principle: Analysis of potential errors in its conventional applications. *J. Appl. Physiol. 5*: 635 (1953).
18. L. L. Huntsman, D. K. Stewart, S. R. Barnes, S. B. Franklin, J. S. Colocousis, and E. A. Hessel. Noninvasive Doppler determination of cardiac output in man: Clinical validation. *Circulation 67*: (1983), pp. 593-602.
19. R. A. Nishimura, F. A. Miller Jr, M. J. Callahan, R. C. Benassi, J. B. Seward, and A. J. Tajik. Doppler echocardiography: Theory, instrumentation, technique and application. *Mayo Clin. Proc. 60*: 321 (1985).
20. J. M. Gardin, J. M. Tobis, A. Dabestani, C. Smith, U. Elkayam, E. Castleman, D. White, A. Allfie, and W. L. Henry. Superiority of two-dimensional measurement of aortic vessels diameter in Doppler echocardiographic estimates of left ventricular stroke volume. *J. Am. Coll. Cardiol. 6*: 66 (1985).
21. J. S. Colocousis, L. L. Huntsman, and P. W. Curreri. Estimation of stroke volume changes by ultrasonic Doppler. *Circulation 56*: 914 (1977).
22. E. H. Starling. *Principles of Human Physiology*, 3rd ed. Philadelphia, Lea & Febiger, 1920, p. 315.
23. D. L. Fry, D. M. Griffs, and F. C. Greenfield. Myocardial mechanics: Tension-velocity-length relationships in heart muscle. *Circ. Res. 14*: 73 (1964).
24. S. E. Downing, and E. H. Sonnenblick. Cardiac muscle mechanics and ventricular performance: Force and time parameters. *Am. J. Physiol. 207*: 705 (1964).
25. E. H. Sonnenblick. Force-velocity relations in mammalian heart muscle. *Am. J. Physiol. 202*: 931 (1962).
26. A. V. Hill. The heat of shortening and the dynamic constants of muscle. *Proc. R. Soc. 126*: 136, (1938).
27. G. Lundin. Mechanical properties of cardiac muscle. *Acta Physiol. Scand. 7 (Suppl. 20)*: (1944).
28. J. Ross, Jr. Assessment of cardiac function and myocardial contractility. In *The Heart*, 5th ed. J. Willis Hurst (ed.). McGraw-Hill, Atlanta, 1982, p. 310.

29. E. Braunwald, S. J. Sarnoff, and W. N. Stainsby. Determinants of duration and mean rate of ventricular ejection. *Circ. Res. 6*: 319 (1958).
30. R. E. Snell, and P. C. Luchsinger. Determination of the external work and power of the left ventricle in intact man. *Am. Heart J. 69*: 529 (1965).
31. W. S. Topham. Comparison of methods for calculation of left ventricular stroke work. *J. Appl. Physiol. 27*: 767 (1969).
32. G. A. H. Miller, J. W. Kirklin, and H. J. C. Swan. Myocardial function and left ventricular volumes in acquired valvular insufficiency. *Circulation 31*: 374 (1965).
33. M. F. O. Rourke. *Arterial Function in Health and Disease*. Churchill Livingstone, New York, p. 34.
34. H. Boudoulas, P. E. Karayannacos, R. P. Lewis, G. S. Kakos, J. W. Kilman, and J. S. Vasko. Influence of lidocaine on ischemic myocardial injury. *Eur. J. Cardiol. 91*: 104 (1978).
35. A. B. Landry, Jr., and A. V. N. Goodyer. Rate of rise of left ventricular pressure: Indirect measurement and physiologic significance. *Am. J. Cardiol. 15*: 660 (1965).
36. W. L. Gleason, and E. Braunwald. Studies on the first derivative of the ventricular pressure pulse in man. *J. Clin. Invest. 41*: 80 (1962).
37. D. T. Mason, E. Braunwald, J. Ross, Jr., and A. G. Morrow. Diagnostic value of the first and second derivatives of the arterial pressure pulse in aortic valve disease and hypertrophic subaortic stenosis. *Circulation 30*: 90 (1964).
38. C. J. Wiggers, and B. Stimson. Studies on the cardiodynamic actions of drugs. III. The mechanism of cardiac stimulation by digitalis and G-strophanthin. *J. Pharmacol. Exp. Ther. 30*: 251 (1927).
39. A. G. Wallace, N. S. Skinner, Jr., and J. H. Mitchell. Hemodynamic determinants of the maximal rate of rise of left ventricular pressure. *Am. J. Physiol. 205*: 30 (1963).
40. D. T. Mason. Usefulness and limitations of the rate of rise of intraventricular pressure (dp/dt) in the evaluation of myocardial contractility in man. *Am. J. Cardiol. 23*: 516 (1969).
41. E. Braunwald, J. Ross, Jr., J. H. Gault, D. T. Mason, C. Mill, I. T. Gabe, and S. E. Epstein. Assessment of cardiac function. *Ann. Intern. Med. 70*: 369 (1969).
42. D. T. Mason, E. H. Sonnenblick, J. W. Covell, J. Ross, Jr., and E. Braunwald. Assessment of myocardial contractility in man: Relationship between the rate of pressure rise and developed pressure throughout isometric left ventricular contraction. *Circulation 36 (Suppl. 2)*: 183 (1967).
43. H. Boudoulas, P. E. Karayannacos, R. P. Lewis, C. V. Leier, and J. S. Vasko. Effect of afterload changes on left ventricular performance: Comparison of the pre-ejection period and other indices of left ventricular performance. In *Recent Advances in Noninvasive Cardiology*. W. J. A. Goedhard, and P. K. Toutouzas (eds.). Staflea's Scientific Publishing Co., Brussels, 1981.
44. H. Boudoulas, P. E. Karayannacos, R. P. Lewis, C. V. Leier, and J. S. Vasko. Effect of afterload on left ventricular performance in experimental animals. Comparison of the pre-ejection period and other indices of left ventricular contractility. *J. Med. 13*: 373-385 (1982).

45. T. J. Reeves, L. L. Hefner, W. B. Jones, Coghlan, G. Prieto, and J. Corrol. The hemodynamic determinants of the rate of change in pressure in the left ventricle during isometric contraction. *Am. Heart J. 60*: 745 (1960).

46. U. P. Veragut, and H. P. Krayenfuhl. Estimation and quantification of myocardial contractility in the closed-chest dog. *Cardiologia 47*: 96 (1965).

47. G. Diamond, J. S. Forrester, K. Chatterjee, S. Wegner, and H. J. C. Swan. Mean electromechanical $\Delta P/\Delta t$. *Am. J. Cardiol. 46*: 291, (1972).

48. D. T. Mason. Usefulness and limitations of the rate of rise of intraventricular pressure (dp/dt) in the evaluation of myocardial contractility in man. *Am. J. Cardiol. 23*: 516 (1969).

49. J. O. Parker, and R. B. Case. Normal left ventricular function. *Circulation 60*: 4-11 (1979).

50. C. E. Rackley, V. S. Behar, R. E. Whalen, and H. D. McIntosh. Biplane cineangiographic determinations of left ventricular function: Pressure-volume relationship. *Am. Heart J. 74*: 766 (1967).

51. R. F. Leighton, S. M. Wilt, and R. P. Lewis. Detection of hypokinesis by a quantitative analysis of left ventricular cineangiograms. *Circulation 50*: 121-127 (1974).

52. H. T. Dodge, H. Sandler, W. A. Baxley, and R. R. Hawley. Usefulness and limitations of radiographic methods for determining left ventricular volume. *Am. J. Cardiol. 18*: 10 (1966).

53. T. M. Bashore, and P. B. Shaffer. Nuclear cardiology. In *Diagnostic Procedures in Cardiology: A Clinician's Guide*. J. V. Warren and R. P. Lewis, (eds.). Year Book Medical Publishers, Chicago, 1985, pp. 143-175.

54. C. A. Boucher. Assessment of left ventricular function. In *Noninvasive Cardiac Imaging*. J. Morgenroth, A. Parisi, and G. M. Pohost (eds.). Year Book Medical Publishers, Chicago, 1983, pp. 71-87.

55. R. L. Popp. Echocardiographic assessment of cardiac disease. In *Reviews of Contemporary Laboratory Methods*. A. M. Weissler (ed.). American Heart Association, Detroit, 1980, p. 197.

56. H. Feigenbaum. Echocardiographic evaluation of cardiac chambers: *Echocardiography*. Lea and Febiger, Philadelphia, 1981, p. 119.

57. J. Hirschleifer, M. Crawford, R. A. O'Rourke, and J. S. Karliner. Influence of acute alterations in heart rate and systemic arterial pressure on echocardiographic measures of left ventricular performance in normal human subjects. *Circulation 52*: 895 (1975).

58. W. S. Aronow. Isovolumic contraction and left ventricular ejection time. *Am. J. Cardiol. 26*: 238 (1970).

59. J. Manolas, W. Rutishauser, P. Wirz, and U. Arbenz. Time relation between apex cardiogram and left ventricular events using simultaneous high fidelity tracings in man. *Br. Heart J. 37*: 1263 (1975).

60. J. Willems, and H. Kesteloot. The left ventricular ejection time: Its relation to heart rate, mechanical systole and some anthropometric data. *Acta Cardiol. 22*: 401 (1967).

61. A. M. Weissler, and C. L. Garrand, Jr. Systolic time intervals in cardiac disease. *Mod. Concepts Cardiovasc. Dis. 40*: 1 (1971).

62. R. C. Talley, J. F. Meyer, and J. L. McNay. Evaluation of the pre-ejection period as an estimate of myocardial contractility in dogs. *Am. J. Cardiol. 27*: 384 (1971).
63. W. S. Aronow, P. R. Harding, V. DeQuattro, and M. Isbell. Diurnal variation of plasma catecholamines and systolic time intervals. *Chest 63*: 722 (1973).
64. H. Boudoulas, P. Geleris, C. A. Bush, R. P. Lewis, P. K. Fulkerson, A. J. Kolibash, and A. M. Weissler. Assessment of ventricular function by combined noninvasive measures: Factors accounting for methodologic disparities. *Int. J. Cardiol. 2*: 493 (1983).
65. E. Braunwald, and A. G. Morrow. Sequence of ventricular contraction in human bundle branch block. *Am. J. Med. 23*: 205 (1957).
66. M. G. Bourassa, G. M. Borteau, and B. J. Allenstein. Hemodynamic studies during intermittent left bundle branch block. *Am. J. Cardiol. 10*: 792 (1962).
67. J. Oravetz, S. Wissner, B. Argano, and A. Luisada. Dynamic analysis of heart sounds in right and left bundle branch blocks. *Circulation 36*: 275 (1967).
68. M. Silei. Etude Phonomecanacardiographique des blocs de branche: A propos de 106 observations. Thesis. Imprimerie Bosc Freres, Lyons, 1969.
69 A. P. Xenakis, V. M. Quarry, and D. H. Spodick. Immediate cardiac response to exercise: Physiologic investigation by systolic time intervals at graded work loads. *Am. Heart J. 89*: 178 (1975).
70. W. S. Harris, C. D. Schoenfeld, R. H. Brooks, and A. M. Weissler. Effect of beta adrenergic blockade on the hemodynamic responses to epinephrine in man. *Am. J. Cardiol. 17*: 484 (1966).
71. W. S. Harris, C. D. Schoenfeld, and A. M. Weissler. Effects of adrenergic receptor activation and blockade on the systolic pre-ejection period, heart rate and arterial pressure in man. *J. Clin. Invest. 46*: 1704 (1967).
72. H. Boudoulas, R. P. Lewis, R. E. Kates, and G. Dalamangas. Hypersensitivity to adrenergic stimulation after propranolol withdrawal in normal subjects. *Ann. Intern. Med. 87*: 433 (1977).
73. H. Boudoulas, P. Geleris, R. P. Lewis, and C. V. Leier. Effect of increased adrenergic activity on the relationship between electrical and mechanical systole. *Circulation 64*: 28 (1981).
74. C. V. Leier, P. T. Heban, P. Huss, C. A. Bush, and R. P. Lewis. Comparative systemic and regional hemodynamic effects of dopamine and dobutamine in patients with cardiomyopathic heart failure. *Circulation 58*: 466 (1978).
75. C. V. Leier, C. E. Desch, R. D. Magorien, D. W. Triffon, D. V. Unverferth, H. Boudoulas, and R. P. Lewis. Positive inotropic effects of hydralazine in human subjects: Comparison with prazosin in the setting of congestive heart failure. *Am. J. Cardiol. 46*: 1039 (1980).
76. H. Boudoulas, S. F. Schaal, R. P. Lewis, T. G. Welch, P. Green, and R. E. Kates. Negative inotropic effect of lidocaine in patients with coronary artery disease and normal subjects. *Chest 71*: 170 (1977).
77. P. Geleris, H. Boudoulas, S. F. Schaal, R. P. Lewis, and J. J. Lima. Effect of procainamide on left ventricular performance in patients with primary myocardial disease. *Eur. J. Clin. Pharmacol. 18*: 311 (1980).

78. J. J. Lima, H. Boudoulas, and M. Blanford. Concentration dependency of disopyramide finding to plasma protein and its influence on kinetics and dynamics. *J. Pharmacol. Exp. Ther. 219*: 741 (1981).

79. H. Boudoulas, B. M. Beaver, R. E. Kates, and R. P. Lewis. Pharmacodynamics of inotropic and chronotropic responses to oral propranolol: Studies in normal subjects and in patients with angina. *Chest 73*: 146 (1978).

80. C. V. Leier, R. D. Magorien, H. Boudoulas, R. P. Lewis, D. Bambach, and D. V. Unverferth. The effect of vasodilator therapy on systolic and diastolic time intervals in congestive heart failure. *Chest 81*: 793 (1982).

81. K. Sagawa. Editorial: The end systolic pressure-volume relation of the ventricle: Definition, modifications and clinical use. *Circulation 63*: 1223-1227 (1981).

82. W. Grossman, E. Braunwald, T. Mann, L. P. McLaurin, and L. H. Green. Contractile state of the left ventricle in man as evaluated from end-systolic pressure-volume relations. *Circulation 56*: 845 (1977).

83. H. C. Mehmel, B. Stockins, K. Ruffmann, K. V. Olshausen, G. Schuler, and W. Kubler. The linearity of the end-systolic pressure-volume relationship in man and its sensitivity for assessment of left ventricular function. *Circulation 63*: 1216-1227 (1981).

84. H. Suga, and K. Sagawa. Instantaneous pressure-volume relationships and their ratio in the excised, supported canine left ventricle. *Circ. Res. 35*: 117 (1974).

85. F. Mahler, J. W. Covell, and J. Ross, Jr. Systolic pressure-diameter relations in the normal conscious dog. *Cardiovasc. Res. 9*: 447 (1975).

86. M. L. Weisfeldt, A. A. Shoukas, J. L. Weiss, N. Dashkoff, P. Come, L. S. C. Griffith, S. C. Achuff, H. Ducci, and K. Sagawa. Emax as a new contractility index in man. (abstr.). *Circulation (Suppl. 2) 54*: 114 (1976).

87. K. Sagawa, H. Suga, A. A. Shoukas, and K. M. Bakalar. End-systolic pressure/volume ratio: A new index of ventricular contractility. *Am. J. Cardiol. 40*: 748 (1977).

88. P. G. Hugenholtz, R. C. Ellison, C. W. Urschel, I. Mirsky, and E. H. Sonnenblick. Myocardial force-velocity relationships in clinical heart disease. *Circulation 41*: 191 (1970).

89. H. Suga, K. Sagawa, and A. A. Shoukas. Load independence of the instantaneous pressure-volume ratio of the canine left ventricle and effects of epinephrine and heart rate on the ratio. *Circ. Res. 32*: 314-322 (1973).

90. J. P. Holt. Regulation of the degree of emptying of the left ventricle by the force of ventricular contraction. *Circ. Res. 5*: 281 (1957).

91. K. M. Borow, L. H. Green, W. Grossman, and E. Braunwald. Left ventricular end-systolic stress-shortening and stress-length relations in humans: Normal values and sensitivity to inotropic state. *Am. J. Cardiol. 50*: 1301 (1982).

92. K. M. Borow, R. Propper, F. Z. Bierman, S. Grady, and A. Inati. Left ventricular end-systolic pressure dimension relation in patients with thalassemia major: A new noninvasive method of assessing contractile state. *Circulation 66*: 980 (1982).

93. B. R. Brodie, L. P. McLaurin, and W. Grossman. Combined hemodynamic-ultrasonic method for studying left ventricular wall stress: comparison with angiography. *Am. J. Cardiol. 37*: 864 (1976).

94. J. D. Marsh, L. H. Green, J. Wynne, P. F. Cohn, and W. Grossman. Left ventricular end-systolic pressure-dimension and stress-length relations in normal human subjects. *Am. J. Cardiol. 44*: 1311 (1979).

95. K. M. Borow, A. Neumann, and J. Wynne. Sensitivity of end-systolic pressure-dimension and pressure-volume relations to the inotropic state in humans. *Circulation 65*: 988-997 (1982).

96. M. A. Stefadouras, M. J. Dougherty, W. Grossman, and E. Craige. Determination of systemic vascular resistance by a noninvasive technique. *Circulation 47*: 101 (1973).

97. M. Takahashi, S. Sasayama, C. Kawai, and H. Kotoura. Contractile performance of the hypertrophied ventricle in patients with systemic hypertension. *Circulation 62*: 116-126 (1980).

98. P. A. Hugenholtz, E. Kaplan, and E. Hall. Determination of left ventricular wall thickness by angiocardiography. *Circulation 45*: 602 (1972).

99. B. Troy, J. F. Pombo, and C. E. Rackley. Measurement of left ventricular wall thickness and mass by echocardiography. *Circulation 45*: 602 (1972).

100. W. Grossman, D. Jones, and L. P. McLaurin. Wall stress and patterns of hypertrophy. *J. Clin. Invest. 56*: 36 (1975).

101. B. R. Brodie, L. P. McLaurin, and W. Grossman. Combined hemodynamic-ultrasonic method for studying left ventricular wall stress: Comparison with angiography. *Am. J. Cardiol. 37*: 864 (1976).

102. S. D. Colan, K. M. Borow, and A. Neumann. Left ventricular end-systolic wall stress-velocity of fiber shortening relation: A load-independent index of myocardial contractility. *J. Am. Coll. Cardiol. 4*: 715 (1984).

103. H. J. Schumann, J. Wagner, A. Knorr, J. Reidemeister, V. Sadony, and G. Schramm. Demonstration in human atrial preparations of A-adrenoreceptors mediating positive inotropic effects. *Arch. Pharmacol. 302*: 333-336 (1978).

104. M. Duke, R. P. Ames, W. H. Abelmann. Hemodynamic effect of methoxamine in normal human subjects. *Am. J. Med. Sci. 246*: 301-307 (1963).

105. L. I. Goldbert, R. D. Bloodwell, E. Braunwald, and A. G. Morrow. The direct effect of norepinephrine, epinephrine, and methoxamine on myocardial contractile force in man. *Circulation 22*: 1125 (1960).

106. B. A. Carabello, S. P. Nolan, and L. B. McGuire. Assessment of preoperative left ventricular function in patients with mitral regurgitation: Value of the end-systolic wall stress-end-systolic volume ratio. *Circulation 64*: 1212 (1981).

107. B. A. Carabello, L. H. Green, W. Grossman, L. H. Cohn, J. K. Koster, and J. J. Collins. Hemodynamic determinants of prognosis of aortic valve replacement in critical aortic stenosis and advanced congestive heart failure. *Circulation 62*: 42 (1980).

108. K. M. Borow, L. H. Green, L. J. Sloss, E. Braunwald, J. J. Collins, L. Cohn, and W. Grossman. End-systolic volume as a predictor of post-operative left ventricular performance in volume overload from valvular regurgitation. *Am. J. Med. 68*: 655 (1980).

109. B. A. Carabello, and J. F. Spann. The uses and limitations of end-systolic indexes of left ventricular function. *Circulation 69*: 1064 (1984).

110. B. A. Carabello, S. P. Nolan, and L. B. McGuire. Assessment of preoperative left ventricular function in patients with mitral regurgitation: Value of the end-systolic wall stress-end-systolic volume ratio. *Circulation 64*: 1212 (1981).

111. R. R. Taylor, J. W. Covell, and J. Ross, Jr. Volume-tension diagrams of ejecting and isovolumic contractions in left ventricle. *Am. J. Physiol. 216*: 1097 (1969).

112. M. E. Goldman. Editorial comment—emerging importance of the right ventricle. *J. Am. Coll. Cardiol. 514*: 925 (1985).

113. C. V. Leier, D. Sahar, J. B. Hermiller, R. D. Magorien, and D. V. Unverferth. Combined systolic time intervals and M-mode echocardiography in the evaluation of central hemodynamics in primary pulmonary hypertension. *Respiration 45*: 422 (1984).

114. A. M. Weissler, A. R. Kamen, R. S. Bornstein, C. D. Schoenfeld, and S. Cohen. Effect of deslanoside on the duration of the phases of ventricular systole in man. *Am. J. Cardiol. 15*: 153 (1965).

115. H. Kestelood, L. Brasseur, J. Carlier, J. C. Demanet, M. Andriange, G. Bataille, P. Collignon, J. Cosyns, J. C. Vancrombreucq, J. P. Van Durme, J. Willems, and J. Foucart. Effect of digitalis on the left ventricular ejection time: A multicenter double blind comparative study of digitoxin and pentaformylgitoxin in normal subjects. *Acta Cardiol. 24*: 409 (1969).

116. A. M. Weissler, R. P. Lewis, R. F. Leighton, and C. A. Bush. Comparative responses to the digitalis glycosides in man. In *Basic and Clinical Pharmacology of Digitalis*. B. H. Marks, and A. M. Weissler (eds.). Charles C Thomas, Springfield, IL 1972.

117. W. F. Forester, R. P. Lewis, A. M. Weissler, and T. A. Wilke. The onset and magnitude of the contractile response to commonly used digitalis glycosides in normal subjects. *Circulation 49*: 517 (1974).

118. A. M. Weissler. Interpreting systolic time intervals in man. *J. Am. Coll. Cardiol 2*: 1019-1020 (1983).

119. N. A. Klein, S. J. Siskind, W. H. Frishman, E. H. Sonnenblick, and T. Le-Jemtel. Hemodynamic comparison of intravenous amrinone and dobutamine in patients with congestive heart failure. *Am. J. Cardiol. 48*: 170 (1981).

120. K. T. Weber, V. Andrews, J. S. Janichi, J. R. Wilson, and A. P. Fishman. Amrinone and exercise performance in patients with chronic heart failure. *Am. J. Cardiol. 48*: 164 (1981).

121. J. R. Benotti, W. Grossman, E. Braunwald, D. D. Davalos, and A. A. Alousi. Hemodynamic assessment of amrinone: A new inotropic agent. *N. Engl. J. Med. 299*: 1373 (1978).

122. J. R. Benotti, W. Grossman, E. Braunwald, and B. A. Carabello. Effects of amrinone on myocardial energy metabolism and hemodynamics in patients with severe congestive heart failure due to coronary artery disease. *Circulation 62*: 28 (1980).

123. J. Wynne, R. F. Malacoff, J. R. Benotti, G. D. Curfman, W. Grossman, B. L. Holman, T. W. Smith, and E. Braunwald. Oral amrinone in refractory heart failure. *Am. J. Cardiol. 45*: 1245 (1980).

124. A. A. Alousi, A. E. Farah, G. Y. Lesher, and C. J. Opalka, Jr. Cardiotonic activity of amrinone-Win 40680 (5-amino-3,4'-bipyridine-6 (1H)-one). *Circ. Res. 45*: 666 (1979).

125. J. R. Benotti, W. Grossman, E. Braunwald, D. D. Davalos, and A. A. Alousi. Hemodynamic assessment of amrinone: A new inotropic agent. *N. Engl. J. Med. 299*: 1373 (1978).

126. T. H. LeJemtel, E. Keung, E. H. Sonnenblick, H. S. Ribner, M. Matsumoto, R. Davis, W. Schwartz, A. A. Alousi, and D. Davalos. Amrinone: A new non-glycosidic, non-adrenergic cardiotonic agent effective in the treatment of intractable myocardial failure in man. *Circulation 59*: 1098 (1979).

127. S. J. Siskind, E. H. Sonnenblick, R. Forman, J. Scheuer, and T. H. LeJemtel. Acute and substantial benefit of inotropic therapy with amrinone on exercise hemodynamics and metabolism in severe congestive heart failure. *Circulation 64*: 966 (1981).

128. C. V. Leier, K. Dalpiaz, P. Huss, J. B. Hermiller, R. Magorien, T. M. Bashore, and D. V. Unverferth. Amrinone therapy for congestive heart failure in outpatients with idiopathic dilated cardiomyopathy. *Am. J. Cardiol. 52*: 304 (1983).

129. J. B. Hermiller, M. E. Leithe, R. D. Magorien, D. V. Unverferth, and C. V. Leier. Amrinone in severe congestive heart failure: Another look at an intriguing new cardioactive drug. *J. Pharmacol. Exp. Ther. 228*: 319-326 (1983).

130. H. Boudoulas, R. P. Lewis, J. A. Sherman, C. A. Bush, G. Dalamangas, and W. F. Forester. Systolic time intervals in atrial fibrillation. *Chest 74*: 629 (1978).

3

Acute Inotropic Support

Intravenously Administered Positive Inotropic Drugs

CARL V. LEIER
Ohio State University College of Medicine, Columbus, Ohio

I. GENERAL INDICATIONS AND CONSIDERATIONS FOR USE

Parenterally administered inotropic drugs are indicated for acute short-term ino-tropic support of a cardiovascular system severely and/or acutely compromised by cardiac-ventricular dysfunction. The clinical setting is generally one of an acute myocardial insult resulting in substantial loss of ventricular contractility and car-diac function with depression of the stroke volume, cardiac output, blood pressure, and peripheral perfusion (reduction in organ blood flow and perhaps organ func-tion), and an increase in ventricular filling pressures. If untreated, the patient's condition frequently deteriorates into cardiovascular shock and, oftentimes, death. Currently in Western societies, myocardial infarction, cardiac surgery, and acute myocarditis are the most common insults to the myocardium resulting in loss of ventricular contractility. Acute inotropic support is commonly used to manage a patient during the course of one of these illnesses (Table 1). Acute inotropic sup-port is also used to transiently improve hemodynamics and the clinical status of patients with chronic heart failure who, for a variety of reasons, are experiencing a sudden deterioration of their already-compromised cardiac function. Patients with stable chronic congestive heart failure occasionally require short-term paren-teral inotropic support while undergoing a major diagnostic or therapeutic proce-dure (such as angiography, abdominal surgery).

It is important for physicians to remember that intravenously administered ino-tropic support is a temporary therapeutic measure. Unless a patient has what is believed to be a transient depression of ventricular function (for example, after cardiac surgery), acute inotropic therapy is just one part of a major therapeutic effort. Therefore, as the physician is starting the intravenous administration of a

TABLE 1 Indications for Intravenously Administered Acute Inotropic Therapy (Dobutamine as Prototype)

I. Short-term inotropic support of a patient with myocardial dysfunction, reduced stroke volume and cardiac output, hypotension, diminished peripheral perfusion, and elevated ventricular filling pressures, secondary to

    A. Acute myocardial insult or injury as seen with acute myocardial infarction or acute myocarditis

    B. Cardiac surgery (immediate and extended postoperative period)

    C. Decompensation of chronic low-output congestive heart failure

II. Short-term inotropic support during major diagnostic and/or surgical procedures (cardiac and noncardiac) for patients with chronic low-output congestive heart failure

---

positive inotrope, the next diagnostic and therapeutic measures (such as cardiac catheterization and surgery) should be entertained.

The administration of acute inotropic therapy is optimized by hemodynamic monitoring. Frequent bedside clinical evaluations and examinations are important, but the limitations of estimating left ventricular filling pressure and the status and change in ventricular function with the bedside clinical examination alone are now well recognized. In the setting of low cardiac output, hypotension, and hypoperfusion, positive inotropes are indicated only when the left ventricular filling pressures are elevated (>15 mmHg); if this clinical setting is accompanied by low-to-normal left ventricular filling pressure, volume expansion by intravenous fluid administration is the first step in therapy. Therefore, knowing the status of the ventricular filling pressures and cardiac function (cardiac output and stroke volume) is pivotal in the proper management of these critically ill patients. Continuous hemodynamic monitoring further assists the clinician in determining whether fluid administration and/or a vasodilator (such as nitroglycerin, nitroprusside) should be added during the course of inotropic therapy. Hemodynamic monitoring is accomplished by the placement of a flow-directed thermodilution pulmonary artery catheter (Swan-Ganz catheter). This catheter provides the measurement of right atrial pressure (as a determination of right ventricular filling pressure), pulmonary capillary wedge pressure (pulmonary artery occlusive pressure, a relatively close approximation of mean left atrial and left ventricular filling pressure), pulmonary artery pressure, and cardiac output. For moderate-to-severe hypotension, placement of an arterial catheter to monitor system blood pressure and to serve as a sampling conduit (blood gas and lactate determinations) is also important. With the aforementioned hemodynamic measurements, the following calculations can be made: cardiac index (liter/min/m^2) = cardiac output/body surface area; stroke volume (ml/beat) = cardiac output/heart rate; stroke volume index (ml/beat/m^2) = stroke volume/body surface area = cardiac index $\times$ 1000/heart rate; stroke work index $(g-m/m^2)$ = stroke volume index $\times$ (mean systemic blood pressure minus pulmonary wedge pressure) $\times$ 13.6/1000; total systemic vascular resistance (resistance units, mmHg/liter/min) = mean system blood pressure/cardiac output; systemic arteriolar resistance (resistance units, mmHg/liter/min) = (mean systemic blood pressure minus mean right atrial pressure)/cardiac output; total pulmonary vascular resistance (resistance units, mmHg/liter/min) = mean pulmonary artery pressure/cardiac output; and pulmonary arteriolar resistance (resistance units, mmHg/liter/min) = (mean pulmonary artery pressure minus pulmonary capillary wedge pressure)/cardiac output. Resistance units (mmHg/liter/min) can be converted to dynes-sec-cm^{-5} by multiplying resistance units by 80.

The catecholamine group of compounds (Fig. 1) are the agents most commonly used to provide acute short-term positive inotropic support. The major thrust of this chapter is therefore directed at this group of compounds. The catechol group includes both naturally (endogenously) occurring catecholamines (such as dopamine and norepinephrine) and the synthetic catechols (such as dobutamine and isoproterenol). The parenteral administration of digitalis, calcium, amrinone, and some of the experimental agents (such as milrinone) will also be discussed.

II. THE CATECHOLAMINES

A. Cardiovascular Site of Action

The most frequently employed catecholamines used to provide acute positive inotropic support are dobutamine, dopamine, and norepinephrine. These three catechols have in common positive inotropy, but otherwise they differ considerably. The differences in the hemodynamic effects of these three catechols are in large part secondary to differences in receptor activation (Table 2). The synthetic catecholamine, dobutamine, is a fairly powerful beta$_1$-adrenoceptor agonist, and as such, augments ventricular contractility with resultant increase in stroke volume and cardiac output (1-4). Recent studies suggest that for dobutamine, some of the positive inotropy may also be mediated through the stimulation of myocardial alpha$_1$-adrenergic receptors (5,6). Its peripheral alpha$_1$-agonist effects (veno- and vasoconstriction) are tempered by concomitant beta$_2$-receptor stimulation (vasodilation). In fact, the beta$_2$-agonist properties tend to override the peripheral alpha$_1$-vasoconstricting effects, giving dobutamine a net effect of mild vasodilation. Because the net peripheral vascular effects of dobutamine are relatively mild, this agent comes closest to being a pure positive inotropic drug. In contrast, the endogenous catecholamine, norepinephrine, is a powerful alpha$_1$-adrenoceptor agonist with relatively mild beta$_2$-stimulating effects (7). Although norepinephrine elicits some positive inotropy, its strong vasoconstricting properties make is a primary vasopressor (7,8). Dopamine stimulates beta$_1$-receptors to cause positive inotropy, but also stimulates peripheral alpha$_1$-receptors (in part, by releasing endogenous norepinephrine [7,9,10]) to provoke considerable vasoconstriction; as such, dopa-

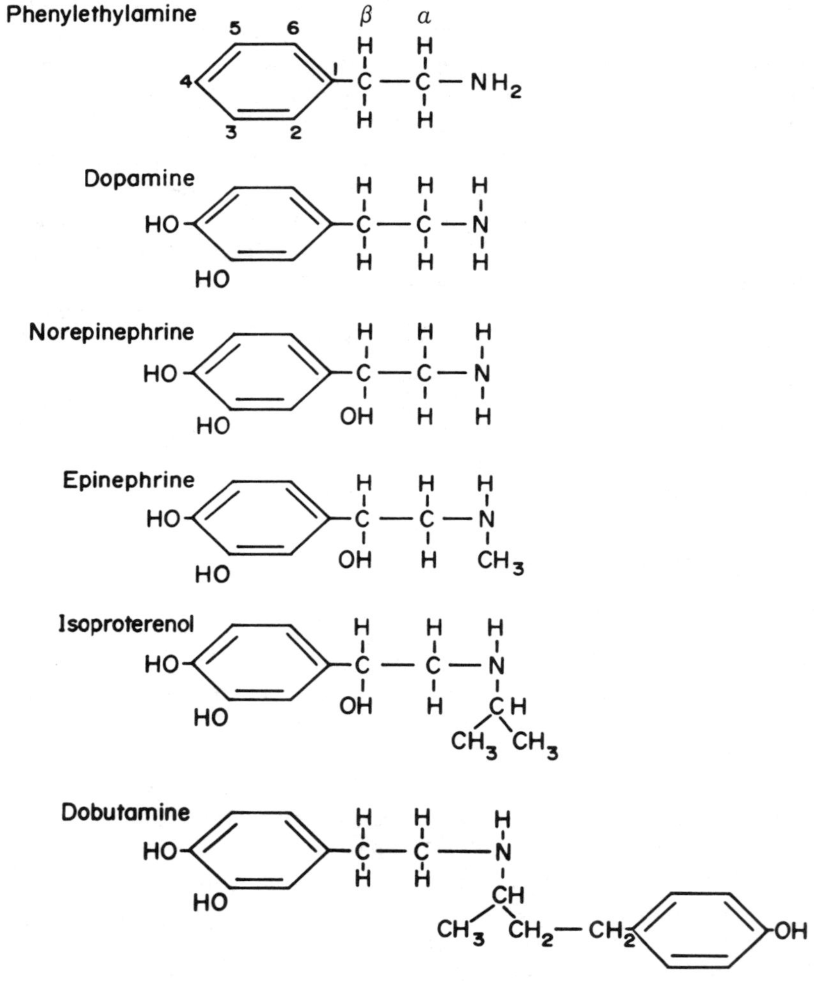

FIGURE 1 The molecular structures of the most commonly employed catecholamines. The addition of 3-OH and 4-OH to phenylethylamine results in the most
basic molecule of the catecholamine group, dopamine.

mine resides between dobutamine and norepinephrine in its hemodynamic effects
(1,7,11). These three catecholamines provide the clinician with a spectrum of drug
therapy which ranges from a primary positive inotropy (dobutamine) to a drug
with combined positive inotropic and vasopressor effects (dopamine) to a primary
vasopressor (norepinephrine). The synthetic catecholamine, isoproterenol, could
be placed to the left of this group as a drug with strong positive inotropic (beta$_1$-
agonist) and vasodilating (beta$_2$-agonist) properties (7).

TABLE 2 Relative Cardiac and Vascular Effects of Parenterally Administered Positive Inotropes

Catecholamine (standard dose)	Positive inotropy (β_1 stimulation, $? \alpha_1, ? \beta_2$)	Positive chronotropy (β_1, β_2 stimulation)	Vasoconstriction (α_1 stimulation)[a]	Vasodilation (β_2 stimulation)	Primary overall cardiovascular effect
Dobutamine	↑↑↑↑	↑	↑	↑↑	Positive inotrope
Dopamine	↑↑↑	↑	↑↑↑	↑ (Dopaminergic agonism)	Positive inotrope *plus* vasopressor
Norepinephrine	↑	0	↑↑↑↑	0	Vasopressor
Isoproterenol	↑↑↑↑	↑↑↑	0	↑↑↑	Positive inotrope *plus* vasodilator

Note: α = alpha-adrenergic receptor, β = beta-adrenergic receptor, ↑ = increases.
[a]Some of the vasoconstriction may also be secondary to stimulation of alpha$_2$-adrenergic receptors located in the arteriole (non-neuronal, extra-junctional).

B. Dobutamine: A Relatively Selective Positive Inotrope

1. Clinical Pharmacology and Application

In the clinical setting of myocardial depression, reduced stroke volume, cardiac output, systemic blood pressure, and peripheral (organ, limb, tissue) perfusion, and elevated ventricular filling pressures, dobutamine improves myocardial contractility, stroke volume, cardiac output, systemic pressure and perfusion, and decreases ventricular filling pressures (12-16) (Fig. 2). Pulmonic and systemic vascular resistances uniformly decrease during dobutamine administration (12-16). Employing current terminology, dobutamine is a positive inotrope with preload-reducing (reduction in ventricular filling pressures) and afterload-reducing (reduction in systemic vascular resistance and ventricular systolic volume) properties. Proper dosage is generally not accompanied by significant positive chronotropy or dysrhythmias, unless these were present prior to the infusion. In low-output heart failure, dobutamine augments renal blood flow by increasing cardiac output rather than activating renal dopaminergic receptors (17). Urine output and urea and sodium clearance generally increase (15). Hepatic-splanchnic blood flow is not greatly altered with standard maintenance doses (17). Dobutamine increases limb blood flow in proportion to cardiac output in patients with low-output congestive heart failure (17).

The hemodynamic effects of dobutamine correlate well and linearly with plasma concentration and dosage (18). Dobutamine is administered as a continuous intravenous infusion at starting doses of 2-3 $\mu g/kg/min$ with 2-3 $\mu g/kg/min$ increments every 10-30 min until the desired hemodynamic effects are attained or undesirable effects appear. During the first 72 hours of dobutamine administration, optimal maintenance dosages usually range between 7.5 and 15 $\mu g/kg/min$. The hemodynamic effects of a continuous infusion may be observed as early as 2 minutes after the onset of the infusion. The maximal (peak-plateau) effects are achieved by 10-14 min. The mean plasma half-life in patients with low-output congestive heart failure is 2.37 ± 0.70 min, indicating that most of the drug is metabolized or eliminated 10-12 min after the infusion is interrupted (19). The short half-life is secondary to rapid redistribution and to metabolism by catechol-O-methyl transferase (20). The major metabolites are 3-O-methyldobutamine glucuronide and dobutamine glucuronide, both pharmacologically inactive. The metabolites are eliminated primarily by the kidney. The short half-life of dobutamine (and other catecholamines) is a favorable feature in the treatment of clinically unstable patients in whom the management of undesirable effects or inadvertent overadministration of a drug is facilitated by rapid elimination. Infusions lasting longer than 72 hours may be accompanied by the development of pharmacodynamic tolerance (21), presumably on the basis of down-regulation of beta-adrenergic receptors. The effects of tolerance development are readily corrected by advancing infusion rates using desired hemodynamic responses and side effects as a guide.

Doses >10 $\mu g/kg/min$ may elicit undesirable effects. These side effects, such as tachycardia, dysrhythmias, headaches, anxiety, tremors, and excessive changes in blood pressure, are relatively uncommon with proper dobutamine doses in the appropriate patient. The characteristics of the "appropriate patient" and the proper dosage schedule have been presented above. Tachycardia and other side effects may occur at doses <10 $\mu g/kg/min$ if the initial dose is too high, advanced too rapidly, or given in the wrong setting (for example, low ventricular filling pressures). Caution during administration is also necessary for patients with a history of dysrhythmias. Dobutamine facilitates conduction over the atrioventricular node (22, 23) and, therefore, may accelerate the ventricular rate in patients with atrial fibrillation or flutter. Patients with a history of systemic hypertension may have an excessive increase in blood pressure with dobutamine (17). Tissue necrosis at an intravenous infiltration site is uncommon, but has been reported for dobutamine (24).

2. Effect on Coronary Blood Flow and Myocardial Oxygen Consumption

Because atherosclerotic coronary artery disease is a common cause of low-output cardiac failure and because many patients, who need acute inotropic support, have acute coronary occlusion with infarction, a brief discussion of the role of acute inotropic therapy (such as dobutamine) in patients with decompensated atherosclerotic heart disease is important. First of all, the patients in whom acute inotropic support is indicated have depressed ventricular function, stroke volume, and cardiac output; hypotension-shock; and high ventricular filling pressures. Although positive inotropy increases myocardial oxygen consumption (MVO_2), a carefully administered positive inotrope (such as dobutamine, low-to-moderate doses of dopamine) may concomitantly elicit changes which tend to decrease MVO_2; these include decreasing wall stress by reducing diastolic and systolic ventricular volumes and ventricular end-diastolic pressure. By increasing diastolic and mean systemic blood pressure and decreasing left ventricular filling pressure, proper inotropic support will increase coronary perfusion pressure. Some of these inotropic agents increase diastolic coronary perfusion time as well (25). The ideal dose of an inotrope is that which elicits the aforementioned hemodynamic changes without causing an increase in heart rate (which $\uparrow MVO_2 \downarrow$ and diastolic coronary perfusion time). Doses which increase heart rate should, therefore, be avoided in patients with occlusive coronary artery disease.

Dobutamine increases coronary blood flow and oxygen delivery equal to or greater than the increase in MVO_2 in patients with congestive heart failure and nonobstructed coronary arteries. In one study, patients with idiopathic dilated cardiomyopathy had an increase in cardiac output of 35% and 65%, coronary blood flow of 35% and 51%, and MVO_2 of 20% and 40% during 5 and 10 $\mu g/kg/min$ (respectively) infusions of dobutamine (26). These findings suggest that in the appropriate hemodynamic setting, proper dosage of a selective positive inotrope may favorably affect myocardial oxygen balance (that is, oxygen supply $\geqslant$ demand).

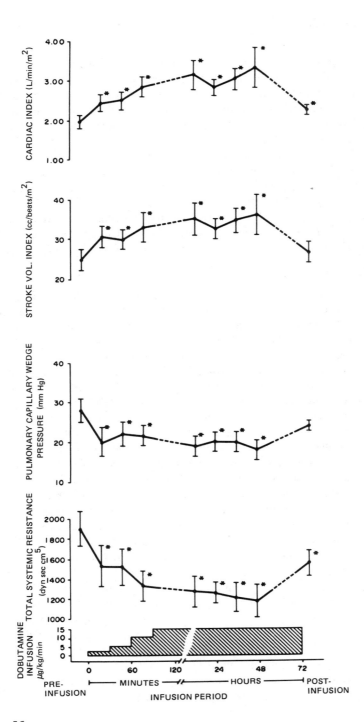

56

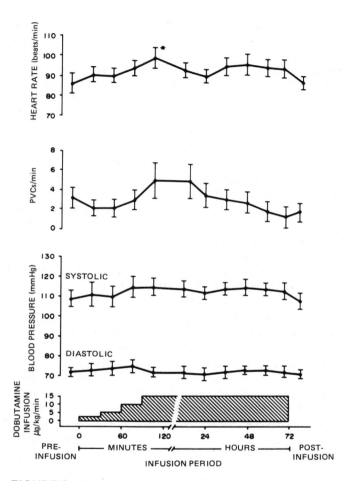

FIGURE 2 The hemodynamic effects of dose-response administration and continuous infusions of dobutamine in patients with severe congestive heart failure. $n = 25$, *$p < 0.05$ versus preinfusion. (Reproduced from Figs. 3 and 4 of Ref. 15, permission granted.)

In patients with chronic myocardial failure secondary to coronary artery disease, Bendersky and colleagues (27) showed that administration of dobutamine at 10 $\mu g/kg/min$ improved cardiac performance; the increase in MVO_2 was accompanied by a comparable increase in coronary blood flow. Although none of the 8 patients had angina or electrocardiographic changes during the infusion, 1 patient demonstrated myocardial lactate production. Pozen and associates (28) showed that dobutamine (up to 15 $\mu g/kg/min$) improved cardiac function including the contractility of ischemic segments. Of their 18 patients, 4 produced myocardial lactate; of these 4, 3 had angina pectoris. These two studies suggest that standard doses of dobutamine improve cardiac function in patients with occlusive coronary artery disease and congestive heart failure at a relatively low risk of developing more ischemia or an infarction. Lactate production, indicating a reduction in cellular oxygenation in one or more regions, occurred in approximately 5 of 26 patients during the infusion; the frequency is likely to be less at lower, but still effective, doses. Kupper et al. (29) found that in patients with occlusive coronary disease and cardiac failure, myocardial lactate production or diminished extraction is primarily related to the degree of tachycardia elicited by dobutamine. Patients with severe triple vessel disease may have a more heterogeneous myocardial blood flow pattern during dobutamine treatment despite an increase in total coronary blood flow (30). Relevant to occlusive coronary artery disease, infusions of dobutamine have been shown to inhibit platelet function (31). Using similar techniques, most other catecholamines generally enhance platelet aggregation.

When mild-to-moderate hypotension and congestive heart failure occur secondary to acute myocardial infarction, dobutamine is the drug of choice. The goals of therapy in this setting are to maintain an adequate systemic and coronary perfusion pressure, improve peripheral perfusion, and decrease left ventricular filling pressure ($\downarrow$ congestion) without greatly increasing MVO_2. In this setting, proper doses of dobutamine augments ventricular performance; increases stroke volume, cardiac output, and peripheral perfusion; and reduces ventricular filling pressure (32-35). Systemic blood pressure increases toward normal levels secondary to the enhancement of pulse pressure by the augmented stroke volume. In contrast, norepinephrine or moderate-to-high doses of dopamine effect much of the increase in systemic pressure by systemic arteriolar vasoconstriction. While the increase in systemic blood pressure with these vasopressors may increase coronary perfusion pressure, systemic vasoconstriction further compromises peripheral tissue perfusion and increases ventricular afterload, filling pressure, and MVO_2. In the clinical setting of acute infarction, mild-to-moderate hypotension, or congestive heart failure, proper dosage of dobutamine has favorable effect on MVO_2 concomitant with an improvement in cardiac-cardiovascular performance. By reducing afterload ($\downarrow$ systemic vascular resistance and ventricular systolic volume) and preload ($\downarrow$ ventricular filling pressure), dobutamine decreases systolic and diastolic wall tension, major determinants of MVO_2. By increasing coronary perfusion pressure ($\downarrow$ or$\rightarrow$systemic mean and/or diastolic arterial pressure and ventricular diastolic filling pressures) and coronary perfusion time (25) and, perhaps, by some coronary vasodilation (36-45), dobutamine may enhance coronary blood flow. The combination of these factors probably offsets much of the increase in MVO_2, which occurs with dobutamine-induced positive inotropy. Again, doses that increase heart rate must be avoided; any increment in heart rate will increase MVO_2 and reduce coronary perfusion time.

Gillespie and colleagues (33), in a controlled study, found that dobutamine did not increase infarct size over predicted values and did not increase the frequency or severity of dysrhythmias. The same laboratory (34) later compared infusions of dobutamine with parenterally administered digitalis in the same clinical setting: dobutamine effected a greater and more predictable improvement in cardiac-cardiovascular performance. Dobutamine effectively improves cardiac function in patients with infarction who had been treated with beta blockade (46).

Clinical and hemodynamic assessment (via flow-directed thermodilution catheter), with proper adjustment of the dobutamine infusion rate, of fluid administration, and of diuretic dosage must occur at frequent and regular intervals. Dopamine is occasionally administered in addition to dobutamine to stimulate dopaminergic receptors in an attempt to improve renal blood flow or to further augment systemic blood pressure. If systemic blood pressure returns toward normal levels or higher for a given individual during the dobutamine infusion, intravenously administered nitroglycerin or nitroprusside may be added to augment hemodynamics, to further reduce systolic and diastolic ventricular wall tension ($\downarrow MVO_2$), and to improve peripheral infusion.

3. Cardiogenic Shock

Cardiogenic shock is a clinical syndrome characterized by a marked reduction in the perfusion (and function) of organ systems and tissues because of inadequate cardiac output secondary to a catastrophic cardiac event. The most common catastrophic event in Western culture is acute myocardial infarction. The syndrome is generally accompanied by marked hypotension, signs and symptoms of reduced organ and tissue perfusion (such as renal dysfunction, cool-pale extremities, lethargy, elevated blood lactate levels), marked reduction in stroke volume, and tachycardia.

The general clinical approach to cardiogenic shock is to proficiently evaluate the clinical and hemodynamic condition of the patient, improve and stabilize the cardiovascular status, and make arrangements for the critical diagnostic studies (for example, cardiac catheterization) and therapeutic interventions (for example, intra-aortic balloon counterpulsation and cardiac surgery). Again, the placement of the flow-directed pulmonary artery catheter is critical to the management of these patients, particularly with respect to fluid and drug administration. In terms of improving and stabilizing the cardiovascular status in cardiogenic shock, the initial objective is to bring systemic blood pressure into a range that will provide adequate coronary perfusion pressure (mean >55-60 mmHg). This is a critical issue in maintaining viability of the noninfarcted myocardium. Dopamine or norepinephrine is generally used in this setting because of the ability of these agents to elicit the vasoconstriction needed to raise systemic blood pressure (7,8,11,47). In essence, peripheral perfusion is temporarily compromised in favor of coronary-myocardial perfusion. The author favors dopamine over norepinephrine as a first-line drug because the former agent probably has a more favorable effect on renal blood flow and function and dopamine increases systemic pressure through a better balance of positive inotropy (↑ contraction, ↑ stroke volume, ↑ pulse pressure) and vasoconstriction. As systemic blood pressure increases into an acceptable range, dobutamine and, occasionally, nitroglycerin or nitroprusside can be added to further improve overall cardiovascular function with the least MVO_2 expended. An occasional patient in cardiogenic shock may have a more favorable initial response to dobutamine compared to dopamine. Rather than starting all patients with cardiogenic shock on dobutamine and adding dopamine or norepinephine if additional augmentation of systemic blood pressure is needed, and because of the critical issue of attaining adequate coronary-myocardial perfusion quickly, the author favors starting with dopamine, adding dobutamine if indicated, then gradually withdrawing dopamine (or norepinephrine) with its accompanying vasoconstricting effects.

Our center and others (48) have found dobutamine useful in improving and maintaining cardiovascular function before, during, and after intra-aortic balloon counterpulsation.

4. Cardiac Surgery and Postoperative Care

The role of dobutamine during and immediately after cardiac surgery requiring cardiopulmonary bypass has not been adequately studied. Hess et al. (49) noted that dobutamine elicited considerable vasopressor activity in some patients undergoing general anesthesia. Piepenbrock and colleagues (50) found that dobutamine provoked an inordinate increase in heart rate in some anesthetized patients, before and during cardiopulmonary bypass. In patients emerging from cardiopulmonary bypass, Steen et al. (51) found only subtle hemodynamic differences between the administration of dobutamine, dopamine, and epinephrine. None of these studies, however, were performed on a uniform population of patients with depressed ventricular systolic function, reduced cardiac output, mild-to-moderate hypotension, and elevated ventricular filling pressures.

In the postoperative period starting 4-6 hr after surgery, Gray et al. (52) and Sakamoto and Yamada (53) found that patients with a depressed cardiac output and high ventricular filling pressures showed considerable improvement of cardiac performance (↑ stroke volume and cardiac output and ↓ ventricular filling pressure) during dobutamine with little positive chronotropy. In the study of Gray et al. (52), optimal doses of dobutamine elicited less tachycardia and reduced ventricular filling pressures more than comparable doses of dopamine. Other studies (54-59) performed after bypass surgery showed varying responses to dobutamine. Again, most of these reports included patients with normal stroke volume, cardiac output, and/or a normal-to-low ventricular filling pressure; these are patients who probably should not be receiving a parenterally administered positive inotropy anyway. Fowler and colleagues (60) compared the cardiac and coronary hemodynamic effects of dobutamine and dopamine in 10 patients at 6, 10, 15, and 24 hours after cardiopulmonary bypass for coronary artery bypass surgery. Both drugs altered hemodynamics similarly; however, only dobutamine increased coronary blood flow commensurate with the increase in MVO_2 (Fig. 3). Tight and associates (61) found that dobutamine, compared to dopamine, caused a greater increase in contractility at lower levels of systolic wall stress and peripheral vascular resistance in patients 16-20 hr after bypass surgery.

More work is needed to define the therapeutic spectrum of dobutamine during and after cardiac surgery. At present, dobutamine should be used primarily in patients whose ventricular dysfunction has caused a reduction in stroke volume and

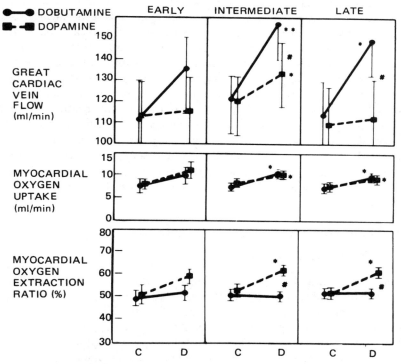

FIGURE 3 A comparison of the effects of dopamine and dobutamine on coronary blood flow and myocardial energetics during the early (first 6 hr), intermediate (10-15 hr), and late (24 hr) postoperative study periods in patients who had undergone cardiopulmonary bypass for coronary artery bypass surgery. (Reproduced from Fig. 4 of Ref. 60, permission granted.)

cardiac output, mild-to-moderate hypotension with diminished peripheral infusion, and an elevation in ventricular filling pressure.

5. Other Indications and Considerations

The hemodynamic guidelines and indications for the intravenous administration of a positive inotrope (such as dobutamine, low-dose dopamine) are the same in cardiac disease states of the pediatric age group as those of adults. Although the conditions causing the loss of myocardial contractility are quite different in the majority of patients (congenital lesions in children versus ischemic events in adults), the overall hemodynamic responses (↑contractility, ↑ stroke volume, ↑ cardiac output, ↓ ventricular filling pressures, ↓ vascular resistances) are similar (62-64). Dobutamine is rarely indicated for noncardiac causes of low output, hypotension and/or shock, such as septic shock. The predominant hemodynamic characteristics of most cases of septic shock are generalized vasodilation, a marked increase in vascular capacitance, and moderate-to-severe systemic hypotension. Dopamine, with its vasopressor properties, is the catecholamine of choice in the treatment of this condition (65,66). The positive inotropic properties of dopamine would also be directed at reversing some of the myocardial depression noted in many patients with septic shock. In this setting, dobutamine's potential for increasing MVO_2 (increased inotropy and possibly increased heart rate) is greater than its capacity to raise myocardial oxygen supply (changes in coronary perfusion pressure and time are unlikely). In septic shock, dobutamine should probably be reserved for patients with concomitant significant ventricular dysfunction and elevated ventricular filling pressures, or used as a second-line drug in instances in which dopamine becomes ineffective (65-67).

C. Dopamine: A Positive Inotrope-Vasopressor

1. Clincal Pharmacology and Application

Dopamine, with its combined positive inotropic and vasoconstricting properties, is used to improve and stabilize the hemodynamic status of patients afflicted with conditions causing myocardial depression, marked hypotension, and/or shock (such as septic shock, initial therapy of cardiogenic shock) (17,68-77). In this clinical setting, infusions of dopamine increase stroke volume, cardiac output, and systemic blood pressure (via augmented stroke volume and arteriolar vasoconstriction). Ventricular filling pressure generally does not change or may increase (at doses >6 μg/kg/min). Systemic vascular resistance usually decreases at low dose (<6 μg/kg/min) and returns to or above baseline at higher doses. Dopamine should, therefore, be regarded as a positive inotrope-vasopressor with variable effects on preload and afterload. Positive chronotropy and dysrhythmias are generally not a problem unless doses exceed 6-8 μg/kg/min.

Dopamine, administered as an infusion, is generally started at 0.5-1.0 μg/kg/min and advanced in 2 μg/kg/min increments every 10-30 min until the desired clinical and hemodynamic effects are attained or undesirable effects appear. Maximal or peak-plateau phase of hemodynamics is achieved 10-14 min after the onset of the infusion. Dopamine is metabolized by catechol-O-methyl transferase, and to a lesser extent, by monoamine oxidase and by conversion to norepinephrine at nerve endings.

Dopamine stimulates $beta_1$-, $alpha_1$-, and dopaminergic-receptors (7,11). Some of dopamine's effects are probably mediated by the release of norepinephrine as well (9,10). Infusions of dopamine elicit a dose-related biphasic hemodynamic response (17). At lower doses, <6 μg/kg/min, dopamine increases stroke volume and cardiac output and decreases vascular resistances with a mild increase in systemic blood pressure; these effects are probably a cumulative result of $beta_1$-, $alpha_1$-, and dopaminergic-receptor agonism. At doses > 6 μg/kg/min, vasopressor effects become dominant, manifested by substantial increase in systemic blood pressure and resistance. It appears that at higher doses, dopamine effects a greater recruitment of alpha-receptor agonism and perhaps a greater release of norepinephrine from nerve endings of vasculature. At these doses, the clinical and hemodynamic effects oftentimes become indistinguishable from those of norepinephrine.

Stimulation of renal "dopaminergic" receptors by dopamine is a rather unique property of this catecholamine (11,78-80). In the proper clinical and hemodynamic setting, dopaminergic-receptor (DA_1) stimulation by dopamine increases renal blood flow, glomerular filtration rate, and sodium clearance (78,79). This dopaminergic-receptor agonism is frequently employed clinically to improve renal function in a variety of conditions (such as states of low renal perfusion, hepatorenal syndrome) and is oftentimes the basis for selecting dopamine over norepinephrine in shock states. The doses most effective in activating dopaminergic receptors generally reside between 2 μg/kg/min and 6 μg/kg/min. Doses > 8 μg/kg/min are often accompanied by considerable $alpha_1$-mediated vasoconstriction (systemic and renal).

The side effects noted with dopamine generally occur at moderate-to-high doses (>6 μg/kg/min), and include those commonly noted with other catecholamines, such as tachycardia, dysrhythmias, headaches, tremor, and anxiety. Although little parenterally administered dopamine is supposed to cross the blood-brain barrier, some patients experience nausea and/or vomiting (17). Local tissue necrosis may occur as a complication of tissue infiltration of dopamine at the infusion site; local injections of phenolamine may be effective in averting tissue necrosis, if employed immediately after the infiltration is detected. Digital necrosis (due to excessive vasoconstriction) may occur with prolonged or high-dose infusions, particularly in patients with pre-existing vascular disease (7,81,82).

2. Comparison of Dopamine and Dobutamine

The drugs most commonly used to provide acute positive inotropic support are dopamine and dobutamine. Several studies (17,76,77) have shown that the clinical and hemodynamic responses of these two catecholamines are different (Fig. 4).

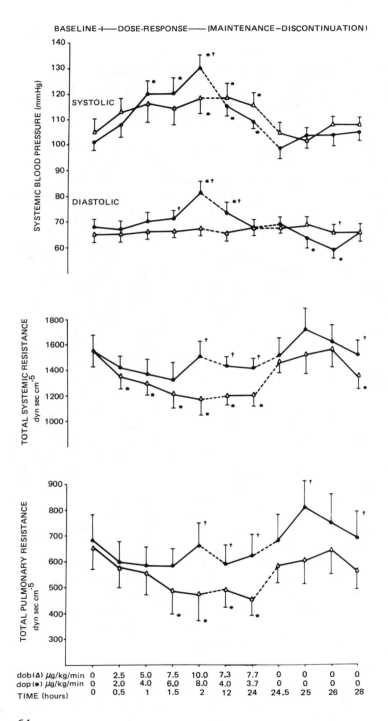

64

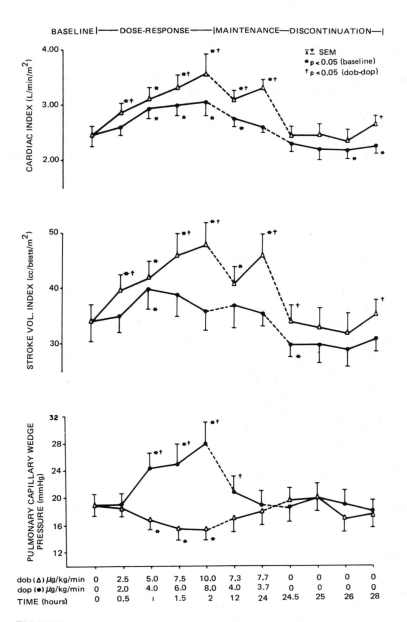

BASELINE |———DOSE-RESPONSE———|MAINTENANCE—DISCONTINUATION—|

FIGURE 4 Graphs comparing the hemodynamic effects of dopamine (dop, ●) and dobutamine (dob, △) in a population of 13 patients with low-output congestive heart failure. (Reproduced from Figs. 1 and 2 of Ref. 17, permission granted.)

The major differences are related to dopamine's ability to elicit greater systemic vasoconstriction. This enhanced vascular tone for dopamine is mediated by its more active and relatively unopposed stimulation of vascular $alpha_1$-receptors and occurs, in part, through dopamine-induced release of endogenous norepinephrine from nerve endings (9,10). Dopamine does not stimulate vascular $beta_2$-adrenoceptors. Dopamine causes a greater increase in systemic blood pressure than comparable doses of dobutamine (17,76). Intense arteriolar vasoconstriction is more likely to be seen with dopamine. Dopamine elicits little or no venodilation, and in contrast to dobutamine, dopamine either does not change or it increases ventricular filling pressures (17,76,77). Parenteral nitroprusside or nitroglycerin is frequently added to dopamine infusions to reverse some of its vasopressor effects. The hemodynamic effects of this combination are similar to those of dobutamine alone without the simplicity and ease of single drug administration (32).

3. Indications and Considerations for Use

Dopamine is the first-line cardiovascular drug for the treatment of cardiogenic shock. Its infusion should be initially directed at bringing blood pressure into a range (>55-60 mmHg mean) capable of adequately perfusing the coronary vascular bed; at this point, another agent (such as dobutamine, nitroglycerin) can be added to effect a further improvement in hemodynamics and organ-tissue perfusion. Because of dopamine's propensity to increase ventricular filling pressures, Richard et al. (83) recommend a combination of dopamine and dobutamine as the initial phase of therapy in cardiogenic shock. Dopamine is also the first-line drug for certain noncardiogenic shock states, particularly those characterized by combined vasodepression and ventricular depression, such as septic shock. Dopamine is a reasonable alternative to norepinephrine in treating hypotension and shock caused by vasodilating events (for example, certain drug intoxications or after resection of pheochromocytoma). Lower doses of dopamine are commonly infused to improve renal blood flow and function (through its dopaminergic-agonist properties) in conditions in which renal blood flow and function are in jeopardy (for example, after aortic aneurysm repair or in the case of hepatorenal syndrome). The reader is referred to Sec. II.B. 3-5 for additional information regarding the pharmacophysiological considerations directing the use of dopamine.

D. Norepinephrine: A Vasopressor

Norepinephrine, an endogenous catecholamine, acts primarily through $alpha_1$-adrenoceptor agonism. The administration of this drug elicits a cardiovascular vasopressor response through dose-related vasoconstriction (7,8,84-87). Norepinephrine should rarely be used as an initial drug for positive inotropic therapy; its powerful vasoconstricting properties may potentially increase afterload to the point of offsetting any positive inotropism and it may possibly increase afterload and preload to levels at which the myocardial oxygen demand to supply ratio is threatened.

The clinical setting, for which norepinephrine could be entertained as a therapeutic intervention, is severe hypotension and/or shock second to a vasodilatory (such as sepsis) and/or a cardiogenic (such as myocardial infarction) mechanism, nonresponsive to dopamine. As mentioned in the sections discussing dopamine and dobutamine, it is critical in these conditions to proficiently bring mean systemic blood pressure to an acceptable level to re-establish and maintain adequate coronary perfusion; norepinephrine may occasionally have to be added to dopamine to accomplish this objective. Some clinicians actually prefer starting with norepinephrine. Once the mean systemic blood pressure has reached >60 mmHg, other interventions (for example, dobutamine, dopamine, and/or intra-aortic balloon counterpulsation) should be entertained in an effort to avoid continuous (>24 hr) maintenance norepinephrine infusions or the necessity to advance the norepinephrine dose. These considerations are directed at averting the complications of prolonged intense vasoconstriction.

Norepinephrine is started at an infusion rate of 0.01-0.02 μg/kg/min and advanced in dose every 10-15 min until the desired effects (generally a systemic pressure response) are achieved or undesirable effects are observed. The plasma half-life is 2-4 min, so that the pharmacologic effects are generally dissipated 10-20 min after discontinuation of the infusion. The undesirable effects are those occasionally seen with other catecholamine infusions (such as tachycardia, dysrhythmias, anxiety, tremor, gastrointestinal distress, myocardial ischemia) and those associated with intense vasoconstriction (for example, reduced organ and tissue perfusion, impairment of renal function, digital gangrene, tissue necrosis at infiltration site). The positive inotropism and chronotropism of norepinephrine are probably a result of its beta$_1$-agonist effects, albeit modest. It is interesting that the positive inotropic effects of norepinephrine may not be mediated by myocardial alpha$_1$-receptor agonism, although stimulation of these receptors by other catecholamines enhances contractility (5,6,88).

E. Isoproterenol, Epinephrine: The "Other" Catecholamines

Because of the spectrum of pharmacological effects provided by dobutamine, dopamine, and norepinephrine, the agents isoproterenol and epinephrine are infrequently used to enhance inotropy. Isoproterenol, a synthetic catecholamine, is a relatively powerful positive intotrope (mediated by beta$_1$ and perhaps some beta$_2$-agonism). The strong unopposed beta$_2$-agonist effects tend to narrow the margin of safety for this drug. Positive inotropism is noted at dosages of 0.007-0.014 μg/kg/min with rather dramatic dose-related recruitment of vasodilation (vascular beta$_2$-agonism), positive chronotropism, and occasionally dysrhythmias at >0.020 μg/kg/min. If both positive inotropy and vasodilation are desired, a dobutamine (or dopamine) and nitroglycerin (or nitroprusside) combination can be used without the hazards of isoproterenol's narrow margin of safety, positive chronotropism, possibly greater dysrhythmic potential, and uncontrolled excessive vasodilation. Epinephrine, an endogenous catecholamine with $beta_1$-, $alpha_1$-, and $beta_2$-agonist effects, has fairly vigorous positive inotropic properties. Unfortunately, its administration as an infusion may provoke a wide range of unpredictable positive inotropic, chrontropic, dysrhythmic, and vascular responses.

The inotropic and cardiovascular effects of isoproterenol and epinephrine are more commonly used in the surgical arena, particularly in the immediate postcardiopulmonary bypass patient (51,55,57,73). A number of patients in this setting often require these particular catechols (occasionally in high doses) to facilitate withdrawal from the cardiopulmonary pump and/or to support the cardiovascular system for a short time thereafter. The therapeutic rationale for this approach is beyond the scope of this treatise and may be gleaned from other sources (51,55, 73,89).

F. Combination Therapy

For optimal clinical and therapeutic effect, it is important to follow certain principles in administering combination catecholamine-vasodilator or catecholamine-catecholamine therapy. First, combination therapy is rarely started as such. Second, the administration of each drug is guided by both clinical and hemodynamic (flow-directed pulmonary artery catheter) monitoring. Last, the endpoints of therapy are generally weighted in favor of those signifying clinical improvement, using hemodynamics as a guide to achieving these endpoints. In other words, once an adequate systemic blood pressure is attained (or is present), therapeutic efforts should be directed at improving peripheral and organ perfusion and renal (and other organ) function, and reducing congestion (such as pulmonary edema) if present.

1. Catecholamine-Vasodilator Combination

For decades now, physicians have realized that in certain clinical situations, drug combinations are oftentimes preferable to the administration of a member of the combination alone. Prior to the availability of dobutamine and dopamine, phentolamine (alpha-adrenoceptor blocker) was occasionally added to norepinephrine infusions for the purpose of blunting the intense vasoconstriction, yet maintaining the positive inotropic properties of this catecholamine (90). As dopamine became available, nitroprusside or nitroglycerin were (and still are) occasionally added to the dopamine administration (91,92). In cardiogenic shock, the vasodilator is added after the dopamine infusion achieves an adequate increase in systemic blood pressure. The combination generally effects a greater improvement in hemodynamics through combined "positive inotropy and afterload reduction" with less hypotension than a vasodilator alone and less vasoconstriction than dopamine alone (19, 92). The hemodynamic effects of dobutamine are similar to those of combination dopamine-vasodilator (nitroprusside or nitroglycerin) (32). Now with the availability of dobutamine, intravenously administered nitroglycerin or nitroprusside occasionally may be added to this inotrope to further improve hemodynamics and peripheral perfusion (93).

Combination catecholamine-vasodilator therapy may be the optimal form of drug intervention in a number of cardiovascular situations. If a patient enters the hospital with myocardial depression, low cardiac output, hypotension, reduced peripheral perfusion, and high ventricular filling pressures, dobutamine is given (dopamine, if hypotension is severe) and advanced in dose until an adequate systemic blood pressure is attained and peripheral and organ perfusion and function improves. If peripheral perfusion remained compromised (for instance, cool hands, reduced capillary filling of fingers and toes, impaired renal function, elevated serum lactate concentrations) despite systemic systolic pressures >100 mmHg (this value may vary from 80 to 110 mmHg) and ventricular filling pressures remain elevated with "congestion," nitroglycerin or nitroprusside can be added to the dobutamine infusion instead of advancing dobutamine to high doses (>15 μg/kg/min). In this setting, the careful concomitant administration of the vasodilator generally effects an improvement in peripheral perfusion and a reduction in elevated ventricular filling pressures. Nitroprusside or nitroglycerin should be the initial agent administered to a patient with myocardial depression, low cardiac output, high ventricular filling pressures, congestion, and normal-to-high systemic blood pressure. If peripheral perfusion and organ (such as renal) function remain compromised at doses which have induced a fall in systemic blood pressure (systolic <100 mmHg) and ventricular filling pressures are adequate or high, dobutamine should probably be added. Low-dose dopamine is a reasonable alternative, particularly if renal dopaminergic agonism is desired.

2. Catecholamine-Catecholamine Combination

Dobutamine is occasionally added to or is used to replace dopamine (or norepinephrine) in the treatment of shock after the vasopressor agents have effected the critical increase in systemic blood pressure. The rationale for the addition or replacement relates to the fact that dobutamine's effects on the myocardial oxygen supply to demand ratio and on overall hemodynamics are generally more favorable than agents with strong vasopressor properties (see Sec. II.B on dobutamine). Dopamine may be administered to a patient receiving dobutamine in order to further augment systemic blood pressure (83) or in an attempt to improve renal function via DA_1 stimulation (11,78-80).

III. NONCATECHOLAMINE POSITIVE INOTROPES

A. Intravenous Administration of Amrinone

The bipyridine derivative, amrinone, increases contractility in normal canine models (94). The mechanism of action itself remains elusive. Amrinone does not act directly on adrenergic or Na-K ATPase receptors. The infusion of amrinone in hu-

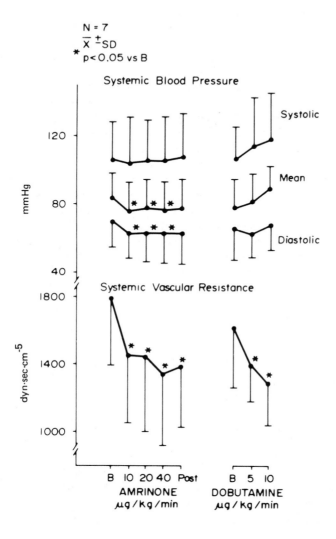

N = 7
$\overline{X} \pm SD$
* p < 0.05 vs B

mans with cardiac failure (95-99) generally effects a reduction in systemic and pulmonic vascular resistances and left ventricular filling pressure (Fig. 5). A decrease in systemic and pulmonic arterial pressures may occur as well. Unless high-dose or bolus amrinone is administered, heart rate usually remains unaltered. Stroke

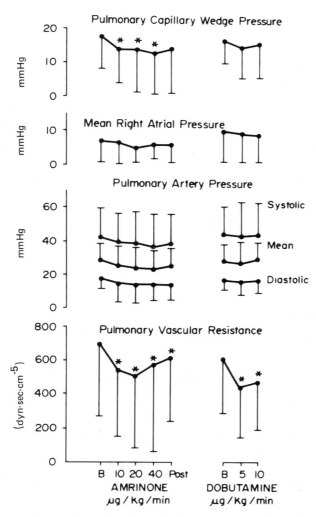

FIGURE 5 Graphs comparing the vascular responses of amrinone to those of dobutamine in patients with low-output congestive heart failure. B = baseline, post = 30 min after the discontinuation of the infusion. (Reproduced from Figs. 2 and 3 of Ref. 98, permission granted.)

volume and cardiac output (Fig. 6) increase secondary to afterload reduction; this response is similar to the response noted with other vasodilators (such as nitroprusside, nitroglycerin) (99).

The use of intravenous amrinone as first-line positive inotropic intervention must be questioned. The reasons for this are severalfold. First, amrinone is primarily

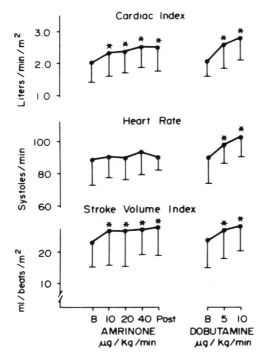

FIGURE 6 Graphs depicting the changes in hemodynamic and inotropic indices during continuous intravenous infusions of amrinone and dobutamine in patients with low output congestive heart failure. B = baseline, post = 30 min after the discontinuation of the infusion, %△D = fractional shortening, △P/△t = isovolumic developed pressure/isovolumic contraction time, PEP/LVET = pre-ejection period/ left ventricular ejection time, VCF = fractional shortening rate. (Reproduced from Figs. 1 and 4 of Ref. 98, permission granted.)

a vasodilator (97-100). Vasodilation is in itself not undesirable in cardiac failure; however, if amrinone is selected for use because of its positive inotropic properties for a patient who is also hypotensive or in shock, further reduction in systemic blood pressure may result. The reported decrease in myocardial oxygen consumption and coronary blood flow observed after amrinone therapy is best explained by the fact that in humans with cardiac failure, this drug is primarily a vasodilator (101). Second, the positive inotropic properties of intravenous amrinone are either nonexistent or modest in patients with heart failure (97-100). An in vitro study examining the effects of amrinone on the contractility of human cardiac muscle showed that the degree of amrinone's positive inotropic response is directly related to the integrity and health of the cardiac muscle (100). Cardiac muscle from patients with severe heart failure did not respond to amrinone; yet these are the

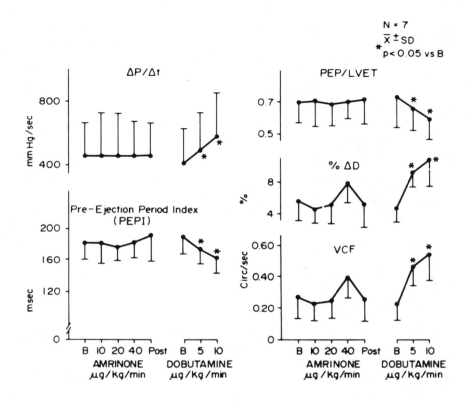

patients who are the most likely to be treated with positive inotropic intervention. Although vasodilator-induced alterations in hemodynamics occur with amrinone, infusions of this drug fail to augment inotropic indices in patients with cardiac failure (Fig. 6) (97-99). Apparently, intravenous bolus administration or high initial infusion rates are required to elicit positive inotropy in the failing human ventricle (95). However, one must question the use of bolus or a high initial dose infusion of a drug to increase contractility because of unpredictable responses in terms of side effects and cardiovascular effects in a critically ill patient population. Third, individual hemodynamic responses to intravenous amrinone are highly variable, and predictable dose-related hemodynamic changes are oftentimes not seen during amrinone infusion (98). Fourth, the elimination half-life of amrinone is long (>2 hr) and highly variable. Compared to dobutamine, dopamine, nitroglycerin, and nitroprusside, the effects of amrinone persist long after the infusion is discontinued; in the author's view, this is a serious disadvantage in acute positive inotropic therapy, because if undesirable effects occur, the clinician must "wait out" or treat the side effects until the drug has dissipated. If side effects or undesirable hemodynamic responses occur with the catecholamines, nitroprusside or intravenous nitroglycerin, these can be corrected within 15 minutes simply by adjusting the dose or discontinuing the drug. It is most difficult to envision a clinical situation in which intravenous amrinone would ever be selected as a first-line drug over one or a combination of the following: dobutamine, dopamine, norepinephrine, nitroglycerin, and nitroprusside.

A hemodynamic effect (vasodilation) can be attained at amrinone infusion rates of 10-40 μg/kg/min. To achieve positive inotropy, an initial infusion rate of 40 μg/kg/min (decrease to 10 μg/kg/min after 1 hr) or an intravenous bolus of 0.5-3.5 μg/kg (over 1 min, repeat in 10 min, if necessary) is probably required. Some of the undesirable effects reported with intravenous amrinone include dysrhythmias, nausea, vomiting, anorexia, abdominal pain, fever, arthralgias, virallike syndromes, chest pain, thrombocytopenia, and elevated serum levels of hepatic enzymes.

B. Intravenous Administration of Digitalis

The intravenous administration of digitalis improves inotropic indices (102,103), and in digitalizing doses, effects some increase in cardiac output as well (104,105). Although the importance of digitalis in managing supraventricular tachycardia, atrial flutter, and atrial fibrillation, particularly in congestive heart failure, is generally appreciated, the use of digitalis as an acute positive inotropic drug is rarely (probably never) indicated. In contrast to dobutamine or dopamine, acute intravenous digitalis therapy has a number of major disadvantages. First, in the setting of myocardial depression and congestive heart failure, its inotropic and hemodynamic effects are relatively mild (105-107). Second, the doses required to achieve a useful hemodynamic response in some patients oftentimes elicit toxic manifestations. Third, the individual hemodynamic responses to acute digitalis (digoxin) administration are highly variable compared to the relatively predictable dose-related hemodynamic responses of dobutamine (18,105-107). Fourth, acute digitalis therapy may elicit severe vasoconstriction of certain vascular beds (108, 109). Fifth, the half-life of the digitalis glycoside preparations (including Cedilanid and ouabain) is long compared to the catecholamines (2-3 min), which indicates that digitalis will remain "on board" for an extended period after the intravenous administration. If side effects (such as dysrhythmias) are noted after administration, the clinician will have to "wait out" the clearance of the drug; if the toxic manifestations are severe, major intervention (such as intravenous antiarrhythmic therapy, hemodialysis) may be necessary. For dobutamine and dopamine, the drug and its side effects are usually cleared within 15 minutes (17-19). This discussion was directed solely at the use of the intravenous administration of digitalis as the initial or primary effort to increase inotropy and improve hemodynamics. The application of oral digitalis preparations in the treatment of chronic congestive heart failure and related issues are presented in Chap. 4.

C. Intravenous Administration of Glucagon

The intravenous administration of glucagon augments cardiac contractility with little positive chronotropy and a paucity of vascular effects. The use of a glucagon infusions has been proposed as a method to increase contractility in patients treated with beta-adrenoceptor blockers, thereby bypassing the blocked beta-receptors (110). In the author's experience, glucagon infusions generally provoke more nausea and vomiting than augmented cardiac output and the hemodynamic responses to this hormone appear to be quite variable. The author has rarely had difficulty in improving contractility and hemodynamics with dobutamine in "beta-blocked" patients, although a mild-to-moderate increase in dosage may be required in some of the patients. The theoretical consequences of stimulating unopposed alpha-receptors (that is, a vasopressor response) has not been observed by the author during dobutamine infusions in patients who had recently been treated with beta-adrenergic blocking agents.

D. Intravenous Administration of Calcium

Although the intravenous administration of calcium chloride or calcium gluconate enhances inotropy, calcium infusions per se are rarely used as a means of reversing low-output cardiac failure. Intravenously administered calcium has been used effectively to reverse the negative inotropy and cardiovascular collapse after the administration of the calcium channel blocker, verapamil (111-114). The myocardial depression noted during anesthesia and after cardioplegia and cardiopulmonary bypass is occasionally approached therapeutically with the intravenous delivery of calcium (115.116).

E. Investigational Agents

Over the past ten years, a considerable number of experimental drugs have been developed and studied for use in low-output heart failure. The largest group examined to date are the sympathomimetic drugs. These drugs are not categorized as catechols because they do not possess the 3-OH,4-OH catechol ring; nevertheless, they act through $beta_1$- and/or $beta_2$-adrenoceptors. In general, the acute hemodynamic effects of these drugs are generally similar to those of isoproterenol or dobutamine. In terms of short-term parenteral therapy, few of the sympathomimetic agents offer any real advantages over the inotrope-to-vasopressor spectrum provided by dobutamine, dopamine, and norepinephrine; this is certainly true if one adds isoproterenol to the dobutamine, dopamine, and norepinephrine group. Most of the sympathomimetic agents studied provoke more positive chronotropy, side effects, and/or undesirable vascular responses (hypotension or vasopressor activity) than does dobutamine. Pirbuterol (117), salbutamol (118), butopamine (119), sulmazol (120), and prenalterol (121,122), are some of the sympathomimetic agents which have been studied for their acute hemodynamic effects.

Phosphodiesterase inhibitors enhance inotropy by retarding the breakdown of cyclic AMP. The agents MDL 17043, an imidazole derivative, and milrinone, a bipyridine derivative and congener of amrinone, effect an acute improvement in hemodynamics when administered intravenously (123-126). An increase in the vascular content of cyclic AMP elicits vasodilation. As a result, the hemodynamic profile of these agents is characterized by positive inotropy and vasodilation. The intensity of the vasodilatory effect appears to reside somewhere between those of dobutamine and isoproterenol. Initial studies suggest that MDL 17043 and milrinone have the potential of becoming reasonable alternatives to dobutamine as acute, short-term, parenteral, positive inotropic agents (125,126).

REFERENCES

1. R. R. Tuttle, and J. Mills. Dobutamine: Development of a new catecholamine to selectively increase cardiac contractility. *Circ. Res. 36*: 185-96 (1975).

2. N. W. Robie, D. O. Nutter, C. Moody, and J. L. McNay. In vivo analysis of adrenergic receptor activity of dobutamine. *Circ. Res. 34*: 663 (1974).

3. R. S. Williams, and T. Bishop. Selectivity of dobutamine for adrenergic receptor subtypes: In vitro analysis by radioligand binding. *J. Clin. Invest. 67*: 1703 (1981).

4. C. V. Leier, and D. V. Unverferth. Dobutamine. *Ann. Intern. Med. 99*: 490 (1983).

5. T. P. Kenakin. An in vitro quantitative analysis of the alpha adrenoceptor partial agonist activity of dobutamine and its relevance to inotropic selectivity. *J. Pharmacol. Exp. Ther. 216*: 210 (1981).

6. R. R. Ruffolo, Jr. On the mechanism of action of dobutamine. *Ann. Intern. Med. 100*: 313 (1984).

7. N. Weiner. Norepinephrine, epinephrine and the sympathomimetic amines. In *The Pharmacological Basis of Therapeutics*, 6th ed. A. G. Gilman, L. S. Goodman, and A. Gilman (eds.). Macmillan, New York, 1980, p. 138.

8. M. J. Allwood, A. F. Cobbold, and J. Ginsburg. Peripheral vascular effects of noradrenaline, isopropyl-noradrenaline, and dopamine, *Br. Med. Bull. 19*: 132 (1963).

9. C. W. Nash, S. A. Wolff, and B. A. Ferguson. Release of tritiated noradrenaline from perfused rat hearts by sympathomimetic amines. *Can. J. Physiol. Pharmacol. 46*: 35 (1968).

10. T. H. Tsai, S. Z. Langer, and V. Trendelenburg. Effect of dopamine and alpha methyldopamine on smooth muscle and on the cardiac pacemaker. *J. Pharmacol. Exp. Ther. 156*: 310 (1967).

11. L. I. Goldberg. Cardiovascular and renal actions of dopamine: Potential clinical applications. *Pharmacol. Rev. 24*: 1 (1972).

12. D. Jewitt, J. Birkhead, A. Mitchell, and C. Doller. Clinical cardiovascular pharmacology of dobutamine, a selective inotropic catecholamine. *Lancet 2*: 363 (1974).

13. J. Beregovich, C. Bianchi, R. D'Angelo, R. Diaz, and S. Rubler. Haemodynamic effects of a new inotropic agent (dobutamine) in chronic cardiac failure. *Br. Heart J. 37*: 629 (1975).

14. N. Akhtar, E. Mikulic, J. Cohn, and M. Chaudry. Hemodynamic effect of dobutamine in patients with severe heart failure. *Am. J. Cardiol. 36*: 202 (1975).

15. C. V. Leier, J. Webel, and C. A. Bush. The cardiovascular effects of the continuous infusion of dobutamine in patients with severe cardiac failure. *Circulation 56*: 468 (1977).

16. J. J. Andy, C. L. Curry, N. Ali, and P. P. Mehrotra. Cardiovascular effects of dobutamine in severe congestive heart failure. *Am. Heart J. 94*: 175 (1977).

17. C. V. Leier, P. Heban, P. Huss, C. A. Bush, and R. P. Lewis. Comparative systemic and regional hemodynamic effects of dopamine and dobutamine in patients with cardiomyopathic heart failure. *Circulation 58*: 466 (1978).

18. C. V. Leier, D. V. Unverferth, and R. E. Kates. The relationship between plasma dobutamine concentrations and cardiovascular responses in cardiac failure. *Am. J. Med. 66*: 238 (1979).

19. R. E. Kates, and C. V. Leier. Dobutamine pharmacokinetics in severe heart failure. *Clin. Pharmacol. Ther. 24*: 537 (1978).

20. P. J. Murphy, T. L. Williams, and D. L. K. Kau. Disposition of dobutamine in the dog. *J. Pharmacol. Exp. Ther. 199*: 423 (1976).

21. D. V. Unverferth, D. M. Blanford, R. E. Kates, and C. V. Leier. Tolerance to dobutamine after a 72 hour continuous infusion. *Am. J. Med. 69*: 262 (1980).

22. C. Bianchi, R. Diaz, C. Gonzales, and J. Beregovich. Effects of dobutamine on atrioventricular conduction. *Am. Heart J. 90*: 474 (1975).

23. A. Masoni, P. Alboni, C. Malacarne, and L. Codeca. Effects of dobutamine on electrophysiological properties of the specialized conduction system in man. *J. Electrocardiol. 12*: 361 (1979).

24. J. V. Hoff, P. A. Beatty, and J. L. Wade. Dermal necrosis from dobutamine (Letter). *N. Engl. J. Med. 300*: 1280 (1979).

25. H. Boudoulas, S. E. Rittgers, R. P. Lewis, C. V. Leier, and A. M. Weissler. Changes in diastolic time with various pharmacologic agents: Implications for myocardial perfusion. *Circulation 60*: 164 (1979).

26. R. D. Magorien, D. V. Unverferth, G. P. Brown, and C. V. Leier. Dobutamine and hydralazine: Comparative influences of positive inotropy and vasodilation on coronary blood flow and myocardial energetics in nonischemic congestive heart failure. *J. Am. Coll. Cardiol. 1*: 499 (1983).

27. R. Bendersky, K. Chatterjee, W. W. Parmley, B. H. Brundage, and T. A. Ports. Dobutamine in chronic ischemic heart failure: Alterations in left ventricular function and coronary hemodynamics. *Am. J. Cardiol. 48*: 554 (1981).

28. R. G. Pozen, R. DiBianco, R. J. Katz, R. Bortz, R. J. Myerburg, and R. D. Fletcher. Myocardial metabolic and hemodynamic effects of dobutamine in heart failure complicating coronary artery disease. *Circulation 63*: 1279 (1981).

29. W. Kupper, D. Waller, P. Hanrath, and W. Bleifeld. Hemodynamic and cardiac metabolic effects of inotropic stimulation with dobutamine in patients with coronary artery disease. *Eur. Heart J. 3*: 29 (1982).

30. S. L. Meyer, G. C. Curry, M. S. Donsky, D. B. Tweig, R. W. Parkey, and J. T. Willerson. Influence of dobutamine on hemodynamics and coronary blood flow in patients with and without coronary artery disease. *Am. J. Cardiol. 38*: 103 (1976).

31. R. E. Smith, B. Briggs, D. V. Unverferth, and C. V. Leier. Dobutamine-induced inhibition of platelet function. *Int. J. Clin. Pharmacol. Res. 2*: 89 (1982).

32. E. C. H. Keung, S. J. Siskind, E. H. Sonnenblick, H. S. Ribner, W. J. Swartz, and T. H. LeJemtel. Dobutamine therapy in acute myocardial infarction. *JAMA 245*: 144 (1981).

33. T. A. Gillespie, H. D. Ambos, B. E. Sobel, and R. Roberts. Effects of dobutamine in patients with acute myocardial infarction. *Am. J. Cardiol. 39*: 588 (1977).

34. R. A. Goldstein, E. R. Passamani, and R. Roberts. A comparison of digoxin and dobutamine in patients with acute infarction and cardiac failure. *N. Engl. J. Med. 303*: 846 (1980).

35. M. Renard and R. Bernard. Clinical and hemodynamic effects of dobutamine in acute myocardial infarction with left heart failure. *J. Cardiovasc. Pharmacol. 2*: 543 (1980).

36. S. F. Vatner, R. J. McRitchie, and E. Braunwald. Effects of dobutamine on left ventricular performance, coronary dynamics, and distribution of cardiac output in conscious dogs. *J. Clin. Invest. 53*: 1265 (1974).

37. C. S. Liang, and W. B. Hood, Jr. Dobutamine infusion in conscious dogs with and without autonomic nervous system inhibition: Effects on systemic hemodynamics, regional flows and cardiac metabolism. *J. Pharmacol. Exp. Ther. 211*: 698 (1979).

38. M. Sakanashi, E. Tomomatsu, and S. Takeo, et al. Effects of dobutamine on coronary circulation and cardiac metabolism of the dog. *Drug Res. 28*: 798 (1978).

39. W. Von Restorff, and E. Bassenge. Effect of dobutamine, a new cardioselective sympathomimetic drug, on myocardial oxygen balance in conscious dogs. *Drug Res. 28*: 990 (1978).

40. C. S. Liang, J. M. Yi, L. G. Sherman, J. Black, H. Gavras, and W. B. Hood, Jr. Dobutamine infusion in conscious dogs with and without acute myocardial infarction. *Circ. Res. 49*: 170 (1981).

41. R. R. Tuttle, G. D. Pollock, G. Todd, B. MacDonald, R. Tust, and W. Dusenberry. The effect of dobutamine on cardiac oxygen balance, regional blood flow, and infarction severity after coronary artery narrowing in dogs. *Circ. Res. 41*: 357 (1977).

42. J. T. Willerson, I. Hutton, J. T. Watson, M. R. Platt, and G. H. Templeton. Influence of dobutamine on regional myocardial blood flow and ventricular performance during acute and chronic myocardial ischemia in dogs. *Circulation 53*: 828 (1976).

43. S. F. Vatner, and H. Baig. Importance of heart rate in determining the effects of sympathomimetic amines on regional myocardial function and blood flow in conscious dogs with acute myocardial ischemia. *Circ. Res. 45*: 793 (1979).

44. D. C. Warltier, M. Zyvoloski, G. J. Gross, H. F. Hardman, and H. L. Brooks. Redistribution of myocardial blood flow distal to a dynamic coronary arterial stenosis by sympathomimetic amines. *Am. J. Cardiol. 48*: 269 (1981).

45. R. E. Rude, C. Izquierdo, L. M. Buja, and J. T. Willerson. Effects of inotropic and chronotropic stimuli on acute myocardial ischemia injury. *Circulation 65*: 1321 (1982).

46. F. Waagstein, I. Malek, and A. C. Hjalmarson. The use of dobutamine in myocardial infarction for reversal of the cardiodepressive effect of metroprolol. *Br. J. Clin. Pharmacol. 5*: 515 (1978).

47. G. S. Francis, B. Sharma, and M. Hodges. Comparative hemodynamic effects of dopamine and dobutamine in patients with acute cardiogenic circulatory collapse. *Am. Heart. J. 103*: 995 (1982).

48. M. Z. Iqbal, and P. R. Liebson. Counterpulsation and dobutamine: Their use in treatment of cardiogenic shock due to right ventricular infarct. *Arch. Intern. Med. 141*: 247 (1981).

49. W. Hess, J. B. Bruckner, J. V. Farber Du Faur, D. Schmidt, and J. Tarnow. Haemodynamische wirkungen von dobutamin und dopamin bei patienten mit koronarer herzkrankheit. *Anaesthesist. 28*: 316 (1979).

50. S. Piepenbrock, G. Hempelmann, W. Reichelt, and T. H. Stegman. Haemodynamische und slektive vaskular effekte von dobutamin wahrend und nach herzchirurgishchen eingriffen. *Anaesthesist. 28*: 307 (1979).

51. P. A. Steen, J. H. Tinker, J. R. Pluth, D. A. Barnhorst, and S. Tarhan. Efficacy of dopamine, dobutamine and epinephrine during emergence from cardiopulmonary bypass in man. *Circulation 57*: 378, (1978).

52. R. Gray, P. K. Shah, B. Singh, C. Conklin, and J. M. Matloff. Low cardiac output states after open heart surgery: Comparative hemodynamic effects of dobutamine, dopamine, and norepinephrine plus phentolamine. *Chest 80*: 16 (1981).

53. T. Sakamoto, and T. Yamada. Hemodynamic effects of dobutamine in patients following open heart surgery. *Circulation 55*: 525 (1977).

54. G. R. J. Lewis, P. A. Poole-Wilson, T. A. Angerpointer, A. E. Farnsworth, B. T. Williams, and D. J. Coltart. Measurement of the circulatory effects of dobutamine, a new inotropic agent, in patients following cardiac surgery. *Am. Heart. J. 95*: 301 (1978).

55. J. H. Chamberlain, J. R. Pepper, and A. K. Yates. Dobutamine, isoprenaline, and dopamine in patients after open heart surgery. *Intensive Care Med. 7*: 5 (1980).

56. N. W. Salomon, J. R. Plachetka, and J. G. Copeland. Comparison of dopamine and dobutamine following coronary artery bypass grafting. *Ann. Thorac. Surg. 33*: 48 (1982).

57. Y. Sato, H. Matsuzawa, and S. Eguchi. Comparative study of effects of adrenaline, dobutamine and dopamine on systemic hemodynamics and renal blood flow in patients following open heart surgery. *Jpn. Circ. J. 46*: 1059 (1982).

58. D. J. Bohn, C. S. Poirier, J. F. Edmonds, and J. A. Barker. Hemodynamic

effects of dobutamine after cardiopulmonary bypass in children. *Crit. Care Med. 8*: 367 (1980).

59. V. J. DiSesa, E. Brown, G. H. Mudge, J. J. Collins, and L. H. Cohn. Hemodynamic comparison of dopamine and dobutamine in the postoperative volume-loaded, pressure-loaded, and normal ventricle. *J. Thorac. Cardiovasc. Surg. 83*: 256 (1982).

60. M. B. Fowler, E. L. Alderman, S. N. Oesterle, G. Derby, G. T. Daughters, E. B. Stinson, N. B. Ingels, R. S. Mitchell, and D. C. Miller. Dobutamine and dopamine after cardiac surgery: Greater augmentation of myocardial blood flow with dobutamine. *Circulation (suppl. 1) 70*: I-103 (1984).

61. P. Van Trigt, T. L. Spray, M. K. Pasque, R. B. Peyton, G. L. Pellom, and A. S. Wechsler. The comparative effects of dopamine and dobutamine on ventricular mechanics after coronary artery bypass grafting: A pressure-dimension analysis. *Circulation (suppl. 1) 70*: I-112 (1984).

62. D. J. Driscoll, P. C. Gillette, and D. F. Duff. Hemodynamic effects of dobutamine in children. *Am. J. Cardiol. 43*: 581 (1979).

63. D. Schranz, H. Stopfkuchen, B-K. Jungst, R. Clemens, and P. Emmrich. Hemodynamic effects of dobutamine in children with cardiovascular failure. *Eur. J. Pediatr. 139*: 4 (1982).

64. R. M. Perkin, D. L. Levin, R. Webb, A. Aquino, and J. Reedy. Dobutamine: A hemodynamic evaluation in children with shock. *J. Pediatr. 100*: 977 (1982).

65. B. Regnier, D. Safran, J. Carlet, and B. Teisseire. Comparative hemodynamic effects of dopamine and dobutamine in septic shock. *Intensive Care Med. 5*: 115 (1979).

66. C. Perret, and F. Depeursinge. Dysfonction mycardique au cours de choc spetique. *Schweiz Med. Wochenschr. 111*: 1799 (1981).

67. F. Jardin, M. Sportiche, M. Bazine, A. Bourobka and, A. Margairaz. Dobutamine: A hemodynamic evaluation in human septic shock. *Crit. Care Med. 9*: 329 (1981).

68. K. L. MacCannell, J. L. McNay, M. B. Meyer and L. I. Goldberg. Dopamine in the treatment of hypotension and shock. *N. Engl. J. Med. 275*: 1389 (1966).

69. R. C. Talley, L. I. Goldberg, C. G. Johnson, and J. L. McNay. A hemodynamic comparison of dopamine and isoproterenol in patients with shock. *Circulation 39*: 361 (1969).

70. H. S. Loeb, E. B. J. Winslow, S. H. Rahimtoola, K. M. Rosen, and R. M. Gunnar. Acute hemodynamic effects of dopamine in patients with shock. *Circulation 44*: 163 (1971).

71. J. Holzer, J. S. Karliner, R. A. O'Rourke, W. Pitt and J. Ross Jr. Effectiveness of dopamine in patients with cardiogenic shock. *Am. J. Cardiol. 32*: 79 (1973).

72. J. Beregovich, C. Bianchi, S. Rubler, E. Lomnitz, N. Cagin, and B. Levitt. Dose-related hemodynamic and renal effects of dopamine in congestive heart failure. *Am. Heart. J. 87*: 550 (1974).

73. E. L. Holloway, E. B. Stinson, G. C. Derby, and D. C. Harrison. Action of drugs in patients early and after cardiac surgery. 1. Comparison of isoproterenol and dopamine. *Am. J. Cardiol. 35*: 656 (1975).

74. S. K. Durairaj, and L. J. Haywood. Hemodynamic effects of dopamine in patients with resistant congestive heart failure. *Clin. Pharmacol. Ther. 24*: 175 (1978).

75. C. E. Ruiz, M. H. Weil, and R. W. Carlson. Treatment of circulatory shock with dopamine. *JAMA 242*: 165 (1979).

76. J. D. Stoner III, J. L. Bolen, and D. C. Harrison. Comparison of dobutamine and dopamine in the treatment of severe heart failure. *Br. Heart. J. 39*: 536 (1977).

77. H. S. Loeb, J. Bredakis, and R. M. Gunnar. Superiority of dobutamine over dopamine for augmentation of cardiac output in patients with chronic low output cardiac failure. *Circulation 55*: 375 (1977).

78. L. I. Goldberg, R. H. McDonald, and A. M. Zimmerman. Sodium diuresis produced by dopamine in patients with congestive heart failure. *N. Engl. J. Med. 269*: 1060 (1963).

79. R. H. McDonald, L. I. Goldberg, J. L. McNay and E. P. Tuttle, Jr. Effects of dopamine in man: Augmentation of sodium excretion, glomerular filtration rate, and renal plasma flow. *J. Clin. Invest. 43*: 1116 (1964).

80. B. K. Yeh, J. L. McNay, and L. I. Goldberg. Attenuation of dopamine renal and mesenteric vasodilation by haloperidol: Evidence for a specific dopamine receptor. *J. Pharmacol. Exp. Ther. 168*: 303 (1969).

81. C. S. Alexander, Y. Sako, and E. Mikulic. Pedal gangrene associated with the use of dopamine. *N. Engl. J. Med. 293*: 591 (1975).

82. S. I. Greene, and J. W. Smith. Dopamine gangrene. *N. Engl. J. Med. 294*: 114 (1976).

83. C. Richard, J. L. Ricome, A. Rimailho, G. Bottineau, and P. Auzepy. Combined hemodynamic effects of dopamine and dobutamine in cardiogenic shock. *Circulation 67*: 620 (1983).

84. J. N. Cohn. Comparative cardiovascular effects of tyramine, ephedrine and norepinephrine in man. *Circ. Res. 16*: 174 (1965).

85. H. Mueller, S. M. Ayres, S. Giannelli, Jr., E. F. Conkin, J. T. Mazzara, and W. J. Grace. Effect of isoproterenol, 1-norepinephrine, and intra-aortic counterpulsation on hemodynamics and myocardial metabolism in shock following acute myocardial infarction. *Circulation 45*: 335 (1972).

86. F. E. Tristani, and J. N. Cohn. Studies in clinical shock and hypotension. VII. Renal hemodynamics before and during treatment. *Circulation 42*: 839 (1970).

87. E. J. Winslow, H. Loeb, S. H. Rahimtoola, S. Kamath, and R. M. Gunnar. Hemodynamic studies and results of therapy in 50 patients with bacteremic shock. *Am. J. Med. 54*: 421 (1973).

88. J. Wagner, H. J. Schumann, A. Knorr, N. Rohm, and J. C. Reidemeister. Stimulation by adrenaline and dopamine, but not by noradrenaline, of myocardial alpha adrenoceptors mediating positive inotropic effects in human atrial preparations. *Arch. Pharmacol. 312*: 99 (1980).

89. J. W. Kirklin, E. H. Blackstone, and J. K. Kirklin. General principles of cardiac surgery. In *Heart Disease*, 2nd ed. E. Braunwald (ed.). Saunders, Philadelphia, 1984, pp. 1797-1814.

90. G. Zucker, and J. Levine. Pressor and diminished local vasoconstrictor effects of levarterenol-phentolamine mixtures. *Arch. Intern. Med. 104*: 607 (1959).

91. D. R. Stemple, J. H. Kleiman, and D. C. Harrison. Combined nitroprusside-dopamine therapy in severe chronic congestive heart failure. Dose-related hemodynamic advantages over single drug infusion. *Am. J. Cardiol. 42*: 267 (1978).

92. R. R. Miller, N. A. Awan, J. A. Joye, K. S. Maxwell, A. N. DeMaria, E. A. Amsterdam, and D. T. Mason. Combined dopamine and nitroprusside therapy in congestive heart failure. *Circulation 55*: 881 (1977).

93. R. M. Gagnon, L. Fortin, R. Boucher, S. Gilbert, M. Morrisette, S. Present, J. Lemire, and A. David. Combined hemodynamic effects of dobutamine and IV nitroglycerin in congestive heart failure. *Chest 78*: 694 (1980).

94. A. Alousi, A. E. Farah, G. Y. Lesher, and C. J. Opalka, Jr. Cardiotonic activity of amrinone-WIN 40680 [5-amino-3,4'-bipyridin-6(1H)-one]. *Circ. Res. 45*: 666 (1979).

95. J. R. Benotti, W. Grossman, E. Braunwald, D. D. Davalos, and A. A. Alousi. Hemodynamic assessment of amrinone: A new inotropic drug. *N. Engl. J. Med. 299*: 1373 (1978).

96. T. H. LeJemtel, E. Keung, E. H. Sonnenblick, H. S. Ribner, M. Matsumoto, R. Davis, W. Schwartz, A. A. Alousi, and D. Davalos. Amrinone: A new non-glycosidic, non-adrenergic cardiotonic agent effective in the treatment of intractable myocardial failure in man. *Circulation 59*: 1098 (1979).

97. P. T. Wilmshurst, D. S. Thompson, B. S. Jenkins, D. J. Coltart, and M. M. Webb-Peploe. Haemodynamic effects of intravenous amrinone in patients with impaired left ventricular function. *Br. Heart J. 49*: 77 (1983).

98. J. B. Hermiller, M. E. Leithe, R. D. Magorien, D. V. Unverferth, and C. V. Leier. Amrinone in severe congestive heart failure: Another look at an intriguing new cardioactive drug. *J. Pharmacol. Exp. Ther. 228*: 319 (1984).

99. P. T. Wilmshurst, D. S. Thompson, S. M. Juul, B. S. Jenkins, D. J. Coltart, and M. M. Webb-Peploe. Comparison of the effects of amrinone and sodium nitroprusside on haemodynamics, contractility and myocardial metabolism in patients with cardiac failure due to coronary artery disease and dilated cardiomyopathy. *Br. Heart J. 52*: 38 (1984).

100. P. T. Wilmshurst, J. M. Walker, C. H. Fry, J. P. Mounsey, C. H. C. Twort, B. T. Williams, M. J. Davies, and M. M. Webb-Peploe. Inotropic and vasodilatoreffects of amrinone on isolated human tissue. *Cardiovasc. Res. 18*: 302 (1984).

101. J. R. Benotti, W. Grossman, E. Braunwald, and B. A. Carabello. Effects of amrinone on myocardial energy metabolism and hemodynamics in patients with severe congestive heart failure due to coronary artery disease. *Circulation 62*: 28 (1980).

102. W. G. Kramer, A. J. Kolibash, R. P. Lewis, M. S. Bathala, J. A. Visconti and R. H. Reuning. Pharmacokinetics of digoxin: Relationship between response intensity and predicted compartmental drug levels in man. *J. Pharmacokinet. Biopharma. 7*: 47 (1979).

103. R. Vogel, J. Frischnecht, and P. Steele. Short- and long-term effects of digitalis on resting and post handgrip hemodynamics in patients with coronary artery disease. *Am. J. Cardiol. 40*: 171 (1977).

104. J. McMichael, and E. P. Sharpey-Schafer. The action of intravenous digoxin in man. *Q. J. Med. 53*: 123 (1944).

105. K. Cohn, A. Selzer, E. S. Kersh, L. S. Karpman, and N. Goldschlager. Variability of hemodynamic responses to acute digitalization in chronic cardiac failure due to cardiomyopathy and coronary artery disease. *Am. J. Cardiol. 35*: 461 (1975).

106. R. A. Goldstein, E. R. Passamani, and R. Roberts. A comparison of digoxin and dobutamine in patients with acute infarction and cardiac failure. *N. Engl. J. Med. 303*: 846 (1980).

107. M. Hodges, G. C. Friesinger, R. C. K. Riggins, and G. Dagenais. Effects of intravenously administered digoxin on mild left ventricular failure in acute myocardial infarction in man. *Am. J. Cardiol. 29*: 749 (1972).

108. H. Garan, T. W. Smith, and W. J. Powell, Jr. The central nervous system as a site of action for the coronary vasoconstrictor effect of digoxin. *J. Clin. Invest. 54*: 1356 (1974).

109. L. L. Shanbaur, and E. D. Jacobson. Digitalis and the mesenteric circulation. *Am. J. Digest Dis. 17*: 826 (1972).

110. E. J. Kosinski, and G. S. Malinzak, Jr. Glucagon and isoproterenol in reversing propranolol toxicity. *Arch. Intern. Med. 132*: 840 (1973).

111. C. M. Perkins. Serious verapamil poisoning: Treatment with intravenous calcium gluconate. *Br. Med. J. 2*: 1127 (1978).

112. R. J. Hariman, L. M. Magiardi, R. G. McAllister, et al. Reversal of the cardiovascular effects of verapamil by calcium and sodium: Differences between electrophysiological and hemodynamic responses. *Circulation 59*: 797 (1979).

113. V. T. Hattori, W. J. Mandel, and T. Peter. Calcium for myocardial depression from verapamil. *N. Engl. J. Med. 306*: 238 (1982).

114. D. L. Morris, and N. Goldschlager. Calcium infusion for reversal of adverse effects of intravenous verapamil. *JAMA 249*: 3212 (1983).

115. A. d'Hollander, G. Primo, D. Hennart, J. L. LeClec, F. E. Deuvaert, and J. Dubois-Primo. Compared efficacy of dobutamine and dopamine in association with calcium chloride on termination of cardiopulmonary bypass. *J. Thorac. Cardiovasc. Surg. 83*: 264 (1982).

116. J. K. Denlinger, J. A. Kaplan, J. H. Lecky, and H. Wollman. Cardiovascular responses to calcium administered intravenously to man during halothane anesthesia. *Anesthesiology 42*: 390 (1975).

117. C. V. Leier, S. Nelson, P. Huss, J. R. Bianchine, A. Y. Olukotun, C. R. Taylor, and D. S. Salzburg. Intravenous pirbuterol. *Clin. Pharmacol. Ther. 31*: 89 (1982).

118. B. Sharma, and J. F. Goodwin. Beneficial effect of salbutamol on cardiac function in severe congestive cardiomyopathy. *Circulation 58*: 449 (1978).

119. M. J. Thompson, P. Huss, D. V. Unverferth, A. F. Fasola, and C. V. Leier. Hemodynamic effects of intravenous butopamine in congestive heart failure. *Clin. Pharmacol. Ther. 28*: 324 (1980).

120. M. Renard, P. Jacobs, P. Dechamps, A. Dresse, and R. Bernard. Hemodynamic and clinical response to three-day infusion of sulmazol (AR-L115BS) in severe congestive heart failure. *Chest 84*: 408 (1983).

121. D. W. Wahr, K. Swedberg, M. Rabbino, M. J. Hoyle, D. Curran, W. W. Parmley, and K. Chatterjee. Intravenous and oral prenalterol in congestive heart failure. *Am. J. Med. 76*: 999 (1984).

122. N. A. Awan, K. E. Needham, M. K. Evenson, A. Win, and D. T. Mason. Hemodynamic actions of prenalterol in severe congestive heart failure due to chronic coronary disease. *Am. Heart J. 101*: 158 (1981).

123. B. F. Uretsky, T. Generalovich, P. S. Reddy, R. B. Spangenberg, and W. P. Follansbee. The acute hemodynamic effects of a new agent, MDL 17043, in the treatment of congestive heart failure. *Circulation 67*: 823 (1983).

124. M. H. Crawford, K. L. Richards, M. T. Sodums, and G. T. Kennedy. Positive inotropic and vasodilator effects of MDL 17043 in patients with reduced left ventricular performance. *Am. J. Cardiol. 53*: 1051 (1984).

125. D. K. Amin, P. K. Shah, F. G. Shellock, S. Hulse, G. Brandon, R. Spangenberg, and H. J. C. Swan. Comparative hemodynamic effects of intravenous dobutamine and MDL 17043, a new cardioactive drug, in severe congestive heart failure. *Am. Heart J. 109*: 91 (1985).

126. D. S. Baim, A. V. McDowell, J. Cherniles, E. S. Monrad, J. A. Parker, J. Edelson, E. Braunwald, and W. Grossman. Evaluation of a new bipyridine inotropic agent—milrinone—in patients with severe congestive heart failure. *N. Engl. J. Med. 309*: 748 (1983).

4

Digitalis

RICHARD P. LEWIS
Ohio State University College of Medicine, Columbus, Ohio

I. HISTORICAL DEVELOPMENT

Digitalis is one of the oldest pharmaceutical agents and still remains one of the most widely prescribed drugs. The year 1985 marks the 200th anniversary of the publication of Withering's remarkable treatise *An Account of the Foxglove, and Some of its Medical Uses* (1). Withering was an astute scientist and clinician, and his observations, particularly of digitalis toxicity, are still applicable today (2). Withering focused on the diuretic action of digitalis but did recognize its important effects on the heart rate. Fourteen years later, Ferriar concluded that the primary effect of digitalis was upon the heart rate (3). Subsequently, knowledge advanced little and digitalis was extensively and inappropriately used for noncardiovascular disorders (4).

By the late nineteenth century, experimental animal studies had demonstrated the positive inotropic effect of digitalis (5). However, led by the thinking of Mackenzie and Lewis, the major beneficial action of digitalis was still considered to be its effect on the heart rate (6,7). In the 1920s Christian focused on the inotropic effect of digitalis, and insisted that digitalis benefited patients in sinus rhythm as well as atrial fibrillation—a concept that was relatively unquestioned for 50 years (8).

During the 1920s the autonomic and peripheral vascular effects of digitalis were demonstrated and were invoked as the explanation for the lack of increase in cardiac output seen in normal subjects (9-11). It was not until after World War II that the beneficial affect of digitalis was measured in humans with congestive heart failure (12,13).

Recognition that digitalis inhibited the active transport of Na^+ and K^+ across cell membranes occurred in the 1950s. Wilbrandt, and subsequently Repke, proposed that inhibition of the enzyme Na^+-K^+ ATPase was responsible for the inotropic action of digitalis probably by increasing intracellular calcium (14,15). Numerous studies since then have supported this hypothesis (16-20).

New techniques, largely developed by Hoffman and co-workers, allowed study of the cellular electrophysiology of digitalis. The effects of digitalis on the action potentials were defined as well as the complex interactions with the autonomic nervous system (21-26). The demonstration in the 1970s of delayed after depolarizations was another important development for understanding the pathophysiology of digitalis toxicity (27-30).

During this period there were significant advances in the clinical pharmacology of digitalis as well. These included the development of isotope labeling and subsequently of the radioimmunoassay which enabled the complex pharmacokinetics of digitalis to be approached in the laboratories of Okita, Doherty, Marcus, and Smith (31-35). At the same time, the development of systolic time intervals by Weissler and colleagues provided a quantitative noninvasive measure of the inotropic effect of digitalis, thus enabling definition of pharmacokinetic-pharmacodynamic interrelationships (36).

Throughout this exciting 40 years of digitalis research there was little questioning of the clinical efficacy of digitalis in heart failure—indeed the concept of "optimal" (as maximal as possible) digitalization was widely advocated. There has never been a large prospective randomized trial of digitalis efficacy.

Introduction of oral diuretic agents in the 1960s resulted in the first effective alternative oral therapy for congestive heart failure (CHF). During the 1970s vasodilator therapy for CHF was introduced as yet another alternative (37). The search for new inotropic agents produced effective synthetic catecholamines for parenteral use in severely ill patients (38). The search for effective new oral inotropes continues but thus far has not been dramatically successful.

In the 1980s a more conservative consensus regarding the role of digitalis in heart failure is once again emerging (39). Several studies questioning its use in patients with heart failure and sinus rhythm, consideration of its potential role in increasing mortality after myocardial infarction, and the introduction of new agents for therapy of CHF and atrial arrhythmias are probably resulting in a decline in digitalis usage. In spite of this, it is likely that digitalis will continue to be widely used. With application of the new knowledge of this agent gained in the last 40 years its future use should be far more circumspect and its toxicity minimized.

The purpose of this chapter is to present an overview of the pathophysiological basis for the use of digitalis in the treatment of heart failure in adult human subjects. It is not intended to be a comprehensive review. The reader is therefore referred to several excellent reviews, textbook chapters, and symposia (40-46).

II. SOURCE OF DIGITALIS

Digitalis glycosides are found naturally in the leaves and seeds of several plant
species and in the venom of certain toads (44). The leaf of the foxglove plant,
Digitalis purpurea, yields digitoxin; the leaf of another species of foxglove, *Digitalis
lanata*, yields digitoxin, digoxin, and deslanoside. Ouabain is derived from the seed
of *Strophanthus gratus*.

Each glycoside contains three portions: a steroid nucleus, a lactone ring, and a
sugar moiety (Fig. 1) (42,47).

The combination of the steroid nucleus and lactone ring is known as an agly-
cone or genin. There are more than 300 chemical variations and isomers of digitalis
glycosides which have varying degrees of cardiac activity and variable polarity. For
cardioactivity the lactone ring must be unsaturated, there must be a B hydroxyl
group at C14, and there must be cis fusion of the C and D rings. From all of these
compounds the four glycosides noted above have become established as the most
useful preparations in the United States. Current technology allows isolation of
purified preparations of each compound.

Cardiac glycosides have essentially the same steroid nucleus as adrenal steroids
and sex hormones (48). Because of this, as well as their ubiquitous distribution in
nature, it has recently been suggested that digitalis glycosides may be a primitive
hormonal substance. This has led to the hypothesis that there may be an endogenous digitalis (49). Although only a hypothesis at this time, it is an intriguing
possibility that might, among other considerations, help explain the variability of
the clinical response to digitalis therapy.

III. CELLULAR BASIS OF DIGITALIS ACTION

Both the inotropic and electrophysiological effects of digitalis are a consequence
(direct or indirect) of inhibition of the cellular membrane enzyme Na^+-K^+ ATPase

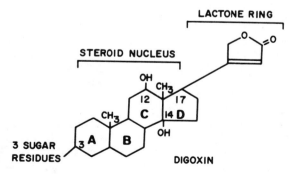

FIGURE 1   The chemical structure of digoxin. Digitoxin differs only by the absence of the hydroxyl group at C-12.

(Fig. 2) (19,20,42-44). This transport enzyme is the "sodium pump," requires Mg^{2+} as a cofactor, and uses energy derived from ATP to transport Na^+ ions from inside to outside the cell against a concentration gradient. Three Na^+ ions (which enter the cell during depolarization) are exchanged for two K^+ ions. The fact that an unequal number of positive ions are exchanged means that an electric current is generated. Thus the transport enzyme is an electrogenic pump. This net outward movement of positive charge helps the cell develop its resting negative intracellular potential. Recent evidence indicates there is an "unstirred layer" immediately adjacent to the cell membrane and a "bulk layer" representing the extracellular fluid (28). The two layers are in equilibrium but the pump responds to the ionic milieu of the unstirred layer. During rapid electrolyte changes the composition of the two layers may be different.

The Na^+-K^+ ATPase enzyme undergoes multiple changes in configuration in the process of transporting Na^+ out of and K^+ into the cell. Digitalis binds more readily to certain configurations (20). Binding is inhibited by K^+. This inhibition by K^+ is no longer considered competitive. Rather, K^+ decreases the proportion

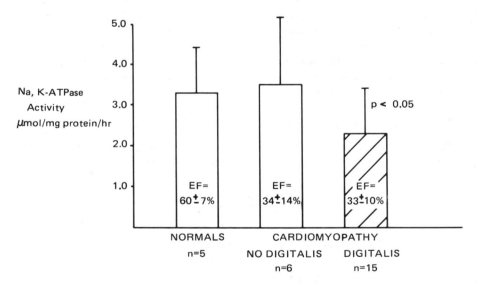

FIGURE 2 The Na^+-K^+ ATPase activity obtained from right ventricular endomyocardial biopsy specimens in 5 normal subjects, 6 patients with cardiomyopathy not receiving digitalis, and 15 patients with cardiomyopathy receiving digitalis. There is a significant reduction in enzyme activity in those receiving digitalis. The mean ejection fraction for each group is listed. There is no significant difference in the cardiomyopathy patients, but both differed significantly from normal. (Courtesy of Donald V. Unverferth.)

of the enzyme in the digitalis-sensitive configuration. Thus hyperkalemia can reverse the inhibitory effects of digitalis and hypokalemia can enhance the effect.

A. Mechanism of the Inotropic Effect

Normally there is an electrochemical gradient favoring entry of Na^+ and Ca^{2+} into the cell. Cardiac contraction is initiated by the action potential which depolarizes the cell surface membrane. The action potential in atrial and ventricular muscle cells is generated by a rapid inward Na^+ current through membrane Na^+ channels. This rapid inflow of Na^+ transiently opens Ca^{2+} channels allowing Ca^{2+} entry into the cell. The entry of Ca^{2+} into the cell triggers release of stored Ca^{2+} from the sarcoplasmic reticulum. The increased cytoplasmic Ca^{2+} interacts with contractile proteins. The Ca^{2+} binds to troponin. This removes the inhibition by tropomyosin of the interaction of actin and myosin, allowing these two proteins to slide over one another (consuming ATP). The Ca^{2+} then dissociates from troponin and undergoes re-uptake into the sarcoplasmic reticulum leading to relaxation. The amount of force generated depends on the size of the inward Ca^{2+} current, the amount of Ca^{2+} released from the sarcoplasmic reticulum, and the sensitivity of the contractile proteins to Ca^{2+} (19).

   In order for the cell to maintain steady state, the Ca^{2+} which enters the cell via the inward Ca^{2+} current must be removed after contraction has occurred. This is accomplished by the electrogenic Na^+-Ca^{2+} exchange mechanism. The Na^+-Ca^{2+} exchange mechanism at the cell membrane is a large capacity system which exchanges three Na^+ ions into the cell for one Ca^{2+} out of the cell. It uses the electrogenic gradient favoring Na entry into the cell. If intracellular Na^+ increases there will be less exchange and intracellular Ca^{2+} will increase.

   It now seems likely that digitalis, by its effect of inhibiting Na^+-K^+ ATPase, results in a net loss of intracellular K^+ and gain in Na^+. A remarkably small increase in intracellular Na^+ (1-2 mM) is all that is required, since this small increase in intracellular Na^+ can double intracellular Ca^{2+} via the Na^+-Ca^{2+} exchange (19).

   Most inotropic agents involve intracellular Ca^{2+} by one mechanism or another (19,50). When heart failure is present there may be altered calcium influx or release from internal stores in part related to depressed cyclic AMP levels. The increase in intracellular Ca^{2+} caused by digitalis increases the amount of Ca^{2+} stored and released from the sarcoplasmic reticulum. There is experimental evidence that the response to digitalis is diminished in the aging heart, though probably by a mechanism distal to the Na^+-K^+ ATPase enzyme (51).

   It is of interest that the effect of digitalis resembles the effect of increasing the heart rate (treppe phenomenon) (19,43,52). Increased heart rate leads to an increase in intracellular Na^+ with resultant increase in intracellular Ca^{2+}. Experimental studies indicate that the inotropic effect of digitalis is augmented at faster stimulation rates (43).

Finally, it should be noted that the inotropic effect of digitalis is minimal in skeletal muscle (53). In vascular smooth muscle there is a direct vasoconstrictor effect probably related to increased intracellular Ca^{2+} (19,54).

B. Electrophysiological Effects

Digitalis has substantial and highly complex electrophysiological actions. As is the case with its hemodynamic effects, the autonomic nervous system plays a significant role. Potassium (both intra- and extracellular) also has a major influence on the electrophysiological effects of digitalis. The direct electrophysiological effects of digitalis will be discussed in this section and the modifying influence of the autonomic nervous system will be discussed in the subsequent section.

The direct electrophysiological effects of digitalis on the heart vary according to the nature of the tissue under consideration (21-26,42). With automatic cells (mostly in the atria) which depend upon the slow calcium channel there is minimal effect at therapeutic levels but enhanced automaticity at toxic levels. In cells which constitute the conduction tissue around the sinoatrial (SA) node and the atrioventricular nodal (AV) cells, the refractory period is prolonged. Conduction is also slowed by decreasing the resting potential (see below). This can produce SA or AV block at toxic levels.

The atrial and ventricular myocardial cells and the Purkinje cells show a similar electrophysiological response to digitalis (26). Therapeutic levels of digitalis have minimal electrophysiological effects on these cells in normal hearts. The most striking effect is a shortening of the plateau phase of repolarization in ventricular myocardial cells. This produces the well-known ST-segment changes and shortening of the QT interval on the surface electrocardiogram (42).

Both atrial myocardial cells and Purkinje cells are more sensitive to the toxic effects of digitalis than are ventricular myocardial cells (21,25). The effect of toxic levels is a direct result of inhibition of Na^+-K^+ ATPase and stimulation of the electrogenic Na^+-Ca^{2+} exchange pump (26,42,44). Intracellular K^+ is depleted, extracellular K^+ (in the unstirred layer) is increased, and intracellular Na^+ and Ca^{2+} are increased. Because of the effects on K^+, the resting membrane potential is decreased. This results in a decrease in maximum velocity of the upstroke (V_{max}) during depolarization, which in turn results in decreased conduction velocity. There is also a decrease in intercellular conduction. Phase 4 depolarization is increased, leading to increased automaticity. These effects are augmented at faster heart rates. It is of interest that in spite of the decreased conduction velocity produced by digitalis, prolongation of the QRS complex seldom occurs.

In addition to the above effects relating to potassium, oscillatory electrical activity appears at toxic levels due to increased intracellular Ca^{2+}. This activity has been termed "delayed afterdepolarizations" (27-30). The mechanism of the oscillatory electrical activity is presumed to be due to oscillatory release of Ca^{2+} from the sarcoplasmic reticulum, which triggers inward Na^+ currents (26). Oscillatory activity is also enhanced at more rapid heart rates (larger amplitude oscillations and greater ease of elicitation).

It is possible that digitalis may effect the electrophysiological properties of the heart by its hemodynamic effects as well. This is particularly true for the atria where reduced stretch as a result of lowered ventricular diastolic pressure can reduce ectopic activity (42). It is not certain whether this phenomenon occurs in the ventricles.

C. Potassium as a Modifier of Digitalis Effects

The level of extracellular fluid (ECF) K^+ affects the extent of digitalis binding to Na^+-K^+ ATPase (55). This effects the magnitude of the inotropic response to digitalis, but is apparently of less clinical significance than the electrophysiological consequences.

Increased extracellular fluid K^+ (in the unstirred layer) reduces the resting membrane potential, leading to electrophysiological effects similar to the toxic effects of digitalis. On the other hand, increased ECF K^+, by reversing the effect of digitalis on Na^+-K^+ ATPase, reduces intracellular Ca^{2+}, which retards delayed afterdepolarizations (26).

Decreased ECF K^+ enhances phase 4 depolarization. This both promotes ectopic activity and reduces conduction velocity (due to lowered initial membrane potential). By enhancing the digitalis effect on Na^+-K^+ ATPase it also enhances oscillatory activity. Thus it can be seen that both hyperkalemia and hypokalemia are undesirable in the presence of digitalis toxicity (26).

Other factors can promote oscillatory activity. These include the presence of catecholamines and hypercalcemia—both of which increase intracellular Ca^{2+} (26).

Digitalis-induced toxic rhythms will be specifically discussed in a later section, but it is clear that their pathophysiology is complex. Mechanisms include re-entry (due to diminished conduction velocity and nonhomogeneous conduction), enhanced automaticity (increased phase 4 depolarization), and triggered rhythms (delayed afterdepolarizations) (26,44). In many cases one or more of these mechanisms may operate simultaneously.

IV. AUTONOMIC NERVOUS SYSTEM EFFECTS

Digitalis has major effects on the autonomic nervous system in addition to its direct effects on the heart and blood vessels (40,42-44,56-58). Many of the effects of digitalis are mediated through stimulation, inhibition, or facilitation of the autonomic nervous system at all levels. These effects vary with dose, metabolic milieu, and nature of the underlying disease. Frequently the "direct" and "indirect" effects of digitalis are opposite but in other instances they may be additive. Proper understanding of both the therapeutic and toxic effects of digitalis requires a thorough understanding of its autonomic effects.

Throughout this and remaining sections of this chapter it should be kept in mind that most experimental animal and human studies of digitalis are necessarily *acute* studies. In view of the complexity of the actions of digitalis, especially its autonomic interactions, it is highly likely that the effects of chronic administration may differ from acute changes. Clearly, future studies must address this problem.

A. Sympathetic-Parasympathetic Interactions

In the past the relationship between the sympathetic and parasympathetic limbs of the autonomic nervous system has been considered to be reciprocal. In general, sympathetic stimulation is stimulatory and parasympathetic stimulation is inhibitory. Although a reciprocal action does in fact occur in response to certain physiological demands (such as exercise), recent evidence indicates that the parasympathetic nervous system can modulate the sympathetic nervous system. Indeed, sympathetic stimulation can be completely overridden (58).

Anatomically the nerve terminals of both systems often lie in close proximity within cardiac structures. Acetylcholine (ACH) release by vagal nerve fibers may inhibit norepinephrine (NE) release from adjacent sympathetic terminals. In addition, ACH can also inhibit the beta-adrenergic receptor response to NE. This is most likely due to inhibition of adenylate cyclase, which is now known to be a dually regulated enzyme (58).

In general, "therapeutic" levels of digitalis result in a net increase in parasympathetic tone, whereas "toxic" levels result in stimulation of the sympathetic nervous system.

B. Parasympathetic Nervous System Effects

Enhancement of parasympathetic tone begins with relatively low doses. Thus in instances where the "direct" effect of digitalis may be opposite from its "indirect" effect of enhancing vagal tone, the indirect effect predominates. A major mechanism of enhanced vagal tone is excitation of ventricular and arterial baroreceptors (afferent enhancement); which is probably achieved by altering sensitivity (40,44). Stimulation of the baroreceptors results in efferent parasympathetic stimulation and reflex sympathetic withdrawal, resulting in sinus bradycardia and arterial and venous dilatation. A similar result occurs with stimulation of the ventricular Bezold-Jarisch reflex and atrial volume receptors. There is also increased renal blood flow (sympathetic withdrawal), inhibition of renin release, and decreased central nervous system antidiuretic hormone (ADH) release (40,44). These neurohumoral effects of digitalis should be beneficial in patients with congestive heart failure (as discussed later).

Digitalis also improves ganglionic transmission in efferent parasympathetic ganglia and potentiates end-organ responsiveness to ACH. As noted earlier, this enhanced efferent activity also inhibits NE release from sympathetic terminals and inhibits adrenergic effects on the beta-receptor (40,44,58).

C. Sympathetic Nervous System Effects

The effects of digitalis on the sympathetic nervous system are less well understood (40,42-44,58). Reflex sympathetic withdrawal and direct inhibition occur with therapeutic levels. At toxic levels sympathetic stimulation can occur, but the precise role of this effect in clinical settings is still not clear.

Increased sympathetic effect at toxic levels can result from both increased central nervous system outflow and enhancement of NE release and inhibition of re-uptake (and hence degradation) by peripheral nerve endings. A recent study suggests that acute digitalis administration may be associated with a greater peripheral sympathetic stimulatory effect than is the case after chronic administration (59). The direct vasoconstrictor effect of digitalis on both the arterial and venous tree may potentiate the effect of NE (40,44). However, in humans, increased sympathetic effects produced by higher doses of digitalis seems to be largely manifested by electrophysiological effects.

D. Autonomic Nervous System Role in Cardiovascular Effects

1. Inotropic Effect

Multiple experimental studies have shown that the positive inotropic effect of digitalis is not mediated by catecholamines (40,42-44). In the experimental animal, the maximum digitalis inotropic effect is less than the maximum inotropic effect of catecholamines (60). In human subjects with an intact autonomic nervous system, the inotropic effect of digitalis can be modified by simultaneous changes in autonomic tone. Therapeutic digitalis levels induce a reflex negative inotropic effect both by vagal stimulation of the atria (and possibly the ventricle) and reflex sympathetic withdrawal. Thus, the positive inotropic effect of digitalis is more pronounced when there is autonomic blockade (42-44,58).

Patients with chronic heart failure often have diminished parasympathetic tone and "down regulation" of cardiac beta-receptors (discussed later) (61,62). In effect these patients are partially denervated. It is possible that this phenomenon may help to explain the experimental observation that the failing heart has a greater hemodynamic response to digitalis (63).

2. Peripheral Vascular Effects

In normal subjects the direct vasoconstrictor effect of digitalis on arteries and veins predominates, since resting sympathetic tone is minimal and parasympathetic dilator effects on the peripheral vessels are minimal (40,64). Digitalis decreases venous return, apparently by its effect on the capacitance bed to increase splanchnic blood volume (40,44). This effect is in marked contrast to that of catecholamines which increase venous return by shifting blood from the peripheral capacitance bed to the central blood volume (65). Digitalis has no direct effects on the pulmonary circulation or pulmonary blood volume (66).

In patients with CHF, the peripheral vascular effects of digitalis appear to be opposite of those which occur in normals. These patients often have high alpha-adrenergic tone in both the arterial and venous system. Digitalis-induced reflex sympathetic withdrawal produces a net arterial and venous dilation which overrides its direct effect (40). The arterial dilation enhances cardiac output by reducing afterload while preload is also reduced. In this sense digitalis assumes some of the salutory effects of vasodilator therapy (discussed later).

The effect of digitalis on the capacitance bed in congestive heart failure is not clear largely because this is a difficult phenomenon to study in humans (67). Theoretically digitalis should reduce the adrenergically mediated increase in central blood volume which occurs in CHF. However, the one experimental study in humans suggests that digitalis decreases the splanchnic volume in patients with CHF (68). Where the splanchnic capacitance volume might be relocated is unknown, as are the hemodynamic implications of this volume shift (in other words, is this important in the increase in cardiac output seen after digitalis administration?).

3. *Electrophysiological Effects*

At therapeutic levels, the autonomic effects of digitalis primarily occur in the atria and AV node due to the fact that there is minimal parasympathetic enervation in the ventricles. At toxic levels of digitalis, the parasympathetic effects may be exaggerated (the usual case in normal hearts), producing disorders of impulse generation and conduction. In diseased hearts, enhanced sympathetic activity may act synergistically with the direct effects of digitalis to produce tachyarrhythmias (28,40, 42-44,57).

Sinus Node.   Therapeutic doses of digitalis have no significant direct effect on the sinus (SA) node. Sinus rate often slows in both normals and patients with heart disease because of parasympathetic stimulation and reflex withdrawal of sympathetic tone. At toxic doses sinus tachycardia may develop because of the direct effect of digitalis to increase automaticity and indirectly by activation of the sympathetic nervous system. The effect of digitalis on the SA node can be altered when SA node disease is present. In this setting digitalis may produce SA exit block by its direct effect, and the depression of automaticity due to increased vagal tone may be exaggerated.

Atria.   Atrial refractory period is decreased by parasympathetic stimulation, which overrides the direct effect of digitalis. Parasympathetic stimulation causes hyperpolarization of automatic cells and atrial fibers, which reduces automaticity but may also improve conduction (42).

Atrioventricular Node.   The refractoriness of the AV node is increased both by direct and indirect effects of digitalis but the indirect autonomic effects are more important (69). Indirect effects are due to a combination of enhanced parasympathetic tone, sympathetic withdrawal, and a decrease in AV node sensitivity to sympathetic stimulation (42-44). These actions account for most of the digitalis effect at rest (70). The direct effect of digitalis is to increase the AV nodal refractory period. When the PR interval is prolonged by digitalis, the increase is exclusively in the AH interval (42).

Digitalis also enhances AV nodal refractoriness in the presence of atrial fibrillation by increasing decremental conduction (71). This occurs because the atrial refractory period is shortened, allowing an increased number of impulses to enter the AV node. In addition, digitalis produces a greater nonuniformity of AV nodal cell refractory periods which augments decremental conduction.

When sympathetic tone is increased, such as with exercise, the direct effect of digitalis is the major mechanism of slowing AV conduction. At toxic levels increased parasympathetic tone and the direct effect can produce AV block. When AV node disease is present, both the direct and indirect effects are exaggerated.

Purkinje System.   Reduced sympathetic tone at therapeutic levels inhibits sympathetic nervous system effects on the Purkinje cells. Thus, for ventricular arrhythmias sensitive to sympathetic stimulation, digitalis can be antiarrhythmic (58).

With toxic concentrations, the direct effects of digitalis on the action potential appear (as discussed earlier). Increased sympathetic tone may be additive in the genesis of tachycardias due either to increased automaticity, delayed afterdepolarizations, or lowering of the threshold for ventricular fibrillation (28,58,72).

V. PHARMACOKINETICS AND PHARMACODYNAMICS

For previous generations of medical students, learning to use digitalis was one of the most difficult and worrisome tasks during medical school. What other commonly used agent was so complex and had such harmful potential if improperly used? The development of radioisotopic-labeled digitalis glycosides in the 1950s and the radioimmunoassay in the 1960s, enabled dramatic advances to be made in understanding the difficult pharmacokinetics of digitalis glycosides. The major differences between the various preparations have been documented. Because of its more widespread use in the United States, digoxin has been the major glycoside studied, and more is known of its kinetics.

With digitalis the distinction between pharmacokinetics (what the body does to the drug) and pharmacodynamics (what the drug does to the body) is extremely important. Unlike digitalis, most other cardiovascular drugs have a rapid equilibration between the plasma and the site of action, and a short elimination half-life. Thus the onset and dissipation of the pharmacodynamic effect is rapid. This makes clinical use of these drugs relatively simple and toxicity less of a problem (73).

TABLE 1 Cardiac Glycosides

Agent	Gastrointestinal absorption	Peak effect	Half-life	Therapeutic range (ng/ml)	Digitalizing dose (mg)	Maintenance dose (mg)
Ouabain	Intravenous only	10-20 min	22 hr		Initial 0.5 up to 1.0	
Deslanoside	Intravenous only	10-20 min	42 hr		Initial 0.5 up to 1.0	0.05-0.20
Digoxin	Tablets 60-75%	4-8 hr	44 hr	1.0-2.0	1.0-1.5	0.125-0.375
	Elixir 75-85%				0.8-1.2	
	Lanoxicaps® 80-90%				0.8-1.0	
	Intravenous	1-2 hr				
Digitoxin	Tablets 95-100%	8-12 hr	4-6 days	15-25	Initial 0.5 up to 1.0	0.05-0.15
	Intramuscular 95-100%					
	Intravenous	4-6 hr			0.6-1.0	

Digoxin became the predominantly used glycoside during the 1960s, replacing digitalis leaf and digitoxin. This was largely because of its shorter half-life, though the half-life is still long by comparison to other cardiovascular agents. Although digoxin absorption was known to be incomplete compared to digitoxin, the clinical significance of this problem was not recognized until the early 1970s. Also, the major effect of renal insufficiency on digoxin elimination was not clearly quantitated until the late 1960s. It is of interest that digitoxin, which does not suffer these problems, has remained the most widely used glycoside in many other countries. Pertinent pharmacokinetic parameters for commonly used glycosides are listed in Table 1.

A. Absorption

Absorption of digitalis glycosides can occur along the entire course of the gastrointestinal tract but mostly occurs in the jejunum (74). The process is complicated by the enterohepatic circulation which may recycle drug already absorbed, producing a prolongation of the absorption process.

Absorption is passive and nonsaturable. Peak plasma levels are reached 1-2 hr after an oral dose (41). The ease of absorption is related to the polarity of the glycoside molecule (74). Glycoside polarity determines lipid solubility. Nonpolar glycosides such as digitoxin are well absorbed (75). Ouabain and deslanoside are highly polar and therefore not significantly absorbed (74). Digoxin is moderately polar and variably absorbed (76). Glycoside polarity also determines the predominant mode of elimination (77). digitoxin is highly bound to serum albumin and thus undergoes minimal glomerular filtration (78). Renal tubular reabsorption of the small amount of digitoxin which is filtered is nearly complete. Thus the drug is predominantly eliminated by metabolism to polar metabolites. This prolongs the elimination half-life.

Because digoxin absorption is incomplete, there is more inter- and intraindividual variation (46,77,79,80). The dose form, state of the gastrointestinal tract, and interference from coadministered agents are also important determinants of digoxin absorption. Poor bioavailability related both to tablet formulation and digoxin content was noted in the early 1970s (81). In 1974, the Food and Drug Administration issued guidelines requiring digoxin manufacturers to establish minimum bioavailability of their tablets. Today's tablets are considered to have 60-75% bioavailability. Digoxin elixir (mostly used in pediatrics) has a 75-85% bioavailability, and a new formulation (Lanoxicaps) is reported to have an 80-90% absorption (82). It is probable that both elixir and Lanoxicaps have greater bioavailability in the presence of congestive failure or gastrointestinal disease (79).

Malabsorption syndromes (including bowel edema from congestive heart failure) or acute diarrhea can decrease digoxin absorption (83-85). Chronic pancreatic insufficiency does not. Concurrent administration of kaolin-pectin, certain nonabsorbable antacids, cholesterol-binding agents, and antineoplastic drugs can reduce absorption by 25-35% (86-88). Antacids and cholesterol-binding agents also affect digitoxin absorption (44). In certain patients an intestinal bacterium (*Eubacterium lentum*) metabolizes digoxin to dihydrodigoxin—a cardioinactive metabolite (46, 89).

B. Distribution and Onset of Activity

A study from our laboratory indicates digoxin distribution follows a three-compartment open pharmacokinetic model with digoxin equilibrating with the third (slow) compartment (90). Digoxin as well as other glycosides are distributed widely throughout the body (in part related to the ubiquitous presence of the enzyme Na^+-K^+ ATPase) but not to fat tissue (33,91-93). After steady-state chronic administra-

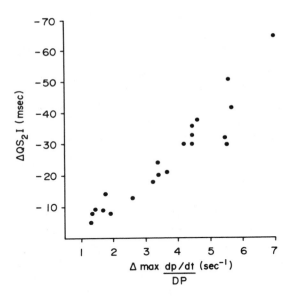

FIGURE 3   Changes in QS2I from baseline (ΔQS2I) and maximum left ventricular dP/dt corrected for developed pressure (maximum dP/dt/DP) obtained serially after administration of 1 mg of intravenous digoxin in five patients. A high-fidelity catheter system was employed. There is a direct relationship between increased rate of pressure development as a result of the inotropic effect of digoxin and shortening of the QS2I. (From R. P. Lewis, The use of systolic time intervals for evaluation of left ventricular function, in *Noninvasive Diagnostic Methods in Cardiology* [N. O. Fowler, ed. and A. N. Brest, ed. in chief, Cardiovascular Clinics], F. A. Davis, Philadelphia, 1983, pp. 335-355. Reproduced with permission.)

tion, the muscle mass contains most of the digoxin (50%) followed by kidney, gastrointestinal tract, and heart. Cardiac binding of digitalis is both specific (to the Na^+-K^+ ATPase receptor on the external surface of the cell membrane) and nonspecific, and is approximately five times greater than for skeletal muscle. The Na^+-K^+ ATPase binding is saturable (93). The nonspecific binding of digoxin (constituting 90% of myocardial digoxin) apparently varies according to the duration of drug administration (42). It is higher for a given serum level after acute administration (94). The significance of this observation with reference to toxicity remains to be determined. As noted earlier, however, acute digitalization may also be associated with greater peripheral sympathetic stimulation. Nonspecific binding is more extensive for digitoxin than digoxin (93). The variable nonspecific binding renders isotope studies of tissue distribution difficult to interpret.

By employing changes in the duration of electromechanical systole ($\Delta QS2I$) from systolic time intervals, the positive inotropic action of digitalis glycosides can be measured (95). The close correlation between $\Delta QS2I$ and the change in left ventricular dP/dt (using high-fidelity catheters) is shown in Figure 3 (96). Subsequently the validity of this approach was shown by demonstrating an excellent correlation

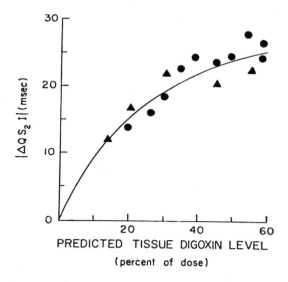

FIGURE 4 Correlation of the change in QS2I ($\Delta QS2I$) and predicted tissue digoxin level derived from serial measurements of plasma digoxin levels after administration of 1 mg of digoxin intravenously in 12 normal subjects. Twenty-two simultaneous QS2I and plasma digoxin levels were obtained over a 96-hour period. Closed circles represent points from onset to peak activity; closed triangles represent the decay portion. The nonlinear correlation was $r = 0.97$ ($P < 0.01$). (From Ref. 97, reproduced with permission.)

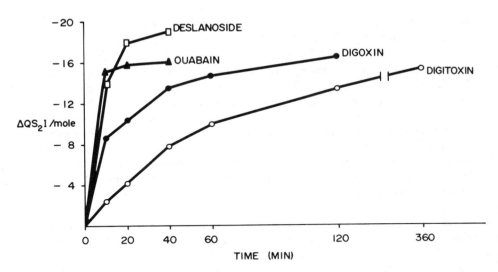

FIGURE 5 Onset of activity of four digitalis glycoside preparations administered intravenously. The inotropic response is shown as the change in the QS2I (ΔQS2I) per mole of glycoside (see text for further details).

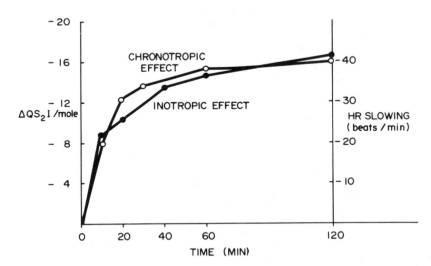

FIGURE 6 Comparison of inotropic and chronotropic effect of intravenous digoxin over a 2-hour period. The chronotropic is calculated from the slowing of the heart rate in patients with atrial fibrillation and the inotropic effect as the shortening of the QS2I (ΔQS2I) per mole (see text for further details).

between changes in the ΔQS2I and the predicted tissue level of digoxin from pharmacokinetic analysis (Fig. 4) (97).

The ΔQS2I can be used to measure the temporal onset of activity of currently employed glycosides in normal subjects (98). The onset of activity follows an exponential pattern typical of drugs binding to a saturable receptor (Fig. 5). From these curves the time constant (63% of maximal response) can be calculated. This allows a comparison of relative rapidity of onset. Ouabain and deslanoside are similar and rapid acting (time constants of 5.8 ± 0.6 min and 7.2 ± 3.3 min, P = ns), while the time constant of digoxin is three times longer (23 ± 2.3 min, $P < 0.01$), and that of digitoxin eight times longer (56 ± 10 min, $P < 0.01$). Thus deslanoside more closely resembles ouabain in its onset of activity and both are significantly more rapid than digoxin. It is of interest that a similar analysis of Gold's (76) original data for the use of intravenous digoxin and digitoxin to slow the ventricular response to atrial fibrillation yields time constants of 25 min for digoxin and 50 min for digitoxin—identical to our data for the inotropic response (Fig. 6) (98).

Figure 7 shows the onset of the inotropic effect after oral doses of digoxin and digitoxin in normal subjects (95). The onset is delayed and the difference between the two drugs is minimal when oral dosing is employed. We have not conducted similar studies in patients with congestive failure, but Gold's studies suggest no significant delay in onset of activity for slowing of the heart rate in atrial fibrillation in patients with heart failure (76).

In our study the intravenous doses selected for each glycoside were based on the empirically derived digitalizing doses in use at that time (95). The maximum effects were not statistically different, indicating the validity of the empiric doses. Table 2 lists currently recommended dosages for oral and intravenous administration for the commonly used glycosides (43). These recommended dosages are approximately one-half of those recommended 20 years ago.

Gold first noted that the dose-response curve for digitalis was nonlinear (76). Subsequently, the same phenomenon was noted by Weissler and co-workers for the inotropic response (ΔQS2I) to graded doses of intravenous deslanoside (Fig. 8) (99). This phenomenon is also seen in Figure 3. Subsequent studies from other laboratories have confirmed this finding (100-102). Thus, increasing the dose yields progressively less pharmacodynamic effect in spite of a linear increase in blood level (44).

Because of the long time for plasma-tissue equilibration, serum digitalis levels fluctuate far more dramatically than do the tissue levels of the drug. The tissue level "peaks and troughs" which complicate class I antiarrhythmic drug therapy are much less of a factor with digitalis (Fig. 9) (46). This is of major importance when a relatively constant drug effect is desired, such as for control of heart rate in atrial fibrillation.

The long equilibration time between plasma and tissue is also of major importance for interpretation of serum digitalis levels. Until equilibration has occurred

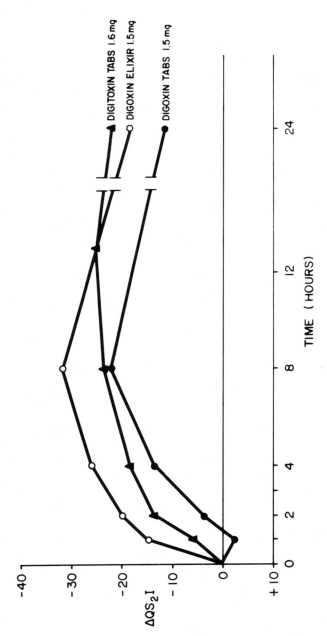

FIGURE 7 Onset of inotropic activity ($\Delta QS2I$) over 12 hours for oral digitoxin tablets, digoxin elixir, and digoxin tablets. Digoxin elixir has the most rapid onset of activity; digoxin tablets have the slowest onset. The lesser extent of effect on the QS2I by digoxin tablets represents incomplete absorption. Digitoxin requires up to 12 hours for full effect to be reached but the onset of activity is similar to digoxin tablets.

TABLE 2 Comparative Efficacy of Agents Used in Congestive Heart Failure

Agent class	Reduce EDP	Reduce SVR	Increase CO	Increase EF
Diuretics	+++	+/o	+/o	o
Positive inotropes				
Digitalis	+	+	++	+
Dobutamine	+	+	+++	++
Vasodilators				
Prazosin	+	++	+	o
ACE inhibitor	++	++	+	o
Hydralazine	+/o	+++	+++	+/o
Oral nitrates	++	+	+/o	o
Nifedipine	+/o	+++	+	o
IV nitroglycerin	+++	++	++	o
IV nitroprusside	+++	+++	++	+/o

Note: ACE = angiotension converting enzyme; EDP = end diastolic pressure; EF = ejection fraction; CO = cardiac output; IV = intravenous; SVR = systemic vascular resistance.

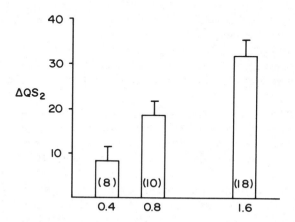

FIGURE 8 The effect of three doses of deslanoside administered intravenously on the $\Delta QS2I$ in normal subjects. Two-thirds of the effect of a full dose is seen with one-half dose (0.8 mg).

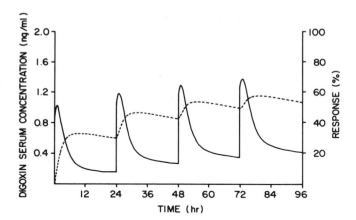

FIGURE 9 Simulated time profile of serum digoxin levels (solid line) and tissue response as judged by QS2I (dashed line) over a 4-day period. The tissue response is plotted as a percentage of maximum response. Pharmacokinetic and pharmacodynamic constants for the simulation were obtained from a single-dose study in normal humans (97). The dosage regimen for the simulation was 0.375 mg digoxin tablets per day with a bioavailability of 0.8. (From Ref. 46, reproduced with permission.)

the plasma level will be "falsely" high. For intravenous digoxin 4-6 hr are required and for intravenous digitoxin 12 hours should be allowed. When oral digoxin is given equilibration is delayed an additional 2-4 hr.

The more polar digoxin exhibits a 20-30% binding to serum albumin while the nonpolar digitoxin has a substantially higher binding to albumin (90-95%) (41). Hypoalbuminemia will raise free drug concentration but this is probably only clinically relevant for digitoxin (82).

As noted earlier, extracellular potassium plays a major role in digitalis binding (and hence effect) (55). Thus, hypokalemia promotes more digitalis binding and the inhibitory effects of digitalis can be partially reversed when extracellular K is increased (20). Hypomagnesemia also potentiates digitalis binding possibly through a similar mechanism (44).

Physical exercise effects digoxin distribution, possibly by altering the Na^+-K^+ ATPase receptor to a high affinity conformation in skeletal muscle. The degree of change is related to the intensity of muscular activity (103). Skeletal muscle digoxin can be increased by 20% and serum level decreased by 40% at a high work load. Even routine physical activity can cause a significant lowering of serum digoxin levels (104).

The volume of distribution of digoxin is reduced in renal failure (105). The mechanism is still unclear, as is the clinical significance (46). This reduction may, in fact, be artifactual due to accumulation of digoxin metabolites.

Because only a small fraction of digitalis glycoside resides in the blood and because of the slow equilibration between the blood and tissue compartments, dialysis is not effective in removing the drug (106).

C. Elimination

1. Metabolism

Polar glycosides (that is, ouabain) are predominantly excreted unchanged in the urine (107). Digitoxin on the other hand is known to undergo extensive hepatic metabolism and these nonpolar metabolites constitute the bulk of renal excretory products (78). Metabolism of digitalis glycosides consists of two major routes (46). The first involves sequential hydrolysis of the sugar moieties producing genins. The intermediates possess some cardioactivity while genins do not. This process begins in the stomach and continues in the liver. The second pathway involves reduction of the lactone double bond to form cardioinactive dihydro compounds. For digoxin, it has been shown that *Eubacterium lentum* in the gastrointestinal tract can perform this reduction, which can be extensive, in up to 10% of subjects (108).

Recent studies have shown that digoxin metabolism may be more extensive than previously thought—especially after oral administration (109). Up to one-third of digoxin activity by plasma immunoassay performed 6 hours after an oral dose can be metabolites. When renal failure is present hepatic metabolism of digoxin plays a more important role in its disposition (110). Metabolism is not affected by liver disease but can be influenced by certain drugs (phenobarbital, phenylbutazone) (42).

2. Excretion

Native glycosides and their metabolites are excreted both by the kidneys and in the stool. It appears that when renal function is impaired, fecal excretion can be augmented. Fecal excretion is from several sources: unabsorbed drug (prominent with polar glycosides), metabolites from gastrointestinal tract degradation, and native drug and metabolites introduced by enterohepatic recycling. Much of the drug secreted in the bile is subsequently reabsorbed. However, apparently not all is reabsorbed, possibly due to hepatic conjugation (46). Normally, fecal excretion is predominant for digitoxin (mostly metabolites) and renal excretion for digoxin, ouabain, and deslanoside (mostly native drug) (41).

Much attention has focused on the renal excretion of digoxin as this is its predominant mode of elimination (46,111-115). Normally, renal digoxin clearance slightly exceeds creatinine clearance owing to net tubular secretion. Tubular secretion is most prominent in the young and in part explains the increased dosage required in children. Physical activity may also increase digoxin excretion by up to 30% (116). When renal failure supervenes renal digoxin clearance parallels creatinine clearance. In this regard it should be remembered that creatinine clearance can be reduced by 50% before the serum creatinine rises. Most patients with heart failure fall into this category, both because of older age and reduced cardiac output. However, compensatory mechanisms (mostly raised fecal excretion) come into play with renal failure such that accurate estimation of total body digoxin clearance from creatinine clearance alone is too inexact for all but a rough guideline (117).

The enterohepatic recycling of digitalis offers a possible mode of increasing the rate of drug elimination. However, this is probably only clinically significant for digitoxin (118). On the other hand, the use of Fab fragments has supplemented this approach (discussed later).

3. Elimination Half-Life

The average elimination half-lives of the commonly employed glycosides are listed in Table 2. The elimination half-life is a function of body clearance of the drug. It is a key pharmacokinetic parameter along with bioavailability and volume of distribution. These three variables determine the steady-state concentration of drug in serum (73).

Elimination half-life determines the time required to reach steady state after a given dose of drug, regardless of dosage interval, route of administration, or amount of drug given. Elimination half-life is measured from analyses of the decay of plasma levels of drug after steady state has been reached. For digitalis glycosides these measurements were first made from tritiated preparations but more recently from immunoassay. Decay of physiological effect (ΔQS2I or ventricular response in atrial fibrillation) measures pharmacodynamic half-life and have yielded similar values (77,95).

A major point to be derived from these studies is that digoxin elimination half-life is significantly increased when creatinine clearance falls (119). The elimination half-life can be doubled from 2 to 4 days with renal insufficiency and as such it approaches the half-life of digitoxin. From available studies it appears that the elimination half-life of digitoxin is unaffected by renal or hepatic disease, and is far more predictable than that of digoxin (78,120).

Elimination half-life of ouabain is approximately 22 hours in normal subjects but is increased to 50 hours in the presence of renal failure (121). Deslanoside elimination is similar to that of digoxin in normal subjects—a reason to consider deslanoside as the drug of choice for rapid digitalization. No studies of the effect of renal failure on deslanoside elimination half-life have been performed, but it is undoubtedly prolonged—probably similar to that of digoxin.

It is of interest that studies of patients who have ingested suicidal doses of digoxin suggest that the elimination half-life is more rapid (10-15 hr) when the body level of digoxin is extremely high (122).

VI. DOSES AND PHARMACOLOGIC INTERACTIONS

The clinical practice of digitalis administration has been dramatically improved by the widespread ability to measure serum digitalis levels by radioimmunoassay. However, the actions of digitalis are extremely complex and variations in autonomic tone and the nature and the severity of the underlying heart disease produce substantial variability in the response of a given patient to a given steady-state serum level. Thus serum levels alone cannot be used to determine the optimum pharmacodynamic effect or to discover whether toxicity is present (46,123,124).

A. Loading Dose

Digitalis was one of the first drugs for which the concept of a loading dose developed. In all likelihood this was due to its long elimination half-life. Normally, in the absence of a loading dose, approximately 85% of steady state is reached within three elimination half-lives (125). With a loading dose, steady state is reached more rapidly. In most instances where rapid digitalis action is needed, a loading or near loading dose is given (usually intravenous) over 24 hours. For elective digitalization it usually matters little whether a loading dose is given for digoxin, but digitoxin with its long elimination half-life is usually started with a loading dose (126).

Determination of the loading dose is primarily related to expected bioavailability and the volume of distribution (mainly determined by lean body mass). The desired body pool of drug at steady state is similar for both digoxin and digitoxin (10 μg/kg or 0.7 mg in a 70 kg individual). Thus the loading dose should be tailored to this figure, with a higher dose for digoxin due to incomplete absorption. When calculating a loading dose it is wise to err on the side of underestimation, particularly for digitoxin.

B. Relationship of Maintenance Dose to Loading Dose

The steady-state digitalis tissue level and serum level depend on the elimination half-life and the bioavailable maintenance dose. When the half-life of digoxin is 2 days, 25% of the loading dose will be excreted daily. For digitoxin with a half-life of 5 days, 10% will be excreted daily. If renal failure is present the elimination half-life of digoxin may increase to 4 days, so the maintenance dose should be halved.

Assuming a constant bioavailability and elimination half-life, a simple relation exists such that

$$\frac{\text{Dose}}{\text{Serum level at steady state } (C_{ss})} = K \ (46)$$

Changes in C_{ss} due to changes in dose can be easily predicted using this formula.

C. Changing Digitalis Preparations

Switching to digitoxin after intravenous digitalization with a rapidly acting glycoside such as ouabain, digoxin, or deslanoside requires a double maintenance dose of digitoxin for 2 days to compensate for the more rapid excretion of the shorter-acting glycoside. Conversely, if one is switching to digoxin from digitoxin, 2-3 days should elapse before starting maintenance digoxin (125).

Intramuscular digoxin is seldom employed due to pain and local tissue injury. If intramuscular administration is required, which would only occur in the postoperative setting in an uncomplicated patient, intramuscular digitoxin is the drug of choice as its bioavailability is similar to oral doses (78).

D. Interactions with Other Pharmacologic Agents

1. Quinidine

Remarkably, the digoxin-quinidine interaction was not discovered until 1977 (127). Since then it has been a subject of great interest and debate (128-132). In spite of the extensive recent literature, significant questions remain. It is likely that this interaction has been a major source of electrophysiological toxicity in the past (for example, the early experience with cardioversion for atrial fibrillation).

Quinidine causes a dose-related increase in serum digoxin concentration, most of which occurs within 24 hours after initiating quinidine and reaches steady state between 2 and 3 days. At usual doses of quinidine the serum digoxin level doubles; this occurs in 90% of patients.

Multiple mechanisms seem to be operative. Both renal and nonrenal digoxin clearance are reduced by up to 50% and elimination half-life doubles. Renal clearance is reduced largely by impaired tubular secretion. However, patients with absent renal function show the same decrease in digoxin clearance as those with intact renal function (133). In this case all reduction in clearance occurs in nonrenal clearance.

Plasma-protein binding of digoxin is unaffected by quinidine. Tissue concentrations of digoxin increase in proportion to the increased serum levels (134). Whether the cardiac effects of digitalis are increased by the higher serum and tissue digoxin level is uncertain. Central nervous system digoxin toxicity manifested by nausea and vomiting increases with the higher serum digoxin level and disappears when the level is lowered by reducing digoxin dosage without changing the quinidine dose (127). It appears that electrophysiological digoxin toxicity is increased (AV conduction delay and ventricular arrhythmias) (135). Most clinical and experimental studies suggest the inotropic effect of digoxin is not as great as would be expected from the digoxin serum level in this setting (134,136-139). Whether this represents the negative inotropic effect of quinidine negating the positive inotropic effect of digoxin, or whether there is less digoxin bound to Na^+-K^+ ATPase is not clear, but evidence favors the former.

The effect of quinidine on digitoxin is even more disputed. Studies either have shown no interaction or have suggested an interaction identical to that seen with digoxin (140-142).

Most studies have shown that if the digoxin dose is halved the serum digoxin level falls to prequinidine levels and apparent toxic symptoms disappear. No dramatic worsening of congestive heart failure has been noted clinically with this approach.

2. Calcium Channel Blocking Agents

Verapamil decreases renal clearance (decreased tubular secretion) and nonrenal clearance in a dose-related manner (143,144). Digoxin levels can increase by 50%. This response is more gradual than with quinidine, stabilizing at 1 week. Electrophysiological toxicity (mostly ventricular) can occur, but disappears when the digoxin dose is reduced. There also may be an enhanced inotropic effect in this interaction (145). Verapamil also inhibits the direct vasoconstrictor response to digitalis (40). It is recommended that digoxin dosage be halved. A small decrease in digoxin renal clearance has been described with diltiazem but none with nifedipine (146).

3. Amiodarone

Amiodarone produces a prompt (< 24 hr) increase in serum digoxin level of 25-50% by a decrease in both renal and nonrenal clearance (147-149). Toxicity consists of bradyarrhythmias. The magnitude of the effect is related to serum amiodarone levels. It is recommended that the digoxin dose be halved.

4. Other Antiarrhythmic Agents

Drugs which do not have significant pharmacokinetic interactions include procainamide, disopyramide, mexilitine, flecanide, and ethmozine (132).

5. Potassium-Sparing Diuretics

Spironolactone can reduce both renal and nonrenal clearance of digoxin and also may reduce the volume of distribution (150). These effects can significantly increase serum digoxin concentration. Amiloride increases renal clearance but reduces nonrenal clearance, with a net result of reduced clearance. Triamterene produces a mild reduction in nonrenal clearance of digoxin.

Because potassium depletion induced by thiazides and loop diuretics enhances digitalis toxicity and oral potassium supplements often have compliance problems, it has been tempting to employ potassium-sparing diuretics in the digitalized patient. A further reason to use these agents is the fact that hypokalemia inhibits digoxin clearance (151). Studies showing reduced digoxin clearance with such agents indicates that serum digoxin levels need to be monitored if this approach is used. On the other hand, one study suggests these potassium-sparing diuretics may also have direct myocardial effects to mitigate myocardial K^+ loss which might reduce myocardial digitalis binding (152). Indeed, attenuation of the positive inotropic effect of digoxin has been reported with spironolactone and amiloride but not triamterene (150).

6. Vasodilator Drugs

Both nitroprusside and hydralazine result in increased tubular secretion of digoxin (153). The clinical significance of this effect or possible similar effects from other vasodilators is unknown.

7. Anti-Inflammatory Agents

Indomethacin can reduce glomerular filtration rate and elevate the serum digoxin level. This has been noted in premature infants and in adults with renal impairment (132). No significant effects from other commonly used anti-inflammatory agents have been reported.

E. Indications for Therapeutic Drug Monitoring with Serum Radioimmunoassay

Before discussing the clinical use of radioimmunoassays of digitalis glycosides, a few issues concerning assay methodology need to be considered (46). First is quality. Numerous commercial kits are available which have variable precision and are performed in clinical laboratories with variable quality control. In ideal circumstances the coefficient of variation for repetitive determinations should be 5-15%. Second, many assays are erroneously ordered prior to tissue equilibration due to inadequate understanding by those ordering the test. Third, gamma-emitting radioisotopes in the blood from other diagnostic tests may interfere—a fact infrequently considered. Fourth is the nonspecificity of the immunoassay itself. Some metabolites are measured in addition to the native drug. This is more likely to be a problem in chronic renal disease and certain gastrointestinal disorders. Fortunately, most cross-reacting metabolites are cardioactive, but the cardioinactive dihydrodigoxin, for instance, is not. It is estimated that from 6-42% of serum digoxin measured by current immunoassays may be metabolites (46). This figure is probably higher for digitoxin. In addition there may be cross-reactivity with endogenous substances, especially in neonates, pregnant women, and patients with hepatic and renal diseases. Finally, digoxin and digitoxin antibodies cross-react (154). This is only of importance in patients treated with digitoxin due to the higher serum concentration of digitoxin (a "toxic" level of digoxin can be found in a patient who has therapeutic levels of digitoxin).

From these considerations it is clear that specificity of serum digitalis assays must be improved. Until that time it might be more appropriate to term serum digitalis assays as monitors of "apparent digitalis concentration" (46).

Serum assays have assumed great clinical importance in the diagnosis and prevention of digitalis toxicity (46,82,123,124). This subject will be considered in detail later. Other indications for serum monitoring include (1) monitoring compliance, (2) investigating an apparent poor response, (3) determining bioavailability, (4) assessing the effects of an individual's renal function, (5) suspected drug interaction, and (6) clinical states in which the response to digitalis is altered (discussed later). Once a satisfactory serum digoxin level has been documented, measurement more often than once a year is seldom indicated.

A final but extremely important point to re-emphasize is that the dose response of the serum digitalis level is linear, but the pharmacodynamic response is *not* linear and begins to diminish just above the empirically derived therapeutic range.

VII. CLINICAL USE OF DIGITALIS AS A POSITIVE INOTROPE

A. Response of the Normal Circulation

The response of the normal circulation to digitalis in many respects is opposite to the response of the failing circulation. A positive inotropic response in normal subjects can be demonstrated by systolic time intervals, echocardiography, left ventricular dP/dt with high-fidelity catheters, and standard hemodynamic parameters (36,155-157). The inotropic response consists of an increased rate of force development for a given end-diastolic fiber stretch, and shortening of the duration of systole by 25-35 msec. The ejection fraction increases 5%, the left ventricular dP/dt increases 25-50%, while ventricular end-diastolic pressure and volume decrease slightly.

The positive inotropic stimulation of normal ventricles is usually not translated into increased cardiac output at rest or during exercise in normal subjects when the drug is administered acutely (158). This undoubtedly relates to reflex sympathetic withdrawal, enhanced vagal tone, and direct constrictor effects on arteries and veins—the net result being a diminished venous return. Venous return is probably mostly reduced by splanchnic pooling (64,159). As noted earlier, digitalis differs considerably from catecholamines which cause increased venous return and cardiac output in the normal circulation.

It has been suggested from animal studies that the inotropic response of the normal heart is not as great as that of the failing heart. Whether this is the case in

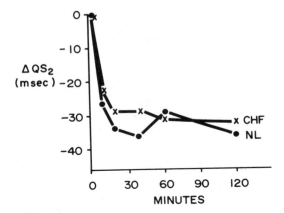

FIGURE 10 Shortening of QS2I (ΔQS2I) in normal subjects (dots) versus subjects with congestive heart failure (Xs) after intravenous administration of 1.6 mg of deslanoside. There is no significant difference in onset or extent of shortening.

humans is not clear. It is of interest that the magnitude of the ΔQS2I response to intravenous deslanoside is the same in normal subjects and patients with left ventricular failure, suggesting a similar inotropic (if not hemodynamic) response (Fig. 10) (160).

B. Response of the Abnormal Circulation

The first demonstration of a positive inotropic response to digitalis in human subjects with congestive heart failure occurred in 1948 (12,13). Subsequently, several studies employing various measurement techniques have confirmed these findings (160-166). In general the response of the failing circulation consists of an increased cardiac output, improved ejection fraction, shortened duration of systole, lowered venous pressure, no significant change in mean arterial pressure (though pulse pressure often increases), lowering of ventricular end-diastolic pressures, and slowing of the heart rate. A diuresis occurs if congestive failure is present, pulmonary edema improves, and gallop sounds may diminish or disappear. The mechanism of these salutory effects is a mixture of direct and autonomic effects involving the heart, vasculature, and other organs.

As noted earlier, many patients with congestive heart failure develop attenuation of arterial and cardiac baroreceptor responses (61). This results in decreased afferent inhibition of brainstem vasomotor centers, producing increased sympathetic outflow and neurohumeral excitation. The latter results in increased circulating norepinephrine, renin, angiotensin, and ADH (167,168). These effects increase arterial and venous tone, producing increases in both preload and afterload.

Digitalis restores baroreceptor and cardiac receptor sensitivity and thereby reduces the excessive sympathetic and other neurohumoral responses (61). This action results in decreased arterial and venous tone, both beneficial effects in CHF, as discussed earlier.

Withering postulated that digitalis had a major effect on renal function (1). Digitalis does induce a natriuresis directly by inhibition of the membrane Na^+-K^+ ATPase system of the distal nephron (43). However, increased renal blood flow due to sympathetic withdrawal and increased cardiac output is probably a more significant effect.

The positive inotropic effect of digitalis can be readily demonstrated in the failing ventricle by various noninvasive and invasive measures of left ventricular function (cardiac output and work, left ventricular dP/dt, ejection fraction, percentage of change in minor axis diameter in M-mode echocardiography, and PEP/LVET).

The major hemodynamic effect of inotropic stimulation is to increase the cardiac output both at rest and during exercise. In many studies the improvement with exercise is more striking than the improvement at rest. Thus, the full benefit of digitalis may not be demonstrable by resting studies. Another consistent effect of digitalis on the failing heart is a fall in the left ventricular end-diastolic pressure. This reduction implies diminished end-diastolic sarcomere stretch and presumably a decrease in end-diastolic volume. This effect has important implications for myocardial energetics (discussed later).

Almost all studies of digitalis in humans have shown significant variability in the response of the failing circulation to digitalis in patients with sinus rhythm. Some patients have a dramatic improvement, while virtually no response is seen in others. Some of this variability can be explained by patient selection, as certain disorders respond less well (discussed later). Autonomic status and the severity of ventricular dysfunction also play important roles in determining the response to digitalis.

An additional factor that may influence the hemodynamic response to digitalis is the contractile state of the atria. Most chronic heart disease results in increased atrial pressure due to altered ventricular compliance or atrioventricular valve regurgitation. Consequently, the atria undergo hypertrophy and dilatation (169). As with the ventricles, atrial wall stress increases. To this burden is often added fibrosis from underlying rheumatic disease or cardiomyopathy. The hypertrophied left atrium can develop atrial systolic pressures ("a" wave) as high as those developed by the normal right ventricle. An effective atrial systole can substantially lower mean left atrial pressure (Fig. 11) (170). In this setting a loud palpable S4 gallop is observed. When the left atrium decompensates, mean left atrial pressure rises and an S3 gallop becomes predominant. Clinical evidence indicates that digitalis therapy may be associated with a shift from a predominant S3 gallop to a predominant S4 gallop, raising the possibility that some of the beneficial effect of digitalis may be to improve atrial contractile performance.

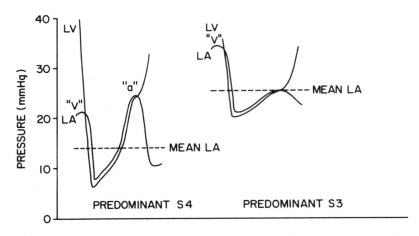

FIGURE 11 Effect of left atrial function upon mean left atrial pressure and gallop sounds in patients with chronic left ventricular disease and elevated left ventricular end-diastolic pressure. On the left, good atrial function with a forceful "a" wave is seen, which raises left ventricular end-diastolic pressure without a commensurate rise in mean left atrial pressure. The "v" wave is of lower amplitude. A loud palpable S4 gallop would be present. On the right, left atrial systolic contraction is nearly nonexistent (due either to atrial failure or atrial fibrillation). There is a large "v" wave and mean left atrial pressure is increased to the same level as left ventricular end-diastolic pressure. A loud S3 gallop would be present.

It has long been recognized that patients with congestive heart failure and atrial fibrillation (or flutter) respond the most favorably to digitalis. At present, few argue the major role of digitalis in congestive heart failure associated with atrial fibrillation or atrial flutter, but over the past two decades several clinical studies have questioned its efficacy in sinus rhythm.

Mulrow et al. recently reviewed all clinical studies of the efficacy of digitalis in patients with heart failure published since 1960 (171). Only 16 studies involving 487 patients were identified. Most studies employed comparison before and after digitalis administration or they were withdrawal studies. Only two were randomized prospective studies using placebo. Thus, from a methodological standpoint most studies were flawed. In addition, inappropriate patient selection and poorly defined patients populations were major problems even in the better studies. Finally, concurrent therapy with other agents may have masked digitalis effect. The authors therefore called for a large prospective randomized trial with long-term follow-up studies and well-defined patient populations to conclusively establish the role of digitalis in heart failure with sinus rhythm.

In spite of the limitations of the available clinical studies, a few broad conclusions seem warranted. First, digitalis has been indiscriminantly employed ever since Withering's time, and many patients with no significant left ventricular disease have been treated—especially the elderly. In such patients little beneficial effect would be anticipated (172). Second, the majority of patients with significant left ventricular dysfunction (especially if associated with an S3 gallop) show favorable short- and long-term benefits although the magnitude varies (173-175). Third, digitalis is not a strikingly useful drug once end-stage heart failure or shock develops (discussed later).

C. Heart Rate and Myocardial Energetics

Myocardial oxygen consumption largely depends on wall stress, heart rate, and inotropic state (176). Wall stress is related to systolic pressure and heart volume. Chronic increases in wall stress produce concentric hypertrophy (new sarcomeres in parallel) for pressure loads, and eccentric hypertrophy (new sarcomeres in series as well as in parallel) for volume loads (177). In myopathic hearts there is both hypertrophy and dilation, and hypertrophy of the remaining viable myocardium occurs after myocardial infarction. Most forms of heart disease produce an increase in cardiac mass. These enlarged hearts require increased resting coronary blood flow which can be up to three times normal (178). The epicardial coronary vessels enlarge and the microcirculation proliferates. In spite of these compensatory mechanisms, subendocardial perfusion may be inadequate in these enlarged hearts, particularly when coronary disease or tachycardia is present (179).

Left ventricular perfusion, particularly subendocardial perfusion, occurs largely in diastole (180). Diastolic perfusion is related to coronary vascular resistance, aortic diastolic pressure, left ventricular diastolic pressure, and diastolic perfusion time. These relationships have led to measurement of the integrated diastolic pressure-time relation as an index of myocardial perfusion (DPTI) (181). Assuming appropriate autoregulation of coronary vascular resistance, it can be shown that under a variety of circulatory perturbations (such as exercise) the major variable effecting DPTI is time (182).

It is not generally appreciated that the relationship of heart rate and diastolic time is not linear (183). The relative duration of diastole falls off rapidly above the normal resting heart rate (Fig. 12). Thus the subendocardium of an hypertrophied heart tolerates tachycardia poorly.

It has been hypothesized that many patients with enlarged hearts suffer from chronic subendocardial ischemia which can become irreversible and lead to fibrosis (179). This abnormality could be ameliorated simply by slowing the heart rate to improve subendocardial blood flow. This may well be a major beneficial effect of digitalis when therapy results in slowing the heart rate.

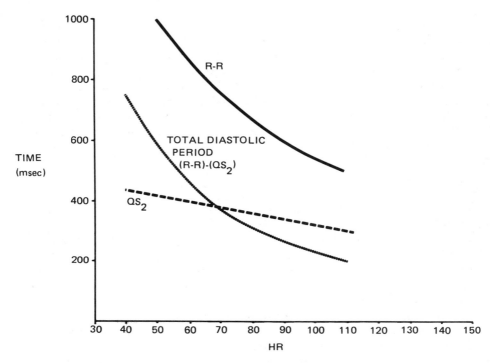

FIGURE 12 Relationship of the duration of systole (QS2) and total diastolic pe-
riod obtained from subtracting QS2 from the RR interval. The relationship of
QS2 to heart rate is linear, while that of the total diastolic period is nonlinear.
(From Ref. 183, reproduced with permission.)

Theoretically digitalis should increase resting myocardial oxygen consumption
by its inotropic stimulation. In normal subjects this may well be the case (158).
However, in the failing heart, myocardial oxygen consumption is usually not significantly increased by digitalis and it may be decreased—most likely because slowing the heart rate and reducing ventricular volume overrides the oxygen-consuming
effect of inotropic stimulation (43).

Experimental studies have indicated that digitalis can cause coronary artery
constriction (184). This effect is generally short-lived and requires rapid intravenous administration of a large dose. However, if digitalis is not given as a rapid intravenous bolus, coronary artery vasoconstriction does not appear to be a clinically
significant problem (discussed later).

D. Comparison of Digitalis to Other Pharmacologic Agents in Congestive Heart Failure

Since the introduction of oral thiazide diuretics 25 years ago, several other new classes of agents used in therapy for congestive heart failure have substantially improved treatment of this disorder. Prior to this time, digitalis, salt restriction, and periodic injection of mercurial diuretics were the mainstay of therapy. Nonetheless, congestive heart failure remained a common cause for hospital admissions. It is now far less common to see such patients on hospital wards. In the author's opinion, oral diuretics are the major reason for this, and these agents are the first-line therapy for congestive heart failure.

In 1964 Rader and associates demonstrated that diuresis alone in patients with congestive heart failure relieved symptoms and reduced intravascular pressures (164). There was, however, no increase in cardiac output. It is for this reason that other agents are used concurrently with diuretics.

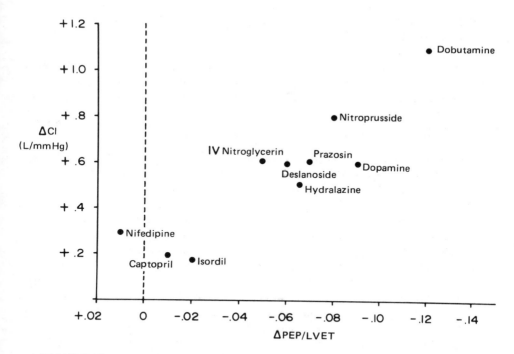

FIGURE 13 Comparison of changes in cardiac index (ΔCI) and PEP/LVET from systolic time intervals (ΔPEP/LVET) with commonly used agents for treatment of congestive heart failure. There is a close relationship between changes in these two variables. Each point represents mean values (see text for further explanation).

Figure 13 compares the changes in cardiac index (ΔCI) with changes in left ventricular performance estimated by the PEP/LVET from systolic time intervals (ΔPEP/LVET). The PEP/LVET was selected because it is sensitive to changes in preload and afterload as well as contractility (96). These studies were conducted in our laboratories (160,185-187). The patient groups consisted of patients with myocardial failure without valve disease. The mean resting cardiac index for the various groups ranged from 1.8 to 2.54 mm/m^2 and PEP/LVET ranged from 0.59 to 0.75 mm/m^2.

There was a strong relationship between ΔCI and ΔPEP/LVET. As expected, dobutamine and nitroprusside are the most potent agents, while nifedipine, oral isordil, and captopril are the least potent. Digitalis (deslanoside) is an intermediate agent, comparable to first-dose prazosin, hydralazine, dopamine, and intravenous nitroglycerin.

Based on the mechanisms of action of various agents used for congestive heart failure and the pathophysiological abnormalities known to occur in congestive heart failure, the relative effects of these agents are compared in Table 2. It is notable that few studies are available wherein digitalis is added to vasodilator therapy (the reverse is usually true) (188). Finally, it should be stressed that because of variability in individual patient adaption to the presence of impaired left ventricular function (that is, degree of fluid retention, excessiveness of neurohumoral response, and so on) there is also variability in the response to oral vasodilators as well as digitalis.

E. Role of the Adrenergic Nervous System

Studies in the past 20 years have improved understanding of the role of the adrenergic nervous system as a primary defense mechanism of the failing circulation (168). Unfortunately our understanding is still incomplete owing to the difficulties of studying adrenergic function. From a teleological point of view an appropriate response to cardiac failure probably never evolved. The adrenergic nervous system is designed to enhance the exercise response and defend against volume loss. When cardiac output declines as a result of left ventricular disease, the response is similar to that which occurs with sudden loss of blood volume. In the patient with heart failure the increased inotropy is desirable, but not the increased afterload. It is of interest that the vascular effects of adrenergic stimulation seem to show little tachyphylaxis (alpha-receptors). However, in the heart, chronic beta-adrenergic stimulation leads to a decreased number (or uncoupling) of beta-receptors and hence to an impaired ability to respond (62). It is possible that part of the benefit of agents that improve circulatory function such as digitalis and vasodilators (or bed rest) is to reduce adrenergic tone and result in "up regulation" of beta-adrenergic myocardial receptors (189). As the inotropic action of digitalis is clearly independent of the beta-adrenergic system—the two can be additive—it is possible that some of the variability in the degree of inotropic response to digitalis is related to the degree of "down regulation" of beta-receptors. Indeed, recent studies suggest that cautious long-term beta-adrenergic blockade may actually improve cardiac function by "up regulating" beta-receptors (190). Could digitalis, by its multiple effects in cardiac failure, do the same? If so, this might account for an apparent diminished benefit from digitalis with the passage of time.

F. Atrial Fibrillation

The beneficial effects of slowing the ventricular response both at rest and during exercise in terms of subendocardial perfusion was discussed earlier. These effects may be of major importance when cardiac hypertrophy and dilation or coronary artery disease are present.

For many years digitalis was the only pharmacologic agent available for treatment of atrial fibrillation. For acute atrial fibrillation associated with marked hemodynamic compromise (such as aortic or mitral stenosis, acute myocardial infarction) direct-current countershock should be considered as the initial treatment of choice. If this modality is not immediately available or successful, then intravenous verapamil or propranolol have a more rapid onset of action than ouabain or deslanoside, which require 10-20 min for maximum effect (191,192). Both verapamil and propranolol are negative inotropes and could potentially produce deleterious effects in patients with significant left ventricular dysfunction. However, the beneficial effect of rapid slowing of the ventricular response usually outweighs the negative inotropic effect of these agents.

In less urgent situations where recent atrial fibrillation has developed, digitalis is still usually the drug of choice because it is the most satisfactory form of chronic therapy. In a recent study, 85% of episodes of acute atrial fibrillation showed reversion to sinus rhythm within 1-96 hr (median 4 hr) after receiving 1.5 mg of digoxin intravenously over 12 hours (193). If sinus rhythm is not restored by 24 hours, additional measures (that is, antiarrhythmic agents) are usually required. However, it must be remembered that the class I antiarrhythmic agents quinidine and disopyramide have anticholinergic properties. Thus, the ventricular rate may transiently increase when such therapy is initiated (42).

The plasma digoxin level required for satisfactory control of the ventricular response both at rest and with exercise in chronic atrial fibrillation is often higher than the usual "optimum level" for patients in sinus rhythm. In some patients, satisfactory control of the ventricular rate is not possible without developing clinical signs of digitalis toxicity. This undoubtedly relates to the fact that exercise normally produces parasympathetic withdrawal and the direct effect of digoxin on AV node refractoriness becomes the major effect on the AV node. In such cases the addition of a beta-blocking agent or verapamil can provide satisfactory heart-rate control provided caution is used to avoid excessive slowing of the heart rate (194-196).

Unusually high digoxin levels needed for adequate heart-rate control suggests four possibilities: hyperthyroidism (increased adrenergic responsiveness), excessive sympathetic tone (acute myocardial infarction, acute pulmonary edema, pulmonary disease, pericardial constriction), densely calcific mitral stenosis, or short digoxin elimination half-life (with "escape" prior to the next dose). For the first two cases, addition of a beta-blocking agent usually results in good control. For calcific mitral stenosis, only mitral valve replacement alleviates the problem (Joseph M. Ryan, M.D., personal observation). For the patient with a short elimination half-life—probably a common cause of failure of digoxin to control the rate—more frequent administration of digoxin or switching to digitoxin usually results in satisfactory control. Experimental studies suggest that digitoxin enhances parasympathetic effect on the AV node more than digoxin does (40).

We have noted patients with "flutter-fibrillation" in whom control of the ventricular rate is highly variable. Many of these patients have "dissimilar" atrial rhythms with areas of both flutter and fibrillation within the atria (197). At varying times either the flutter or fibrillation determines the input into the AV junction. This results in marked variability of the ventricular response (fast with flutter, slow with fibrillation). In these patients a pacemaker is usually required for satisfactory rate control.

Another major source of variability of the digitalis dose required to achieve heart-rate control in atrial fibrillation is the state of the AV node. Many patients with atrial fibrillation have diffuse conduction disease which also involves the AV node. The diseased AV node may be unusually sensitive to small doses of digitalis and in some cases digitalis need not be given. In these cases, the correlation between the serum digoxin concentration and slowing of the ventricular rate is poor (198-199).

Digitalis toxicity in atrial fibrillation often consists of regularization of the ventricular response due to junctional tachycardia or complete AV block with a junctional pacemaker (200). To avoid toxicity during therapy for atrial fibrillation or flutter, digitalis should never be "pushed." Rather, another agent (that is, a beta blocker or verapamil) can be added. The Wolff-Parkinson-White syndrome represents a special problem (201-202). Digitalis may decrease the refractoriness of the accessory pathway in one-third of such patients. In these patients rapid conduction in the presence of atrial fibrillation can lead to ventricular fibrillation.

In atrial fibrillation with a rapid ventricular response, there is markedly poor systolic contractile performance of beats preceded by short RR intervals (Fig. 14) (203). Such beats have both inadequate preload and excessive afterload compared to a sinus tachycardia beat at the same rate (204). Thus little blood is ejected (pulse deficit) but myocardial energy is required nonetheless. Below heart rate 75 there is minimal hemodynamic difference between a sinus beat or one in atrial fibrillation—atrial contraction is less critical when diastolic time is long (204). The therapeutic goal should be to achieve a resting heart rate in the 70s rising to no more

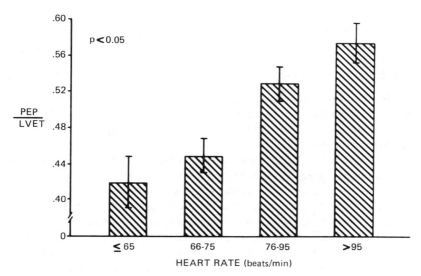

FIGURE 14 Effect of atrial fibrillation on left ventricular performance in relation to the effective heart rate for the beat under consideration (obtained from the preceding RR interval). Each bar represents mean values of beats from five patients at the various heart rates. As the heart rate increases, there is a dramatic drop off in left ventricular performance, particularly above heart rate 75 (see text for further explanation). (From Ref. 203, reproduced with permission.)

than 110-120 with exercise. This is especially important in patients with impaired left ventricular function.

G. Tolerance

Few long-term studies have been performed with the specific goal of determining whether tolerance to digitalis develops. Short-term studies of the inotropic effect in humans employing noninvasive parameters (systolic time intervals, echocardiography) and experimental animal studies have not suggested that tolerance develops (205-208). Experience in patients with chronic atrial fibrillation also does not suggest tolerance. Indeed, there have been patients who have been successfully treated with digitalis for more than 40 years.

One interpretation of studies in which digitalis was stopped without apparent clinical deterioration is that tolerance had developed. However, many such individuals did not have significant ventricular dysfunction at the time digitalis was initially given (171). Thus, all but major changes would have been undetectable in the short term. Furthermore, as noted earlier, autonomic adjustments may cause the chronic effects of digitalis to differ from acute effects. Nonetheless, the lack of tolerance to the inotropic effect of digitalis is an advantage over several other types of agents used for treatment of chronic CHF (adrenergic blocking agents, nitrates).

H. Prophylactic Digitalis

Prophylactic digitalization in patients with pressure or volume loads and intact left ventricular function (hypertension and valvular disease) remains an attractive but unproved practice (158,209-213). Experimental studies support this concept although human studies are limited.

Routine preoperative digitalization in patients with heart disease has lost favor as better anesthetics and monitoring techniques have become available for surgical patients and as effective new pharmacologic agents (that is, beta-blocking agents after cardiac surgery) have been discovered to treat postoperative complications. There is often a heightened sensitivity to digitalis in the postoperative period primarily due to metabolic disturbances but possibly due to a higher myocardial concentration in acutely digitalized patients (as discussed earlier) (214). Patients receiving chronic digitalis therapy before cardiac surgery, particularly valvular surgery, do appear to have a reduced incidence of postoperative supraventricular arrhythmias (215). If preoperative digitalization is performed, ideally it should be done several weeks before surgery. Digitalis is usually required for managing postoperative atrial fibrillation.

There is merit in prophylactic digitalization of patients with nonsurgical mitral stenosis and sinus rhythm. Such patients are at risk for developing atrial fibrillation, and this arrhythmia can have devastating consequences when the ventricular rate is rapid.

I. Contraindications

Digitalis allergy apparently occurs but is *extremely* unusual (216). This infrequency may be due to the fact that digitalis is structurally similar to endogenous substances. Factors that increase sensitivity to digitalis (and therefore represent relative contraindications) have been summarized by Surawicz (216).

Digitalis is generally contraindicated in patients with obstructive cardiomyopathy in which digitalis may aggravate outflow tract obstruction. Digitalis is contraindicated in patients with advanced AV conduction disease. Digitalis can usually be safely (albeit cautiously) administered to patients with first-degree AV block but should not be given when second-degree or third-degree AV block is present. As noted earlier, digitalis is contraindicated in up to one-third of patients with the Wolff-Parkinson-White syndrome.

The use of digitalis in patients with the sick sinus syndrome is controversial (217-220). Variable effects on sinus rate (depending on baseline vagal tone and SA conduction abnormalities) have been reported. In many patients no effect on sinus rate or an actual increase have been noted. However, excessive slowing of the sinus rate can occur. If digitalis is required for control of paroxysmal atrial fibrillation or flutter, patients with sick sinus syndrome often require concomitant pacemaker therapy.

Patients with significant ventricular arrhythmias generally should not be treated with digitalis. Indeed, digitalis should always be stopped in such patients to observe the effect. There are, however, some patients in whom digitalis reduces ventricular ectopy as noted earlier (221,222).

Digitalis is generally contraindicated in cardiogenic shock, where its efficacy is not striking and adverse effects such as increased arterial resistance (if given as an intravenous bolus) or ventricular arrhythmias may occur. It should be considered only if atrial fibrillation with a rapid ventricular response is present. In patients with decompensated pulmonary disease who exhibit multifocal atrial tachycardia, digitalis seldom is effective and the chance of toxic ventricular arrhythmias is high (200).

Digitalis is not the first-line drug in obstructive diseases such as aortic and mitral stenosis and pericardial constriction unless accompanied by problematic atrial fibrillation. In these patients surgical correction is the procedure of choice.

In patients with various forms of "high-output failure" (including left-to-right shunts), treating the cause is the most effective approach (223). Nonetheless, beneficial effects of digitalis may be noted if treating the underlying cause is not feasible.

J. Heart Failure in the Elderly

Many older patients with congestive failure and cardiac enlargement have relatively good systolic function (224). Abnormal diastolic compliance seems to be the major component of this syndrome. Generally, digitalis is not dramatically effective in this setting. The senescent heart may be less responsive to the inotropic effect of digitalis (discussed earlier). In addition, the elderly are more likely to have a decreased body mass and impaired renal function, making toxicity more likely to occur (225). Central nervous system side effects of digitalis are more common in the elderly.

K. Chronic Pulmonary Disease

It has long been believed that patients with chronic pulmonary disease are susceptible to digitalis-induced toxic arrhythmias at therapeutic doses (216,226). This is probably true, but in these patients there are often additional factors which can aggravate the arrhythmogenic effects of digitalis. These include acute hypoxemia, hypokalemia from diuretics or aggressive ventilation therapy, and concurrent bronchodilator therapy with adrenergic agents and/or theophylline.

When chronic pulmonary disease has resulted in chronic pulmonary hypertension and right-sided congestive heart failure, digitalis is often employed. Although an inotropic effect on the right ventricle can be demonstrated, there appears to be minimal hemodynamic benefit (226). The most effective therapy is to reduce the right ventricular afterload by improving pulmonary function. In this setting the major role of digitalis is to control atrial flutter or fibrillation, which are often present (beta-blockers are usually contraindicated in this setting). However, these patients require careful monitoring for possible digitalis toxic ventricular arrhythmias.

A recent study has suggested that digitalis is of hemodynamic benefit only in those patients with associated left ventricular dysfunction (227). In this setting the right ventricle may be unloaded by a reduction of left atrial pressure due to improved left ventricular performance.

L. Thyroid Disease

The effects of thyroid disease on digitalis are still incompletely understood (34, 41,216). Hypothyroidism appears to reduce digoxin clearance, necessitating lowered dosage. There may also be increased sensitivity. Hyperthyroidism is associated with lower-than-expected serum digoxin levels and a lesser clinical response (such as slowing the heart rate in atrial fibrillation). Experimental studies suggest there is an increase in myocardial Na^+-K^+ ATPase activity (43). Finally, increased sensitivity to adrenergic stimulation occurs in hyperthyroidism. Beta-blocking agents are usually also required for slowing the heart rate when atrial fibrillation occurs.

M. Clinical End Points

A simple, reliable pharmacodynamic end point for the inotropic effect of digitalis does not exist. When atrial fibrillation or flutter are being treated, the ventricular rate is a useful pharmacodynamic guide, as is the prevention of recurrent episodes when the arrhythmia is paroxysmal.

In part the end-point problem relates to two outmoded concepts. First, the pharmacodynamic dose-response curve is linear until toxicity supervenes; second, digitalis is the cornerstone of therapy for congestive heart failure. As noted earlier, recent evidence indicates that the inotropic response to digitalis substantially diminishes as the dose is "pushed" above empirically derived dose guidelines. Because the pharmacodynamic dose-response curve is not linear, two-thirds of the inotropic effect of full dosage is achieved at half dosage. Thus therapeutic benefits diminish as the dose is increased, while toxic effects increase (Fig. 15). This fact, along with the relatively modest inotropic effect of digitalis, dictates that the drug should be used conservatively in patients with sinus rhythm—a practice that seems to be increasing over the past 10 years.

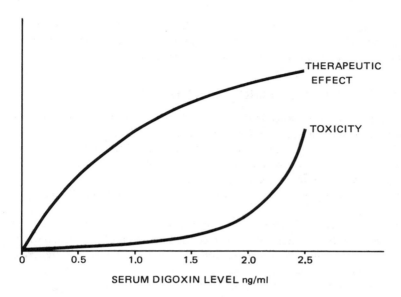

THERAPEUTIC
EFFECT

TOXICITY

SERUM DIGOXIN LEVEL ng/ml

FIGURE 15   Schematic illustration of the relation between the therapeutic effect of digoxin, the toxic effect, and the serum digoxin level. Above a level of 2.0 ng/ml there is minimal further therapeutic effect but a dramatic increase in the toxic effect.

The widespread availability of serum digitalis levels (a pharmacokinetic measure) has provided an invaluable quantitative end point to ensure appropriate digitalis doses—provided it is recognized that the serum digitalis level is not a pharmacodynamic parameter.

End points that rely on the appearance of arrhythmic toxicity are no longer indicated under any circumstances. Acetylstrophanthidin testing is an experimental procedure which does employ arrhythmic end points (221,228). It has provided extremely useful clinical information regarding the arrhythmogenic and antiarrhythmic effects of digitalis. This procedure is not available for routine clinical use. As discussed later in this chapter, in the future, Fab fragments may be useful.

Although systolic time intervals are a helpful measure of the acute inotropic effect of digitalis, their use in chronic therapy remains to be established. Echocardiography has also been employed for acute evaluation with favorable results under well-controlled conditions. Radionuclide angiography has not been clearly useful (173,229). Thus, the value of noninvasive measurements for assessing chronic digitalis therapy needs to be determined.

In the absence of atrial fibrillation, assessment of the inotropic effect of digitalis must therefore be accomplished by clinical observation (symptoms, gallops, increased exercise tolerance, and so on) in combination with a serum digitalis level showing a concentration of drug in the "therapeutic range." In this regard it is note-worthy that the variable bioavailability of digoxin often results in subtherapeutic serum levels in spite of an apparently adequate dose regimen.

VIII. DIGITALIS IN ISCHEMIC HEART DISEASE

Experimental and clinical evidence indicates that digitalis does not usually aggravate ischemia during an acute myocardial infarction, provided it is not given as an intra-venous bolus (229-233). Also, it does not usually aggravate exertional ischemia in patients with angina. The increased oxygen demand resulting from the inotropic effect is apparently counterbalanced by decreased oxygen demand from decreased wall stress (43). Perhaps improved coronary flow (increased diastolic time) also plays a role.

The arrhythmic effect of digitalis in ischemic heart disease is another issue. There is increasing concern that digitalis may enhance the likelihood of ventricular ar-rhythmias in patients who have recovered from myocardial infarction. Adrenergic tone is often raised in patients with ischemic heart disease, especially with acute ischemia (234,235). This combination could enhance the possibility of digitalis-induced ventricular arrhythmias. On the other hand, many such patients are now receiving beta-adrenergic blocking agents. These agents appear to reduce the lethal potential of such arrhythmias (235,236). Whether beta-adrenergic blocking agents can mitigate the arrhythmogenic effects of digitalis is not known.

A. Angina Pectoris

Most studies have shown little effect of digitalis on exercise capacity of patients with angina pectoris and normal resting left ventricular function (238-245). An-gina appears at the same rate-pressure product. However, most studies have shown left ventricular performance during exercise is improved in spite of the apparent lack of clinical benefit. As most patients with angina now receive beta-blocking agents and/or calcium channel blocking agents, it is possible that combining digit-alis with these agents may be useful—especially when extensive myocardial scar-ring is not present. Further studies of combination therapy are required.

B. Acute Myocardial Infarction

Most patients with acute myocardial infarction tolerate the hemodynamic insult without the need for digitalis—probably because of increased sympathetic tone. The increased sympathetic tone makes it difficult to demonstrate a benefit of the inotropic effect of digitalis, though most studies have shown modest improvement in contractile performance (246-248). Increased sympathetic tone can also poten-tiate toxic digitalis effects on the Purkinje system. However, studies do not suggest that patients with acute myocardial infarction are more sensitive to the arrhythmogenic effects of digitalis (249). Thus, the use of digitalis, while not contraindicated, should probably be reserved for overt congestive failure or atrial arrhythmias. The only indication in cardiogenic shock is for atrial fibrillation (250).

C. Digitalis for Long-Term Management after Acute Myocardial Infarction

Digitalis can produce an objective improvement of resting or exercise ventricular performance in patients who have had an infarction(s) (251-254). Left ventricular end-diastolic pressure is lowered and the contractile performance of noninfarcted segments improves, though the function of infarcted segments may deteriorate. Whether these effects translate into significant clinical improvement in the absence of symptoms of congestive heart failure remains to be determined.

Three studies have suggested that administration of digitalis may in fact increase mortality in the years after myocardial infarction (255-257). Two other studies did not find digitalis to be an independent risk factor for mortality (258-259). None of these were prospective controlled studies specifically examining the role of digitalis, however. The presumed adverse effect is due to death from ventricular arrhythmias. Ventricular arrhythmias in patients who have had myocardial infarctions demonstrate two separate mechanisms (260). Some are related to transient ischemia, which requires viable myocardium with impaired blood flow ("jeopardized myocardium"). The second and probably more common type is related to the presence of scar tissue from old infarction (261). Whether digitalis can enhance both types of arrhythmias (which probably have differing electrophysiological mechanisms) requires elucidation.

In view of these studies, caution should probably be used in the administration of digitalis to patients with previous myocardial infarction. The need for controlled studies to define the role of digitalis therapy in patients who have sustained a myocardial infarction is obvious. In the interim it would appear prudent to limit maintenance digitalis therapy in patients with previous myocardial infarction to those with obvious manifestations of congestive heart failure or atrial arrhythmia not controlled by other measures. Employing the lowest possible dosage is also indicated.

IX. DIGITALIS TOXICITY

Neither digitalis nor the physician's art guarantees immortaility, but the excessive use of drugs as if immortality could be thus obtained, may well lead to an untimely and premature end (262).

A. Changing Spectrum

For many years digitalis intoxication was the most serious drug toxicity in clinical medicine. The mortality was up to 10% when recognized, and much higher when unrecognized (263,264). Studies in the early 1970s employing the newly available serum digoxin assay noted an incidence of toxicity averaging 20% in hospitalized patients receiving digoxin (265-268).

Since the advent of the serum digitalis assay the incidence of toxicity appears to have substantially decreased (269-271). A Scandinavian study of digitoxin therapy in 1977 showed an incidence of toxicity of only 5.8%. A study of digoxin toxicity after introduction of routinely available serum digoxin levels revealed an incidence of 4% (264,270). The major reason for a lower incidence of toxicity, however, is that smaller digitalis doses are now being employed. In the Scandinavian study, the toxic group had the highest average dose but this was still below the usual recommended dose prior to 1970.

For digoxin there has also been a lowering of the usual dosages. In addition, awareness is more widespread of the danger of diuretic-induced hypokalemia as well as the effects of impaired renal function and antiarrhythmic drug interactions on digoxin elimination half-life (272). Monitoring of serum digoxin levels in these settings is becoming the rule (271). Indeed, several institutions have begun computerized surveillance of digoxin dosing; these programs appear to reduce the incidence of toxicity (273,274).

Another important reason for the lowered incidence of digitalis toxicity has been the introduction of alternative approaches to therapy of congestive heart failure or atrial fibrillation.

Nonetheless, digitalis toxicity has not and most likely will not disappear. It must be remembered that digitalis is usually administered to individuals with heart disease and therefore toxicity can develop at "therapeutic" levels of drug. Indeed, a universal finding of studies of digitalis toxicity is the wide overlap in serum levels between toxic and nontoxic patients in spite of the fact that the toxic group virtually always has a mean serum level significantly higher than the nontoxic group (44).

Digitalis toxicity consists of abnormalities of cardiac rhythm and central nervous system toxicity—both in part reflecting impaired function of Na^+-K^+ ATPase. The autonomic nervous system plays a key role, as do metabolic factors.

Neurologic manifestations of toxicity are probably more common than cardiac symptoms and are often overlooked (275). Profound fatigue and visual disturbances (often nonspecific) occur in 90% of patients with toxicity, followed closely by anorexia and nausea. Mild psychiatric disturbances are common but serious symptoms such as delirium, hallucinations, and seizures occur in up to 10% of patients with toxicity.

B. Electrophysiological Manifestations

The manifestations of cardiac toxicity in large part depend upon the nature and extent of the underlying heart disease. In normal subjects who ingested suicidal doses of digitalis, the major arrhythmias are bradyarrhythmias, sinus arrest, and AV block (276). Bradyarrhythmias can occur in the presence of heart disease as well, but tachyarrhythmias frequently dominate the clinical picture in such patients (277,278).

The electrophysiological effects of digitalis and the complex interactions with the autonomic nervous system and the serum potassium were discussed earlier. The toxic effects on major sites of the specialized conduction tissues will only be summarized here.

1. Sinoatrial Node

Toxic levels of digitalis may increase sinus rate, probably by the direct effect on automaticity as well as by enhanced sympathetic effect (277). This manifestation is most likely to occur in patients with concurrent acute illnesses which result in high adrenergic tone. In other patients, sinus bradycardia, SA arrent, or SA exit block may develop, especially is sinus node disease is present.

2. Atrial Muscle

The toxic effects of digitalis on atrial muscle cells are similar to those which occur in the Purkinje cells. These effects can produce tachyarrhythmias either by increased automaticity, triggered rhythms from delayed after depolarizations, or by re-entry. Notably, both of the first two mechanisms may produce depression of conduction under certain circumstances and thus lead to re-entrant rhythms. The most common toxic atrial rhythm is atrial tachycardia which behaves as an automatic rhythm (200,278). It is nearly always associated with AV block. Atrial flutter and fibrillation are rare manifestations of digitalis toxicity. As noted earlier, atrial fibrillation in the Wolff-Parkinson-White syndrome may be associated with a more rapid ventricular response and the induction of ventricular fibrillation.

3. Atrioventricular Node

Increase in AV node refractoriness and further slowing of conduction occur with toxicity as the direct depressant effect of digitalis on AV node cells is added to the autonomic effects. When atrial fibrillation is present, complete AV block is manifested as a slow regular ventricular response (278).

Junctional tachycardia is one of the more common and most specific of digitalis toxic rhythms (200,278). It is believed to be an automatic tachycardia. It is manifested by "regularization" of the ventricular response with atrial fibrillation and AV dissociation (when SA slowing has occurred), and occasionally is manifested as a reciprocal tachycardia.

4. Purkinje System

The autonomic interactions with digitalis and the Purkinje system are minimal at therapeutic concentrations. With toxicity, enhanced sympathetic outflow may be additive to the direct effect of digitalis. Abnormalities of the serum potassium, hypomagnesemia, and hypoxia are also additive (43,216).

Premature ventricular contractions are the most common manifestation of toxicity in the Purkinje system. Ventricular tachycardia and fibrillation can develop, and they are the major cause of death from digitalis toxicity. The mechanism is believed to be re-entry, but it could also be triggered rhythms or automatic tachycardias (26,200). Torsade de pointes seems to be a rare form of digitalis-induced ventricular tachycardia.

C. Clinical Diagnosis

The diagnosis of digitalis toxicity may be difficult since arrhythmias may be due to the underlying disease (279). In more obscure cases the diagnosis is established only by determining the response to *withdrawal* of the drug. Even the noncardiac toxic symptoms have relatively low specificity in patients with chronic congestive failure. The overriding principle in the diagnosis of toxicity is to assume toxicity until proven otherwise. Digitalis toxicity is potentially lethal and digitalis is seldom necessary for survival regardless of the clinical situation.

Determination of the serum digitalis level is very useful but not diagnostic (44, 271,279). Many patients with high glycoside serum levels do not have toxicity and toxicity can occur with normal or even low serum levels. In general, however, 80% of patients with digitalis toxicity have serum glycoside levels above the recommended therapeutic range (2.0 ng/ml for digoxin, 25 ng/ml for digitoxin).

Studies have proposed the utility of low-level exercise testing to elicit latent toxicity by uncovering arrhythmias (280). Carotid sinus massage to look for the appearance of complex ventricular ectopy has also been employed (277). Acetyl-strophanthadin testing may be the most specific test but it is still an investigative tool (277).

When a patient seems intolerant of digitalis, a common problem in end-stage myocardial disease, it is best to avoid the agent. In most cases an alternative form of therapy is now available. However, many such patients can tolerate low-dose digitalis which, as noted earlier, can still provide significant inotropic effect.

D. Treatment

The initial therapy for toxicity is obviously to stop administering digitalis. In most cases this is all that need be done. When marked bradyarrhythmias are the problem, a temporary pacemaker may be needed, but often periodic atropine and careful observation will suffice. When tachyarrhythmias are the problem (including frequent premature ventricular contractions) the judicious administration of potassium frequently abolishes the arrhytmia even though the initial serum K is normal. Potassium, particularly by the intravenous route, should *never* be administered for bradyarrhythmias (41).

If potassium therapy and correction of other metabolic abnormalities (including a low serum Mg^{2+}) is ineffective for tachyarrhythmias, then lidocaine should be used. Other measures that can be effective include beta-blocking agents, phenytoin, overdrive pacing, and verapamil (41). Experimentally, verapamil is the only agent effective for triggered tachyarrhythmias (26).

In the early days of cardioversion, apparent digitalis toxic arrhythmias were commonly seen after reversion and were occasionally fatal (281). This led to the recommendation that digitalis be stopped several days before cardioversion. More recent experience has indicated that in the absence of overt digitalis intoxication before cardioversion, discontinuing digitalis (often with adverse effect on the ventricular rate) is not necessary (282). It is possible that the digitalis-quinidine interaction was complicating the earlier experience.

E. Overdose

Occasionally, suicidal doses of digitalis are ingested or severe cardiac toxicity develops in the course of routine therapy and is not responsive to standard measures. In suicide attempts, severe hyperkalemia may be a major factor in lethal arrhythmias (usually bradyarrhythmias) (276). The recently developed Fab fragments of digitalis antibodies have been shown to rapidly bind digitalis in the extracellular fluid to make it inactive. This reverses toxicity, as a concentration gradient is thereby established for release of digitalis bound to receptors (276,283). The Fab-digitalis complex then undergoes renal excretion. The Fab fragments will soon be commercially available and represent an apparently safe and effective treatment for a formerly lethal disorder. If further clinical experience continues to show safety and efficacy, and the cost is low, it is possible that administration of Fab fragments could be useful for routine clinical evaluation of suspected digitalis toxicity or to help assess the hemodynamic efficacy of digitalis (124).

X. CONCLUSIONS

Digitalis is one of the most complex and fascinating drugs in the pharmacopeia, as the voluminous literature attests. Unfortunately, much of this literature deals with its complex mechanisms of action and is not helpful for determining *who* should be given the drug. Digitalis has been accorded little attention by current clinical investigators exploring the new pharmacologic approaches to heart failure. Notably, digitalis is usually not discontinued. It could be argued that this has been a significant mistake.

The fact that digitalis has been used for 200 years in spite of its well-known toxicity suggests a priori that it is a useful drug. Digitalis has never been subjected to an appropriate large randomized double-blind clinical trial. Unfortunately such a trial will probably never occur. The clinician is faced with the decision to use or not use digitalis but lacks rigorous scientific guidelines.

This being the case, the author considers that the following guidelines and concepts are reasonable on this 200th anniversary of the introduction of digitalis for the treatment of heart failure.

1. Because the therapeutic effect (inotropic or chronotropic) has a nonlinear dose-response curve, the smallest possible dose should be employed. This will minimize toxicity and also provide most of the effect of traditional full doses.
2. The role of digitalis for control of ventricular rate in atrial fibrillation is secure, with the caveat that if full-dose therapy is not completely effective, other agents (beta-blockers or verapamil) should be added rather than "pushing" digitalis.
3. When digitalis is used for its inotropic property in patients with sinus rhythm, it is useful to categorize the patient according to the severity of the clinical and laboratory presentation.
   a. *Latent or mild myocardial dysfunction.* These patients are NYHA functional class I or II and includes those with pressure loads (that is, hypertension) or volume loads (that is, valvular regurgitation, shunts, or certain high-output states) in whom surgery is not indicated. Patients with prior small infarctions would also fit this category. Experimental evidence suggests digitalis may improve exercise performance in these patients as well as enhance the heart's adaptation to the hemodynamic load. However, the expected benefits are not striking. Thus, the indication for digitalis in these patients is "soft."
   b. *Clinically overt left ventricular decompensation.* These patients are generally NYHA class III prior to therapy and usually have an S3 gallop. This category of patients represent those most likely to benefit from digitalis. It includes patients with prior large infarction(s), cardiomyopathy, mitral regurgitation, long-standing hypertensive heart disease, and some congenital heart diseases. Such patients may or may not have fluid retention, but if it is present, diuretics are the first line of therapy. If a satisfactory clinical response to diuretics does not occur, digitalis is indicated, provided significant ventricular arrhythmias are not present. If no response is apparent, a trial of vasodilators should be considered. Digitalis is selected prior to vasodilators largely because of cost, relative simplicity of its administration, and low incidence of side effects.
   c. *End-stage left ventricular dysfunction* (NYHA Class IV). Unfortunately, these patients often have a minimal response to digitalis and the chance of toxicity, even at therapeutic levels, is high. Vasodilators would appear to be the best initial choice in this group. The role of digitalis in cardiogenic shock is confined to use for atrial fibrillation.
   d. *Acute myocardial injury* (infarction, myocarditis). Aside from treatment of atrial arrhythmias, digitalis should be used, with caution, only when overt congestive heart failure is present.

4. Therapy of paroxysmal atrial tachycardia, while not discussed in this chapter, remains an indication for digitalis. It is not uniformly effective, however, and efficacy should be documented.
5. The best way to prevent digitalis toxicity is to thoroughly understand the factors that may produce it. Of these, dose in relation to body size and renal function are the most important. However, maintaining a normal body potassium and understanding interactions with other cardiovascular agents, especially for digoxin, are equally important. The wide availability of serum glycoside monitoring greatly facilitates this task.
6. Recognition that in patients with ischemic heart disease digitalis may cause death (presumably by facilitating ventricular arrhythmias) requires caution in this group. At present it is not known, but needs to be determined, whether there are definable high-risk subsets. We also need to discover whether the same problem might exist in patients with dilated cardiomyopathy who also have a high incidence of sudden death.
7. All things considered, the switch from digitoxin to digoxin in the United States may not have been wise (284). Digoxin is a more difficult glycoside to use on a chronic basis because of its variable absorption and elimination. Its major advantage is a shorter elimination half-life, but this may be a disadvantage when control of the ventricular rate in atrial fibrillation is the goal of therapy. Furthermore, in most patients with low cardiac output (and therefore diminished cretinine clearance) the elimination half-life of digoxin approaches that of digitoxin.

If the clinician regards digitalis for what it is—a moderate inotropic agent that also possesses desirable neurohumoral actions and effects on preload, afterload, and atrial fibrillation—and uses it with appropriate indications and caution, it is likely that a beneficial clinical result with a low risk of toxicity can be achieved in many patients with chronic congestive heart failure (285).

REFERENCES

1. W. Withering. *An Account of the Foxglove, and Some of its Medical Uses: With Practical Remarks on Dropsy, and other Diseases.* G. G. J. and J. Robinson, London, 1785.
2. C. Fisch. Introduction. William Withering: An account of the foxglove and some of its medical uses 1785-1985. *J. Am. Coll. Cardiol. 5*: 1A-2A (1985).
3. J. Ferriar. *An Essay of the Medical Properties of Digitalis Purpurea or Foxglove.* Cadell and Davies, London, 1799.
4. D. M. Krikler. The foxglove, "The old woman from Shropshire" and William Withering. *J. Am. Coll. Cardiol. 5*: 3A-9A (1985).
5. J. M. Fothergill. *Digitalis: Its Mode of Action.* London, 1871.
6. J. Mackenzie. *Diseases of the Heart*, 2nd ed. Oxford, London, 1910.
7. T. Lewis. On cardinal principles in cardiological practice. *Br. Med. J. 2*: 621 (1919).

8. M. H. Christian. Digitalis therapy: Satisfactory effects in cardiac cases with regular pulse rate. *Am. J. Med. Sci. 157*: 593-602 (1919).

9. C. S. Burwill, D. W. Neighbors, and E. M. Regan. The effect of digitalis upon the output of the heart in normal man. *J. Clin. Invest. 5*: 125 (1928).

10. W. Dock, and M. L. Tainter. The circulatory changes after full therapeutic doses of digitalis, with a critical discussion of views on cardiac output. *J. Clin. Invest. 8*: 467-484 (1929).

11. L. N. Katz, S. Rodbard, M. Friend, and W. Rottersman. The effect of digitalis on the anesthetized dog. I. Action on the splanchnic bed. *J. Pharmacol. Exp. Ther. 62*: 1 (1938).

12. E. C. Stead, Jr., and J. V. Warren. Effect of lanatoside C on the circulation of patients with congestive heart failure. *Arch. Intern. Med. 81*: 282-287 (1948).

13. R. A. Bloomfield, B. Rappoport, J. P. Melnor, et al. The effects of the cardiac glycosides upon the dynamics of the circulation in congestive heart failure. *J. Clin. Invest. 27*: 588-599 (1948).

14. W. Wilbrandt. Zum wirkungmechanismus des herzglykoside. *Schweiz. Med. Wochenschr. 85*: 315-320 (1955).

15. K. R. H. Repke. Ueber den biochemischen wirkungsmodus von digitalis. *Klin. Wochenschr. 42*: 157-165 (1964).

16. T. Akera, F. S. Larsen, and T. M. Brody. Correlation of cardiac sodium-and-potassium-activated adenosine triphosphatase activity with ouabain induced inotropic stimulation. *J. Pharmacol. Exp. Ther. 173*: 145-151 (1970).

17. T. J. Hougen, and T. W. Smith. Inhibition of myocardial cation active transport by subtoxic doses of ouabain in the dog. *Circ. Res. 42*: 856-863 (1978).

18. L. H. Michael, A. Schwartz, and E. T. Wallick. Nature of the transport adenosine triphosphatase-digitalis complex: XIV inotropy and cardaic glycoside interaction with Na^+, K^+-ATPase of isolated cat papillary muscles. *Mol. Pharmacol. 16*: 135-146 (1979).

19. H. A. Fozzard, and M. F. Sheets. Cellular mechanism of action of cardiac glycosides. *J. Am. Coll. Cardiol. 5*: 10A-15A (1985).

20. A. M. Katz. Effects of digitalis on cell biochemistry. Sodium pump inhibition. *J. Am. Coll. Cardiol. 5*:16A-21A (1985).

21. M. Vassalle, J. Karis, and B. F. Hoffman. Toxic effects of ouabain on Purkinje fibers and ventricular muscle fibers. *Am. J. Physiol. 203*: 433-439 (1962).

22. D. G. Kassebaum. Electrophysiological effects of strophanthin in the heart. *J. Pharmacol. Exp. Ther. 140*: 329-338 (1963).

23. P. Muller. Ouabain effects on cardiac contraction, action potential and cellular potassium. *Circ. Res. 17*: 46-56 (1965).

24. M. R. Rosen, H. Gelband, and B. F. Hoffman. Correlation between effects of ouabain on the canine electrocardiogram and transmembrane potentials of isolated Purkinje fibers. *Circ. Res. 47*: 65-72 (1973).

25. A. J. Hordof, A. Spotnitz, L. Mary-Rabine, R. N. Edie, and M. R. Rosen. The cellular electrophysiologic effects of digitalis on human atrial fibers. *Circulation 57*: 223-229 (1978).

26. M. R. Rosen. Cellular electrophysiology of digitalis toxicity. *J. Am. Coll. Cardiol. 5*: 22A-34A (1985).

27. G. R. Ferrier, J. H. Saunders, and C. Mendez. A cellular mechanism for the generation of ventricular arrhythmias by acetylstrophanthidin. *Circ. Res. 32*: 600-609 (1973).
28. L. D. Davis. Effect of changes in cycle length on diastolic depolarization produced by ouabain in canine Purkinje fibers. *Circ. Res. 32*: 206-214 (1973).
29. M. R. Rosen, H. Gelband, C. Merker, and B. F. Hoffman. Mechanism of digitalis toxicity: Effects of ouabain on phase 4 of canine Purkinje fiber transmembrane potential. *Circ. Res. 47*: 681-689 (1973).
30. K. Hashimoto, and G. K. Moe. Transient depolarizations induced by acetylstrophanthidin in specialized tissues of dog atrium and ventricle. *Circ. Res. 32*: 618-624 (1973).
31. E. M. K. Geiling, and B. J. McIntosh. Biosynthesis of radioactive drugs using carbon-14. *Science 108*: 558 (1948).
32. G. T. Okita. Distribution, disposition and excretion of digitalis glycosides. In *Digitalis*. C. Fisch, and B. Surawicz (eds.). Grune and Stratton, New York, 1969, pp. 13-26.
33. J. E. Doherty. The clinical pharmacology of digitalis glycosides: A review. *Am. J. Med. Sci. 255*: 382-414 (1968).
34. F. I. Marcus, G. J. Kapadia, and G. G. Kapadia. The metabolism of digoxin in normal subjects. *J. Pharmacol. Exp. Ther. 145*: 203 (1964).
35. T. W. Smith, V. P. Butler, Jr., and E. Haber. Determination of therapeutic and toxic serum digoxin concentrations by immunoassay. *N. Engl. J. Med. 281*: 1212-1217 (1969).
36. A. M. Weissler, J. R. Snyder, C. D. Schoenfeld, and S. Cohen. Assay of digitalis glycosides in man. *Am. J. Cardiol. 17*: 768-780 (1966).
37. R. R. Miller, L. A. Vismara, D. O. Williams, et al. Pharmacological mechanisms for left ventricular unloading in clinical congestive heart failure: Differential effects of nitroprusside, phentolamine, and nitroglycerin on cardiac function and peripheral circulation. *Circ. Res. 39*: 127-133 (1976).
38. C. V. Leier, J. Webel, and C. A. Bush. The cardiovascular effects of the continuous infusion of dobutamine in patients with severe cardiac failure. *Circulation 56*: 468-472 (1977).
39. A. Selzer. Digitalis in cardiac failure: Do benefits justify the risks? *Arch. Intern. Med. 141*: 18-19 (1981).
40. R. A. Gillis, and J. A. Quest. The role of the nervous system in the cardiovascular effects of digitalis. *Pharmacol. Rev. 31*: 19-97 (1980).
41. J. E. Doherty. Digitalis 1982: Over 200 years of clinical use, research, and opinion. *Cardiol. Ser. 5*: 5-27 (1982).
42. B. F. Hoffman, and J. T. Bigger, Jr. Digitalis and allied cardiac glycosides. In *The Pharmacologic Basis of Therapeutics*, 2nd ed. A. G. Gilman, L. S. Goodman, and A. Gilman (eds.). Macmillan, New York, 1980, pp. 729-760.
43. T. W. Smith, and E. Braunwald. The management of heart failure. In *Heart Disease: A Textbook of Cardiovascular Medicine*, 2nd ed. E. Braunwald (ed.). Saunders, Philadelphia, 1984, pp. 503-559.
44. T. W. Smith, E. M. Antman, P. L. Friedman, C. M. Blatt, and J. D. Marsh. Digitalis glycosides: Mechanisms and manifestations of toxicity. *Prog. Cardiovasc. Dis. 26*: 413-441; *26*: 495-523; *27*: 21-56 (1984).

45. C. Fisch, ed. William Withering: An account of the foxglove and some of its medical uses 1785-1985. *J. Am. Coll. Cardiol. 5*: 1A-123A (1985).

46. R. H. Reuning, and D. R. Geraets. Digoxin. In *Applied Pharmacokinetics,* 2nd ed. W. E. Evans, J. J. Schentag, and W. J. Jusko (eds.). Applied Therapeutics, San Francisco, 1986 (in press).

47. F. G. Henderson. Chemistry and biologic activity of the cardiac glycosides. In *Digitalis.* C. Fisch, and B. Surawicz (eds.). Grune and Stratton, New York, 1969.

48. E. B. LeWinn. The steroidal actions of digitalis. *Perspect. Biol. Med. 27*: 183-199 (1984).

49. A. Schwartz, K. Whitmer, G. Grupp, I. Grupp, R. J. Adams, and S. W. Lee. Mechanism of action of digitalis: Is the Na, K-ATPase the pharmacological receptor? *Ann. N.Y. Acad. Sci. 402*: 253-271 (1982).

50. H. Scholz. Inotropic drugs and their mechanisms of action. *J. Am. Coll. Cardiol. 4*: 389-397 (1984).

51. T. Guarnieri, H. Spurgeon, J. P. Froehlich, M. L. Weisfeldt, and E. G. Lakatta. Diminished inotropic response but unaltered toxicity to acetylstrophanthidin in the senescent beagle. *Circulation 60*: 1548-1554 (1979).

52. S. F. Vatner, and E. Braunwald. Effects of chronic heart failure on the inotropic response of the right ventricle of the conscious dog to a cardiac glycoside and to tachycardia. *Circulation 50*: 728-734 (1974).

53. H. Smulyan, and R. H. Eich. Effect of digitalis on skeletal muscle in man. *Am. J. Cardiol. 37*: 716-723 (1976).

54. J. C. Longhurst, and J. Ross, Jr. Extracardiac and coronary vascular effects of digitalis. *J. Am. Coll. Cardiol. 5*: 99A-105A (1985).

55. R. H. Goldman, D. J. Coltart, J. P. Friedman, G. T. Nola, D. K. Berke, E. Schweizer, and D. C. Harrison. The inotropic effects of digoxin in hyperkalemia: Relation to (Na^+, K^+)-ATPase inhibition in the intact animal. *Circulation 48*: 830-838 (1973).

56. G. H. Mudge, B. L. Lloyd, D. J. Greenblatt, and T. W. Smith. Inotropic and toxic effects of a polar cardiac glycoside derivative in the dog. *Circ. Res. 43*: 847-854 (1978).

57. R. A. Gillis, D. L. Pearle, and B. Levitt. Digitalis: A neuroexcitatory drug. *Circulation 52*: 739-742 (1975).

58. A. M. Watanabe. Digitalis and the autonomic nervous system. *J. Am. Coll. Cardiol. 5*: 35A-42A (1985).

59. L. S. Cook, J. E. Doherty, R. C. Elkins, and K. D. Straub. Comparison of the canine tissue distribution of digoxin after acute and chronic administration: Implications for digitalis therapy. *Am. J. Cardiol. 53*: 1703-1706 (1984).

60. G. D. Beiser, S. E. Epstein, R. E. Goldstein, M. Stempfer, and E. Braunwald. Comparison of the peak inotropic effects of a catecholamine and a digitalis glycoside in the intact canine heart. *Circulation 42*: 805-813 (1970).

61. D. W. Ferguson, F. M. Abboud, and A. L. Mark. Selective impairment of baroreflex-mediated vasoconstrictor responses in patients with ventricular dysfunction. *Circulation 69*: 451-460 (1984).

62. M. R. Bristow, R. Ginsburg, W. Minobe, R. S. Cubicciotti, W. S. Sageman, K. Lurie, M. E. Billingham, D. C. Harrison, and E. B. Stinson. Decreased catecholamine sensitivity and beta-adrenergic-receptor density in failing human hearts. *N. Engl. J. Med. 307*: 205-211 (1982).

63. S. F. Vatner, and E. Braunwald. Effects of chronic heart failure on the inotropic response of the right ventricle of the conscious dog to a cardiac glycoside and tachycardia. *Circulation 50*: 728-734 (1974).

64. D. T. Mason, and E. Braunwald. Studies on digitalis X: Effects of ouabain on forearm vascular resistance and venous tone in normal subjects and patients with heart failure. *J. Clin. Invest. 43*: 532-543 (1964).

65. R. M. Fuchs, D. L. Rutlen, and W. J. Powell, Jr. Effect of dobutamine on systemic capacity in the dog. *Circ. Res. 46*: 133-138 (1980).

66. G. W. Murphy, B. F. Schreiner, Jr., and P. N. Yu. Effects of acute digitalization on the pulmonary blood volume in patients with heart disease. *Circulation 43*: 145-153 (1971).

67. J. Ross, Jr. Cardiac function and myocardial contractility: A perspective. *J. Am. Coll. Cardiol. 1*: 52-62 (1983).

68. M. I. Ferrer, S. E. Bradley, H. O. Wheeler, Y. Enson, R. Preisig, and R. M. Harvey. The effect of digoxin in the splanchnic circulation in ventricular failure. *Circulation 32*: 524-537 (1965).

69. D. J. Goodman, R. M. Rossen, D. S. Cannom, A. K. Rider, and D. C. Harrison. Effect of digoxin on atrioventricular conduction. *Circulation 51*: 251-256 (1975).

70. Y. I. Kim, R. J. Noble, and D. P. Zipes. Dissociation of the inotropic effect of digitalis from its effect on atrioventricular conduction. *Am. J. Cardiol. 36*: 459-467 (1975).

71. F. L. Meijler. An "account" of digitalis and atrial fibrillation. *J. Am. Coll. Cardiol. 5*: 60A-68A (1985).

72. A. George, J. F. Spear, and E. N. Moore. The effects of digitalis glycosides on the ventricular fibrillation threshold in innervated and denervated canine hearts. *Circulation 50*: 353-358 (1974).

73. H. Boudoulas, J. J. Lima, and R. P. Lewis. Monitoring drug therapy: Pharmacologic response and use of plasma levels. In *Diagnostic Procedures in Cardiology: A Clinician's Guide*. J. V. Warren, and R. P. Lewis (eds.). Year Book, Chicago, 1985, pp. 317-339.

74. N. J. Greenberger, and J. H. Caldwell. Studies on the intestinal absorptions of ^{3}H-digitalis glycosides in experimental animals and man. In *Basic and Clinical Pharmacology of Digitalis*. B. H. Marks, and A. M. Weissler (eds.). Charles C Thomas, Springfield, Ill., 1972, pp. 15-47.

75. B. Beermann, K. Hellstrom, and A. Rosen. Fate of orally administered ^{3}H-digitoxin in man with special reference to the absorption. *Circulation 43*: 852-861 (1971).

76. H. Gold, McK. Cattell, T. Greiner, L. W. Hanlon, N. T. Kwit, W. Modell, E. Cotlove, J. Benton, and H. L. Otto. Clinical pharmacology of digoxin. *J. Pharmacol. Exp. Ther. 109*: 45-57 (1953).

77. J. E. Doherty. The metabolism of digitalis glycosides in man. In *Basic and Clinical Pharmacology of Digitalis*. B. H. Marks, and A. M. Weissler (eds.). Charles C Thomas, Springfield, Ill., 1972, pp. 230-242.
78. D. S. Lukas. Some aspects of the distribution and disposition of digitoxin in man. *Ann. N.Y. Acad. Sci. 179*: 338-361 (1971).
79. E. Astorri, G. Bianchi, G. La Canna, D. Assanelli, O. Visioli, and A. Marzo. Bioavailability and related heart function index of digoxin capsules and tablets in cardiac patients. *J. Pharmaceut. Sci. 68*: 104-106 (1979).
80. B. F. Johnson, and C. Bye. Maximal intestinal absorption of digoxin, and its relation to steady state plasma concentration. *Br. Heart J. 37*: 203-208 (1975).
81. J. Lindenbaum, M. H. Mellow, M. O. Blackstone, and V. P. Butler, Jr. Variation in biologic availability of digoxin from four preparations. *N. Engl. J. Med. 285*: 1344-1347 (1971).
82. T. W. Smith. Pharmacokinetics, bioavailability and serum levels of cardiac glycosides. *J. Am. Coll. Cardiol. 5*: 43A-50A (1985).
83. W. D. Heizer, T. W. Smith, and S. E. Goldfinger. Absorption of digoxin in patients with malabsorption syndromes. *N. Engl. J. Med. 285*: 257-259 (1971).
84. W. H. Hall, and J. E. Doherty. Tritiated digoxin XXII. *Am. J. Med. 56*: 437-442 (1974).
85. A. J. Kolibash, W. G. Kramer, R. H. Reuning, and J. H. Caldwell. Marked decline in serum digoxin concentrations during an episode of severe diarrhea. *Am. Heart J. 94*: 806-807 (1977).
86. D. D. Brown, and R. P. Juhl. Decreased bioavailability of digoxin due to antacids and kaolin-pectin. *N. Engl. J. Med. 295*: 1034-1037 (1976).
87. D. D. Brown, R. P. Juhl, and S. L. Warner. Decreased bioavailability of digoxin due to hypochelesterolemic interventions. *Circulation 58*: 164-172 (1978).
88. J. Kuhlmann, W. Ziely, and J. Wilke. Effects of cytostatic drugs on plasma level and renal excretion of B-acetyl digoxin. *Clin. Pharmacol. Ther. 30*: 518-527 (1981).
89. J. Lindenbaum, D. G. Rund, V. P. Butler, Jr., D. Tse-Eng, and J. R. Saha. Inactivation of digoxin by the gut flora: Reversal by antibiotic therapy. *N. Engl. J. Med. 305*: 789-794 (1981).
90. W. G. Kramer, R. P. Lewis, T. C. Cobb, W. F. Forester, J. A. Visconti, L. A. Wanke, H. G. Boxenbaum, and R. H. Reuning. Pharmacokinetics of digoxin: Comparison of a two- and a three-compartment model in man. *J. Pharmacokin. Biopharm. 2*: 299-312 (1974).
91. C. E. Harrison, Jr., R. O. Brandenburg, P. A. Ongley, A. L. Orvis, and C. A. Owen, Jr. The distribution and excretion of tritiated substances in experimental animals following the administration of digoxin-[3]H. *J. Lab. Clin. Med. 67*: 764-777 (1966).
92. G. A. Ewy, B. M. Groves, M. F. Ball, L. Nimmo, B. Jackson, and F. Marcus. Digoxin metabolism in obesity. *Circulation 44*: 810-814 (1971).
93. B. H. Marks. Factors that affect accumulation of digitalis glycosides in the heart. In *Basic and Clinical Pharmacology of Digitalis*. B. H. Marks, and A. M. Weissler (eds.). Charles C Thomas, Springfield, Ill., 1972, pp. 69-93.

94. R. W. Krasula, A. R. Hastreiter, S. Levitsky, R. Yanagi, and L. F. Soyka. Serum, atrial, and urinary digoxin levels during cardiopulmonary bypass in children. *Circulation 49*: 1047-1052 (1974).

95. A. M. Weissler, R. P. Lewis, R. F. Leighton, and C. A. Bush. Comparative responses to the digitalis glycosides in man. In *Basic and Clinical Pharmacology of Digitalis*. B. H. Marks, and A. M. Weissler (eds.). Charles C Thomas, Springfield, Ill., 1972, pp. 260-280.

96. R. P. Lewis, R. F. Leighton, W. F. Forester, and A. M. Weissler. Systolic time intervals. In *Noninvasive Cardiology*. A. M. Weissler (ed.). Grune and Stratton, New York, 1974, pp. 301-368.

97. W. G. Kramer, A. J. Kolibash, R. P. Lewis, M. S. Bathala, J. A. Visconti, and R. H. Reuning. Pharmacokinetics of digoxin: Relationship between response intensity and predicted compartmental drug levels in man. *J. Pharmacokinet. Biopharm. 7*: 47-61 (1979).

98. W. Forester, R. P. Lewis, A. M. Weissler, and T. A. Wilke. The onset and magnitude of the contractile response to commonly used digitalis glycosides in normal subjects. *Circulation 49*: 517-521 (1974).

99. A. M. Weissler, A. R. Kamen, R. S. Bornstein, C. D. Schoenfeld, and S. Cohen. The effect of deslanoside on the duration of the phases of ventricular systole in man. *Am. J. Cardiol. 15*: 153-161 (1965).

100. G. G. Belz, R. Erbel, K. Shumann, H. J. Gilfrich. Dose-response relationships and plasma concentrations of digitalis in man. *Eur. J. Clin. Pharmacol. 13*: 103-111 (1978).

101. D. Lampe, H. Lampe, K. Berwing. On the problem of optimal digitalization in man. *Int. J. Clin. Pharmacol. Biopharmacol. 16*: 380-383 (1978).

102. J. Buch, and S. Waldorff. Classical concentration-response relationship between serum digoxin level and contractility indices. *Dan. Med. Bull. 27*: 287-290 (1980).

103. T. Joreteg, and T. Jogestrand. Physical exercise and digoxin binding to skeletal muscle: Relation to exercise intensity. *Eur. J. Clin. Pharmacol. 25*: 585-588 (1983).

104. T. Jogestrand. Influence of everyday physical activity on the serum digoxin concentration in digoxin treated patients. *Clin. Physiol. 1*: 209-214 (1981).

105. R. H. Reuning, R. A. Sams, and R. E. Notari. Role of pharmacokinetics in drug dosage adjustment. I. Pharmacologic effect kinetics and apparent volume of distribution of digoxin. *J. Clin. Pharmacol. 13*: 127-141 (1973).

106. W. J. F. Van der Vijgh, and P. L. Oe. Pharmacokinetic aspects of digoxin in patients with terminal renal failure. *Int. J. Clin. Pharmacol. 15*: 249-259 (1977).

107. R. Selden, and T. W. Smith. Ouabain pharmacokinetics in dog and man: Determination by radioimmunoassay. *Circulation 45*: 1176-1182 (1972).

108. J. F. Dobkin, J. R. Saha, V. P. Butler, H. C. Neil, and J. Lindenbaum. Digoxin-inactivating bacteria: Identification in human gut flora. *Science 220*: 325-327 (1983).

109. M. H. Gault, L. L. Longerich, J. C. K. Loo, P. T. H. Ko, A. Fine, S. C. Vasdev, and M. A. Dawe. Digoxin biotransformation. *Clin. Pharmacol. Ther. 35*: 74-82 (1984).

110. F. I. Marcus, A. Peterson, A. Salel, J. Scully, G. G. Kapadia. The metabolism of tritiated digoxin in renal insufficiency in dogs and man. *J. Pharmacol. Exp. Ther. 152*:372-382 (1966).

111. J. E. Doherty, W. H. Perkins, and M. C. Wilson. Studies with tritiated digoxin in renal failure. *Am. J. Med. 37*: 536-544 (1964).

112. F. I. Marcus. Metabolic factors determining digitalis dosage in man. In *Basic and Clinical Pharmacology of Digitalis*. B. H. Marks, and A. M. Weissler (eds.). Charles C Thomas, Springfield, Ill., 1972, pp. 243-259.

113. E. Steiness. Renal tubular secretion of digoxin. *Circulation 50*: 103-107 (1974).

114. R. D. Okada, W. D. Hager, P. E. Graves, M. Mayersohn, D. G. Perrier, and F. I. Marcus. Relationship between plasma concentration and dose of digoxin in patients with and without renal impairment. *Circulation 58*: 1196-1203 (1978).

115. T. Risler, J. C. Somberg, R. D. Blute, Jr., and T. W. Smith. The effect of altered renal perfusion pressure on clearance of digoxin. *Circulation 61*: 521-525 (1980).

116. K. E. Pedersen, J. Madsen, K. Kjaer, N. A. Klitgaard, and S. Hvidt. Effects of physical activity and immobilization on plasma digoxin concentration and renal digoxin clearance. *Clin. Pharmacol. Ther. 34*: 303-308 (1983).

117. R. W. Jelliffe, and G. Brooker. A nomogram for digoxin therapy. *Am. J. Med. 57*: 63-68 (1974).

118. J. H. Caldwell, C. A. Bush, and N. J. Greenberger. Interruption of the enterohepatic circulation of digitoxin by cholestyramine. II. Effect on metabolic disposition of tritium-labeled digitoxin and cardiac systolic intervals in man. *J. Clin. Invest. 50*: 2638-2644 (1971).

119. F. O. Finkelstein, J. A. Goffinet, E. D. Hendler, and J. Lindenbaum. Pharmacokinetics of digoxin and digitoxin in patients undergoing hemodialysis. *Am. J. Med. 58*: 525-531 (1975).

120. K. Rasmussen, J. Jewell, L. Storstein, and K. Gjerdrum. Digitoxin kinetics in patients with impaired renal function. *Clin. Pharmacol. Ther. 13*: 6-14 (1972).

121. R. Selden, and G. Haynie. Ouabain plasma level kinetics and removal by dialysis in chronic renal failure: A study in fourteen patients. *Ann. Intern. Med. 83*: 15-19 (1975).

122. J. D. Hobson, and A. Zettner. Digoxin serum half-life following suicidal digoxin poisoning. *JAMA 223*: 147-149 (1973).

123. A. Selzer. Role of serum digoxin assay in patient management. *J. Am. Coll. Cardiol. 5*: 106A-110A (1985).

124. E. Haber. Antibodies and digitalis: The modern revolution in the use of an ancient drug. *J. Am. Coll. Cardiol. 5*: 111A-117A (1985).

125. F. I. Marcus. Digitalis pharmacokinetics and metabolism. *Am. J. Med. 58*: 452-459 (1975).

126. F. I. Marcus, L. Burkhalter, C. Cuccia, J. Pavlovich, and G. G. Kapadia. Administration of tritiated digoxin with and without a loading dose. *Circulation 34*: 865-874 (1966).

127. E. B. Leahey, Jr., J. A. Reiffel, R. E. Drusin, R. H. Heissenbuttel, W. P. Lovejoy, and J. T. Bigger, Jr. Interaction between digoxin, quinidine. *JAMA 240*: 533-534 (1978).

128. E. B. Leahey, Jr., J. A. Reiffel, E-G. V. Giardina, and J. T. Bigger, Jr. The effect of quinidine and other oral antiarrhythmic drugs on serum digoxin. *Ann. Intern. Med. 92*: 605-608 (1980).

129. D. R. Mungall, R. P. Robichaux, W. Perry, J. W. Scott, A. Robinson, T. Burelle, and D. Hurst. Effects of quinidine on serum digoxin concentration. *Ann. Intern. Med. 93*: 689-693 (1980).

130. E. B. Leahey, Jr., J. T. Bigger, Jr., V. P. Butler, Jr., J. A. Reiffel, G. C. O'Connell, L. E. Scaffidi, and J. N. Rottman. Quinidine-digoxin interaction: Time course and pharmacokinetics. *Am. J. Cardiol. 48*: 1141-1146 (1981).

131. J. T. Bigger, Jr. The quinidine-digoxin interaction. *Mod. Concepts Cardiovasc. Dis. 51*: 73-78 (1982).

132. F. I. Marcus. Pharmacokinetic interactions between digoxin and other drugs. *J. Am. Coll. Cardiol. 5*: 82A-90A (1985).

133. P. E. Fenster, W. D. Hager, D. Perrier, J. R. Powell, P. E. Graves, and U. F. Michael. Digoxin-quinidine interaction in patients with chronic renal failure. *Circulation 66*: 1277-1280 (1982).

134. N. J. Warner, J. T. Barnard, and J. T. Bigger, Jr. Tissue digoxin concentrations and digoxin effect during the quinidine-digoxin interaction. *J. Am. Coll. Cardiol. 5*: 680-686 (1985).

135. E. B. Leahey, Jr., J. A. Reiffel, R. H. Heissenbuttel, R. E. Drusin, W. P. Lovejoy, and J. T. Bigger, Jr. Enhanced cardiac effect of digoxin during quinidine treatment. *Arch. Intern. Med. 139*: 519-521 (1979).

136. E. Steiness, S. Waldorff, P. B. Hansen, H. Kjaergard, J. Buch, and H. Edgblad. Reduction if digoxin-induced inotropism during quinidine administration. *Clin. Pharmacol. Ther. 27*: 791-795 (1980).

137. P. D. Hirsch, H. J. Weiner, and R. L. North. Further insights into digoxin-quinidine interaction: Lack of correlation between serum digoxin concentration and inotropic state of the heart. *Am. J. Cardiol. 46*: 863-868 (1980).

138. J. F. Williams, Jr., and B. Mathew. Effect of quinidine on positive inotropic action of digoxin. *Am. J. Cardiol. 47*: 1052-1056 (1981).

139. S. Goldman, W. D. Hager, M. Olajos, D. Perrier, and M. Mayersohn. Effect of the ouabain-quinidine interaction on left ventricular and left atrial function in conscious dogs. *Circulation 67*: 1054-1058 (1983).

140. H. R. Ochs, J. Pabst, D. J. Greenblatt, and H. J. Dengler. Noninteraction of digitoxin and quinidine. *N. Engl. J. Med. 303*: 672-674 (1980).

141. P. E. Fenster, J. R. Powell, P. E. Graves, K. A. Conrad, W. D. Hager, S. Goldman, and F. I. Marcus. Digitoxin-quinidine interaction: Pharmacokinetic evaluation. *Ann. Intern. Med. 93*: 698-701 (1980).

142. M. Garty, P. Sood, and D. E. Rollins. Digitoxin elimination reduced during quinidine therapy. *Ann. Intern. Med. 94*: 35-37 (1981).

143. H. O. Klein, R. Land, E. Weiss, E. Di Segni, C. Libhaber, J. Buerrero, and E. Kaplinsky. The influence of verapamil on serum digoxin concentration. *Circulation 65*: 998-1002 (1982).

144. K. E. Pedersen, A. Dorph-Pedersen, S. Hvilt, N. A. Klitgaard, and F. Nielsen-Kudsk. Digoxin-verapamil interaction. *Clin. Pharmacol. Ther. 30*: 311-316 (1981).

145. K. E. Pederen, P. Thayssen, N. A. Klitgaard, B. P. Christiansen, and F. Nielsen-Kudsk. Influence of verapamil on the inotropism and pharmacokinetics of digoxin. *Eur. J. Clin. Pharmacol. 25*: 199-206 (1983).

146. Y. Oyama, S. Fujii, K. Kanda, E. Akino, H. Kawasaki, M. Nagata, and K. Goto. Digoxin-diltiazem interaction. *Am. J. Cardiol. 53*: 1480-1481 (1984).

147. W. J. Oetgen, S. M. Sobol, T. B. Fri, W. H. Heydorn, and L. Rakita. Amiodarone-digoxin interaction, clinical and experimental observations. *Chest 86*: 75-79 (1984).

148. K. Nademanee, R. Kannan, J. Hendrickson, M. Ookhtens, I. Kay, and B. N. Singh. Amiodarone-digoxin interaction: Clinical significance, time course of development, potential pharmacokinetic mechanisms and therapeutic implications. *J. Am. Coll. Cardiol. 4*: 111-116 (1984).

149. P. E. Fenster, N. W. White, Jr., and C. D. Hanson. Pharmacokinetic evaluation of the digoxin-amiodarone interaction. *J. Am. Coll. Cardiol. 5*: 108-112 (1985).

150. S. Waldorff, P. B. Hansen, H. Egeblad, et al. Interactions between digoxin and potassium-sparing diuretics. *Clin. Pharmacol. Ther. 33*: 418-423 (1983).

151. E. Steiness. Suppression of renal excretion of digoxin in hypokalemic patients. *Clin. Pharmacol. Ther. 23*: 511-514 (1978).

152. R. H. Seller, J. Greco, S. Banach, and R. Seth. Increasing the inotropic effect and toxic dose of digitalis by the administration of antikaliuretic drugs —further evidence for a cardiac effect of diuretic agents. *Am. Heart J. 90*: 56-67 (1975).

153. J. J. Cogan, M. H. Humphreys, C. J. Carlson, N. L. Benowitz, and E. Rapaport. Acute vasodilator therapy increases renal clearance of digoxin in patients with congestive heart failure. *Circulation 64*: 973-976 (1981).

154. T. T. Edmonds, P. L. Howard, and T. D. Trainer. Measurement of digitoxin and digoxin. *N. Engl. J. Med. 286*: 1266 (1972).

155. D. T. Mason, and E. Braunwald. Studies on digitalis. IX. Effects of ouabain on the non failing heart. *J. Clin. Invest. 42*: 1105-1111 (1963).

156. M. H. Crawford, J. S. Karliner, and R. A. O'Rourke. Favorable effects of oral maintenance digoxin therapy on left ventricular performance in normal subjects: Echocardiographic study. *Am. J. Cardiol. 38*: 843-847 (1976).

157. E. Braunwald. Effects of digitalis on the normal and the failing heart. *J. Am. Coll. Cardiol. 5*: 51A-59A (1985).

158. D. G. Kassebaum, and H. E. Griswold. Digitalis in non-failing cardiac diseases. *Prog. Cardiovasc. Dis. 12*: 484-492 (1970).

159. J. Ross, Jr., E. Braunwald, and J. A. Waldhausen. Studies on digitalis. II. Extracardiac effects on venous return and the capacity of the peripheral vascular bed. *J. Clin. Invest. 39*: 937 (1960).

160. A. M. Weissler, and C. D. Schoenfeld. Effect of digitalis on systolic time intervals in heart failure. *Am. J. Med. Sci. 259*: 4-20 (1970).

161. H. Lagerlof, and L. Werko. Studies on circulation in man; the effect of Cedilanid (lanatoside C) on cardiac output and blood pressure in pulmonary circulation in patients with compensated and decompensated heart disease. *Acta Cardiol. 4*: 1 (1949).

162. R. M. Harvey, M. I. Ferrer, R. T. Cathcart, D. W. Richards, and A. Cornand. Some effects of digoxin upon the heart and circulation in man: Digoxin in left ventricular failure. *Am. J. Med. 7*: 439 (1949).

163. R. I. S. Bayliss, M. J. Etheridge, A. L. Hyman, H. G. Kelly, J. McMichael, and E. A. S. Reid. The effect of digoxin on the right ventricular pressure in hypertensive and ischemic heart failure. *Br. Heart J. 12*: 317 (1950).

164. B. Rader, W. W. Smith, A. R. Berger, and L. W. Eichna. Comparison of the hemodynamic effects of mercurial diuretics and digitalis in congestive heart failure. *Circulation 29*: 328-345 (1964).

165. G. W. Murphy, B. F. Schreiner, P. L. Bleakley, and P. N. Yu. Left ventricular performance following digitalization in patients with and without heart failure. *Circulation 30*: 358-369 (1964).

166. N. A. Yankopoulos, C. Kawai, E. E. Federici, L. N. Adler, and W. H. Abelmann. The hemodynamic effects of ouabain upon the diseased left ventricle. *Am. Heart J. 76*: 466-480 (1968).

167. C. Chedsey, E. Braunwald, and A. G. Morrow. Catecholamine excretion and cardiac stores of norepinephrine in congestive heart failure. *Am. J. Med. 39*: 442 (1965).

168. G. S. Frances, S. R. Goldsmith, T. B. Levine, M. T. Glivari, and J. N. Cohn. The neurohumoral axis in congestive heart failure. *Ann. Intern. Med. 101*: 370 (1984).

169. H. J. Sauter, H. T. Dodge, R. R. Johnston, and T. P. Graham. The relationship of left atrial pressure and volume in patients with heart disease. *Am. Heart J. 67*: 635-642 (1964).

170. P. M. Shah, R. Grameak, D. H. Kramer, and P. N. Yu. Determinants of atrial (S4) and ventricular (S3) gallop sounds in primary myocardial disease. *N. Engl. J. Med. 278*: 753-758 (1968).

171. C. D. Mulrow, J. R. Feussner, and R. Velez. Reevaluation of digitalis efficacy. *Ann. Intern. Med. 101*: 113-117 (1984).

172. J. L. Fleg, S. H. Gottlieb, and E. G. Lakatta. Is digoxin really important in treatment of compensated heart failure? *Am. J. Med. 73*: 244-250 (1982).

173. S. B. Arnold, R. C. Byrd, W. Meister, K. Melmon, M. D. Cheitlin, J. D. Bristow, W. W. Parmley, and K. Chatterjee. Long-term digitalis therapy improves left ventricular function in heart failure. *N. Engl. J. Med. 303*: 1443-1448 (1980).

174. R. G. Murray, A. C. Tweddel, W. Martin, D. Pearson, I. Hutton, and T. D. V. Lawrie. Evaluation of digitalis in cardiac failure. *Br. Med. J. 284*: 1526-1528 (1982).

175. D. C-S. Lee, R. A. Johnson, J. B. Bingham, M. Leahy, R. E. Dinsmore, A. H. Goroll, J. B. Newell, H. W. Strauss, and E. Haber. Heart failure in outpatients:

A randomized trial of digoxin versus placebo. *N. Engl. J. Med. 306*: 699-705 (1982).

176. E. Braunwald, and B. E. Sobel. Coronary blood flow and myocardial ischemia. In *Heart Disease. A Textbook of Cardiovascular Medicine*. E. Braunwald (ed.). Saunders, Philadelphia, 1984, pp. 1235-1262.

177. A Linzbach. Heart failure from the point of view of quantitative anatomy. *Am. J. Cardiol. 5*: 370 (1960).

178. E. L. Fallen, W. C. Elliott, and R. Gorlin. Mechanisms of angina in aortic stenosis. *Circulation 36*: 480-488 (1967).

179. D. V. Unverferth, R. D. Magorien, R. P. Lewis, and C. V. Leier. The role of subendocardial ischemia in perpetuating myocardial failure in patients with nonischemic congestive cardiomyopathy. *Am. Heart J. 105*: 176-179 (1983).

180. R. Rubio, and R. M. Berne. Regulation of coronary blood flow. *Prog. Cardiovasc. Dis. 18*: 105 (1975).

181. J. I. E. Hoffman, and G. D. Budkberg. The myocardial supply:demand ratio —A critical review. *Am. J. Cardiol. 41*: 327 (1978).

182. G. D. Buckberg, D. E. Foxler, J. P. Archie, and J. I. E. Hoffman. Experimental subendocardial ischemia in dogs with normal coronary arteries. *Circ. Res. 30*: 67-81 (1972).

183. H. Boudoulas, S. E. Rittgers, R. P. Lewis, and A. M. Weissler. Changes in diastolic time with various pharmacologic agents. Implications for myocardial perfusion. *Circulation 60*: 164-169 (1979).

184. H. DeMots, S. H. Rahimtoola, E. L. Kremkau, W. Bennett, and D. Mahler. Effects of ouabain on myocardial oxygen supply and demand in patients with chronic coronary artery disease: A hemodynamic, volumetric, and metabolic study in patients without heart failure. *J. Clin. Invest. 58*: 312-319 (1976).

185. C. V. Leier, P. T. Heban, P. Huss, C. A. Bush, and R. P. Lewis. Comparative systemic and regional hemodynamic effects of dopamine and dobutamine in patients with cardiomyopathic heart failure. *Circulation 58*: 466-475 (1978).

186. C. V. Leier, R. D. Magorien, H. Boudoulas, R. P. Lewis, D. Bambach, and D. V. Unverferth. The effect of vasodilator therapy on systolic and diastolic time intervals in congestive heart failure. *Chest 81*: 723-729 (1982).

187. C. V. Leier, T. J. Patrick, J. Hermiller, K. D. Pacht, P. Huss, R. D. Magorien, and D. V. Unverferth. Nifedipine in congestive heart failure: Effects on resting and exercise hemodynamics and regional blood flow. *Am. Heart J. 108*: 1461-1468 (1984).

188. I. Cantelli, P. C. Pavesi, C. Parchi, F. Naccarella, and D. Bracchetti. Acute hemodynamic effects of combined therapy with digoxin and nifedipine in patients with chronic heart failure. *Am. Heart J. 106*: 308-315 (1983).

189. J. A. Thomas, and B. H. Marks. Plasma norepinephrine in congestive heart failure. *Am. J. Cardiol. 41*: 233 (1978).

190. R. S. Engelmeier, J. B. O'Connell, R. Walsh, N. Rad, P. J. Scanlon, and R. M. Gunnar. Improvement in symptoms and exercise tolerance by Metoprolol in patients with dilated cardiomyopathy: A double-blind, randomized placebo-controlled trial. *Circulation 72*: 536-546 (1985).

191. J.C.J.L. Bath. Treatment of cardiac arrhythmias in unanesthetized patients: Role of adrenergic beta receptor blockade. *Am. J. Cardiol. 18*: 415-425 (1966).

192. L. Shamroth, D. M. Krickler, and C. Garrett. Immediate effects of intravenous verapamil in cardiac arrhythmias. *Br. Med. J. 1*: 660 (1972).

193. P. Weiner, M. M. Bassan, J. Jarchovsky, S. Iusim, and L. Plavnick. Clinical course of acute atrial fibrillation treated with rapid digitalization. *Am. Heart J. 105*: 223-227 (1983).

194. D. David, E. Di Segni, H. O. Klein, and E. Kaplinsky. Inefficacy of digitalis in the control of heart rate in patients with chronic atrial fibrillation: Beneficial effect of an added beta adrenergic blocking agent. *Am. J. Cardiol. 44*: 1378-1382 (1979).

195. J. B. Schwartz, D. Keefe, R. E. Kates, E. Kirsten, and D. C. Harrison. Acute and chronic pharmacodynamic interaction of verapamil and digoxin in atrial fibrillation. *Circulation 65*: 1163-1170 (1982).

196. I. P. Panidis, J. Morganroth, and C. Baessler. Effectiveness and safety of oral verapamil to control exercise-induced tachycardia in patients with atrial fibrillation receiving digitalis. *Am. J. Cardiol. 52*: 1197-1201 (1983).

197. C. V. Leier, T. M. Johnson, and R. P. Lewis. Uncontrolled ventricular rate in atrial fibrillation: A manifestation of dissimilar atrial rhythms. *Br. Heart J. 42*: 106-109 (1979).

198. D. A. Chamberlain, R. J. White, M. R. Howard, and T. W. Smith. Plasma digoxin concentrations in patients with atrial fibrillation. *Br. Med. J. 3*: 429-432 (1970).

199. A. Redfors. Plasma digoxin concentration—its relation to digoxin dosage and clinical effects in patients with atrial fibrillation. *Br. Heart J. 34*: 383-391 (1972).

200. C. Fisch, and S. B. Knoebel. Digitalis cardiotoxicity. *J. Am. Coll. Cardiol. 5*: 91A-98A (1985).

201. H. J. Wellens, and D. Durrer. Effects of digitalis on atrioventricular conduction and circus movement tachycardias in patients with Wolff-Parkinson-White syndrome. *Circulation 47*: 1229-1233 (1973).

202. T. D. Sellers, Jr., T. M. Bashore, and J. J. Gallagher. Digitalis in the pre-excitation syndrome: Analysis during atrial fibrillation. *Circulation 56*: 260-270 (1977).

203. H. Boudoulas, S. Dervenagas, P. K. Fulkerson, C. A. Bush, and R. P. Lewis. Effect of heart rate on diastolic time and left ventricular performance in patients with atrial fibrillation. In *Noninvasive Cardiovascular Diagnosis*. E. G. Diethrich (ed.). PSG Publishing Co., Littleton, Mass., 1981, pp. 433-445.

204. H. Boudoulas, R. P. Lewis, J. A. Sherman, C. A. Bush, G. Dalamangas, and W. F. Forester. Systolic time intervals in atrial fibrillation. *Chest 74*: 629-634 (1978).

205. F. Mahler, J. S. Karliner, and R. A. O'Rourke. Effects of chronic digoxin administration on left ventricular performance in the normal conscious dog. *Circulation 50*: 720-727 (1974).

206. N. H. Carliner, C. A. Gilbert, A. W. Pruitt, and L. I. Goldberg. Effects of maintenance digoxin therapy on systolic time intervals and serum digoxin concentrations. *Circulation 50*: 94-98 (1974).

207. J. H. Kleiman, N. B. Ingels, G. Daughters II, E. B. Stinson, E. L. Alderman, and R. H. Goldman. Left ventricular dynamics during long-term digoxin treatment in patients with stable coronary artery disease. *Am. J. Cardiol. 41*: 937-942 (1978).

208. B. E. Griffiths, W. J. Penny, M. J. Lewis, and A. H. Henderson. Maintenance of the inotropic effect of digoxin on long-term treatment. *Br. Med. J. 284*: 1819-1822 (1982).

209. H. A. Christian. The use of digitalis other than in the treatment of cardiac decompensation. *JAMA 100*: 789 (1933).

210. R. M. Harvey, M. I. Ferrer, R. T. Cathcart, and J. K. Alexander. Some effects of digoxin on the heart and circulation in man: Digoxin in enlarged hearts not in clinical congestive failure. *Circulation 4*: 366-371 (1951).

211. A. Selzer, and R. O. Malmborg. Hemodynamic effects of digoxin in latent cardiac failure. *Circulation 25*: 695-702 (1962).

212. R. L. Kahler, Jr., H. Thompson, E. R. Buskirk, R. L. Frye, and E. Braunwald. Studies on digitalis. VI. Reduction of the oxygen debt after exercise with digoxin in cardiac patients without heart failure. *Circulation 27*: 397-405 (1963).

213. J. F. Williams, Jr., and R. D. Potter. The effect of chronic digitoxin administration on the contractile state of normal and nonfailing hypertrophied myocardium. *J. Clin. Invest. 56*: 71-78 (1975).

214. J. Morrison, and T. Killip. Serum digitalis and arrhythmia in patients undergoing cardiopulmonary bypass. *Circulation 47*: 341-352 (1973).

215. T. P. Chee, N. Sri Prakash, K. B. Desser, and A. Benchimol. Postoperative supraventricular arrhythmias and the role of prophylactic digoxin in cardiac surgery. *Am. Heart J. 104*: 974-977 (1982).

216. B. Surawicz. Factors affecting tolerance to digitalis. *J. Am. Coll. Cardiol. 5*: 69A-81A (1985).

217. T. R. Engel, and S. F. Schaal. Digitalis in the sick sinus syndrome: The effects of digitalis on sinoatrial automaticity and atrioventricular conduction. *Circulation 48*: 1201-1207 (1973).

218. R. C. Dhingra, F. Amat-y-Leon, C. Wyndham, D. Wu, P. Denes, and K. Rosen. The electrophysiological effect of ouabain on sinus node and atrium in man. *J. Clin. Invest. 56*: 555-562 (1975).

219. Z. Vera, R. R. Miller, D. McMillin, and D. T. Mason. Effects of digitalis on sinus nodal function in patients with sick sinus syndrome. *Am. J. Cardiol. 41*: 318-323 (1978).

220. J. A. Reiffel, J. T. Bigger, Jr., and M. Cramer. Effects of digoxin on sinus nodal function before and after vagal blockage in patients with sinus nodal dysfunction. *Am. J. Cardiol. 43*: 983-989 (1979).

221. B. Lown, T. B. Graboys, P. J. Podrid, B. H. Cohen, M. B. Stockman, and C. E. Gaughan. Effect of a digitalis drug on ventricular premature beats. *N. Engl. J. Med. 296*: 301-306 (1977).

222. A. H. Gradman, M. Cunningham, M. A. Harbison, H. J. Berger, and B. L. Zaret. Effects of oral digoxin on ventricular ectopy and its relation to left ventricular function. *Am. J. Cardiol. 51*: 765-769 (1983).

223. W. Berman, Jr., S. M. Yabek, T. Dillon, C. Niland, S. Corlew, and D. Christensen. Effects of digoxin in infants with a congested circulatory state due to a ventricular septal defect. *N. Engl. J. Med. 308*: 363-366 (1983).

224. R. J. Luchi, E. Snow, J. M. Luchi, C. L. Nelson, and F. J. Pircher. Left ventricular function in hospitalized geriatric patients. *J. Am. Geriatr. Soc. 30*: 700-705 (1982).

225. G. A. Ewy, G. G. Kapadia, L. Yao, M. Lullin, and F. I. Marcus. Digoxin metabolism in the elderly. *Circulation 39*: 449-453 (1969).

226. L. H. Green, and T. W. Smith. The use of digitalis in patients with pulmonary disease. *Ann. Intern. Med. 87*: 459-465 (1977).

227. P. N. Mathur, A. C. P. Powles, S. O. Pugsley, M. P. McEwan, and E. J. M. Campbell. Effect of digoxin on right ventricular function in severe chronic airflow obstruction: A controlled clinical trial. *Ann. Intern. Med. 95*: 283-288 (1981).

228. M. D. Klein, B. Lown, I. Barr, F. Hagemeijer, H. Garrison, and P. Axelrod. Comparison of serum digoxin level measurement with acetylstrophanthidin tolerance testing. *Circulation 49*: 1053-1062 (1974).

229. M. Gheorghiade, and G. A. Beller. Effects of discontinuing maintenance digoxin therapy in patients with ischemic heart disease and congestive heart failure in sinus rhythm. *Am. J. Cardiol. 51*: 1243-1250 (1983).

230. S. F. Vatner, H. Baig, W. T. Manders, and P. A. Murray. Effects of a cardiac glycoside in combination with propranolol on the ischemic heart of conscious dogs. *Circulation 57*: 568-574 (1978).

231. S. F. Vatner, and H. Baig. Comparison of the effects of ouabain and isoproterenol on ischemic myocardium of conscious dogs. *Circulation 58*: 654-662 (1978).

232. V. S. Banka, H. Yamazaki, J. B. Agarwal, M. M. Bodenheimer, and R. H. Helfant. Effects of digitalis on subendocardial and subepicardial dysfunction during acute ischemia. *Circulation 65*: 1315-1320 (1982).

233. H. DeMots, S. H. Rahimtoola, J. H. McAnulty, and G. A. Porter. Effects of ouabain on coronary and systemic vascular resistance and myocardial oxygen consumption in patients without heart failure. *Am. J. Cardiol. 41*: 88-93 (1978).

234. R. P. Lewis, H. Boudoulas, W. F. Forester, and A. M. Weissler. Shortening of electromechanical systole as a manifestation of excessive adrenergic stimulation in acute myocardial infarction. *Circulation 46*: 856-862 (1972).

235. H. Boudoulas, M. K. Lewis, G. L. Snyder, and R. P. Lewis. Adrenergic activity in patients with heart disease. *IRCS Med. Sci. 13*: 380 (1985).

236. The Norwegian Multicenter Study Group. Timolol-induced reduction in mortality and reinfarction in patients surviving acute myocardial infarction. *N. Engl. J. Med. 304*: 801-807 (1981).

237. Beta-Blocker Heart Attack Study Group. The beta-blocker heart attack trial. *JAMA 246*: 2073-2074 (1981).

238. J. O. Parker, R. O. West, J. R. Ledwich, and S. Di Giorgi. The effect of acute digitalization on the hemodynamic response to exercise in coronary artery disease. *Circulation 40*: 453-462 (1969).

239. D. L. Glancy, L. M. Higgs, K. P. O'Brien, and S. E. Epstein. Effects of ouabain on the left ventricular response to exercise in patients with angina pectoris. *Circulation 43*: 45-56 (1971).

240. L. M. Higgs, D. L. Glancy, K. P. O'Brien, and S. E. Epstein, Effects of ouabain on the left ventricular response to atrial pacing in patients with angina pectoris. *Am. J. Cardiol. 28*: 17-24 (1971).

241. B. Sharma, P. A. Majid, M. K. Meeran, W. Whitaker, and S. H. Taylor. Clinical, electrocardiographic, and haemodynamic effects of digitalis (ouabain) in angina pectoris. *Br. Heart J. 34*: 631-637 (1972).

242. M. Niederberger, R. A. Bruce, R. Frederick, F. Kusumi, and A. Marriott. Reproduction of maximal exercise performance in patients with angina pectoris despite ouabain treatment. *Circulation 49*: 309-315 (1974).

243. H. S. Loeb, N. Streitmatter, D. Braunstein, W. R. Jacohs, R. P. Croke, and R. M. Gunnar. Lack of ouabain effect on pacing-induced myocardial ischemia in patients with coronary artery disease. *Am. J. Cardiol. 43*: 995-1000 (1979).

244. B. G. Firth, G. J. Dehmer, J. R. Corbett, S. E. Lewis, R. W. Parkey, and J. T. Willerson. Effect of chronic oral digoxin therapy on ventricular function at rest and peak exercise in patients with ischemic heart disease: Assessment with equilibrium gated blood pool imaging. *Am. J. Cardiol. 46*: 481-490 (1980).

245. R. Vogel, J. Frischknecht, and P. Steele. Short- and long-term effects of digitalis on resting and posthandgrip hemodynamics in patients with coronary artery disease. *Am. J. Cardiol. 40*: 171-176 (1977).

246. M. Hodges, G. C. Friesinger, R. C. K. Riggins, and G. R. Dagenais. Effects of intravenously administered digoxin on mild left ventricular failure in acute myocardial infarction in man. *Am. J. Cardiol. 29*: 749-756 (1972).

247. R. A. Goldstein, E. R. Passamani, and R. Roberts. A comparison of digoxin and dobutamine in patients with acute infarction and cardiac failure. *N. Engl. J. Med. 303*: 846-850 (1980).

248. J. Morrison, J. Coromilas, M. Robbins, et al. Digitalis and myocardial infarction in man. *Circulation 62*: 8-16 (1980).

249. B. Lown, J. D. Klein, I. Barr, F. Hagemeijer, B. D. Kosowsky, and H. Garrison. Sensitivity to digitalis drugs in acute myocardial infarction. *Am. J. Cardiol. 30*: 388-395 (1972).

250. J. N. Cohn, F. E. Tristani, and I. M. Khatri. Cardiac and peripheral vascular effects of digitalis in clinical cardiogenic shock. *Am. Heart J. 78*: 318-330 (1969).

251. S. H. Rahimtoola, M. Z. Sinno, R. Chugquimia, H. S. Loeb, K. M. Rosen, and R. M. Gunnar. Effects of ouabain on impaired left ventricular function in acute myocardial infarction. *N. Engl. J. Med. 287*: 527-531 (1972).

252. S. H. Rahimtoola, and R. M. Gunnar. Digitalis in acute myocardial infarction: Help or hazard? *Ann. Intern. Med. 82*: 234-240 (1975).

253. R. A. O'Rourke, H. Henning, P. Theroux, M. H. Crawford, and J. Ross, Jr. Favorable effects of orally administered digoxin on left heart size and ven-

tricular wall motion in patients with previous myocardial infarction. *Am. J. Cardiol. 37*: 708-715 (1976).

254. J. H. Kleiman, E. L. Alderman, R. H. Goldman, N. B. Ingels, G. T. Daughters II, and E. B. Stinson. Effects of digitalis on normal and abnormal left ventricular segmental dynamics. *Am. J. Cardiol. 43*: 1001-1008 (1979).

255. A. J. Moss, H. T. Davis, D. L. Conard, J. J. DeCamilla, and C. L. Odoroff. Digitalis-associated cardiac mortality after myocardial infarction. *Circulation 64*: 1150-1156 (1981).

256. H. Boudoulas, Y. H. Sohn, W. O'Neill, and A. M. Weissler. Evidence that therapy with digitalis is a risk factor in patients with coronary artery disease. *J. Terapevticheskii Arkhiv 54*: 45-47 (1982).

257. J. T. Bigger, Jr., J. L. Fleiss, L. M. Rolnitzky, J. P. Merab, and K. J. Ferrick. Effect of digitalis treatment on survival after acute myocardial infarction. *Am. J. Cardiol. 55*: 623-630 (1985).

258. T. J. Ryan, K. R. Bailey, C. H. McCabe, S. Luk, L. D. Fisher, M. B. Mock, and T. Killip. The effects of digitalis on survival in high-risk patients with coronary artery disease: The coronary artery surgery study (CASS). *Circulation 67*: 735-742 (1983).

259. E. B. Madsen, E. Gilpin, H. Henning, S. Ahnve, M. LeWinter, J. Mazur, R. Shabetai, D. Collins, and J. Ross, Jr. Prognostic importance of digitalis after acute myocardial infarction. *J. Am. Coll. Cardiol. 3*: 681-689 (1984).

260. R. P. Lewis, J. T. Bigger, Jr., N. E. Davies, E. W. Hancock, J. O. Humphries, F. E. Kloster, A. S. Nies, and R. C. Schlant. Cardiovascular diseases. *Am. Coll. Phys. MKSAP 6*: 483-527 (1983).

261. Y. Iesaka, K. Aonuma, A. J. Gosselin, T. Pinakatt, W. Stanford, J. Benson, R. Sampsell, J. J. Rozanski, and J. W. Lister. Susceptibility of infarcted canine hearts to digitalis-toxic ventricular tachycardia. *J. Am. Coll. Cardiol. 2*: 45-51 (1983).

262. C. K. Friedberg. Epilogue. In *Digitalis*. C. Fisch, and B. Surawicz (eds.). Grune and Stratton, New York, 1969, pp. 174-183.

263. G. A. Beller, T. W. Smith, W. H. Abelmann, E. Haber, and W. B. Hood, Jr. Digitalis intoxication: A prospective clinical study with serum level correlations. *N. Engl. J. Med. 284*: 989-997 (1971).

264. O. Storstein, V. Hansteen, L. Hatle, L. Hillestad, and L. Storstein. Studies on digitalis. XIII. A prospective study of 649 patients on maintenance treatment with digitoxin. *Am. Heart J. 93*: 434-443 (1977).

265. S. Shapiro, D. Slone, G. P. Lewis, and H. Jick. The epidemiology of digoxin. *J. Chronic Dis. 22*: 361 (1969).

266. N. Hurwitz, and O. L. Wade. Intensive hospital monitoring of adverse reactions to drugs. *Br. Med. J. 1*: 531 (1969).

267. D. C. Evered, and C. Chapman. Plasma digoxin concentrations and digoxin toxicity in hospital patients. *Br. Heart J. 33*: 540 (1971).

268. D. Howard, C. I. Smith, G. Stewart, M. Vadas, D. J. Filler, W. J. Hensley, and J. G. Richards. A prospective survey of the incidence of cardiac intoxication with digitalis in patients being admitted to hospital and correlation with serum digoxin levels. *New Zealand Med. J. 2*: 279 (1973).

269. T. W. Smith, and E. Haber. Digoxin intoxication: The relationship of clinical presentation to serum digoxin concentration. *J. Clin. Invest. 49*: 2377-2386 (1970).

270. D. W. Duhme, D. J. Greenblatt, and J. Koch-Weser. Reduction of digoxin toxicity associated with measurement of serum levels. *Ann. Intern. Med. 80*: 516-519 (1974).

271. T. W. Smith. Digitalis toxicity: Epidemiology and clinical use of serum concentration measurements. *Am. J. Med. 58*: 470-476 (1975).

272. W. Shapiro. Correlative studies of serum digitalis levels and the arrhythmias of digitalis intoxication. *Am. J. Cardiol. 41*: 852-859 (1978).

273. L. B. Sheiner, H. Halkin, C. Peck, B. Rosenberg, and K. L. Melmon. Improved computer-assisted digoxin therapy: A method using feedback of measured serum digoxin concentrations. *Ann. Intern. Med. 82*: 619-627 (1975).

274. K. S. White, A. Lindsay, T. A. Pryor, W. F. Brown, and K. Walsh. Application of a computerized medical decision-making process to the problem of digoxin intoxication. *J. Am. Coll. Cardiol. 4*: 571-576 (1984).

275. A. H. Lely, and C. H. J. van Enter. Non-cardiac symptoms of digitalis intoxication. *Am. Heart J. 83*: 149-152 (1972).

276. T. W. Smith, V. P. Butler, Jr., E. Haber, H. Fozzard, F. I. Marcus, W. F. Bremner, I. C. Schulman, and A. Phillips. Treatment of life-threatening digitalis intoxication with digoxin-specific Fab antibody fragments: Experience in 26 cases. *N. Engl. J. Med. 207*: 1357-1362 (1982).

277. B. Lown, G. Hagemeijer, I. Barr, and M. Klein. Digitalis intoxication: Clinical and experimental assessment of the degree of digitalization. In *Basic and Clinical Pharmacology of Digitalis*. B. H. Marks, and A. M. Weissler (eds.). Charles C Thomas, Springfield, Ill., 1972, pp. 299-318.

278. H. J. J. Wellens. The electrocardiogram in digitalis intoxication. In *Progress in Cardiology*. P. N. Yu, and J. F. Goodwin (eds.). Lea & Febiger, Philadelphia, 1976, pp. 271-290.

279. J. A. Ingelfinger, and P. Goldman. The serum digitalis concentration—Does it diagnose digitalis toxicity? *N. Engl. J. Med. 294*: 867-870 (1976).

280. A. S. Gooch, G. Natarajan, and H. Goldberg. Influence of exercise on arrhythmias induced by digitalis-diuretic therapy in patients with atrial fibrillation. *Am. J. Cardiol. 33*: 230-237 (1974).

281. R. Kleiger, and B. Lown. Cardioversion and digitalis. II. Clinical studies. *Circulation 33*: 878-887 (1966).

282. R. V. Ditchey, and J. S. Karliner. Safety of electrical cardioversion in patients without digitalis toxicity. *Ann. Intern. Med. 95*: 676-679 (1981).

283. T. L. Wenger, V. P. Butler, Jr., E. Haber, and T. W. Smith. Treatment of 63 severely digitalis-toxic patients with digoxin-specific antibody fragments. *J. Am. Coll. Cardiol. 5*: 118A-123A (1985).

284. D. S. Lukas. Of toads and flowers. *Circulation 46*: 1-4 (1972).

285. M. T. Sodums, R. A. Walsh, and R. A. O'Rourke. Digitalis in heart failure: Farewell to the foxglove? *JAMA 246*: 158-160 (1981).

5

Nonparenteral Sympathomimetics

PHILIP C. KIRLIN
Michigan State University, East Lansing, Michigan

I. INTRODUCTION

Nonparenteral (orally administered) sympathomimetics are a heterogeneous class of cardiotonics currently under investigation for potential therapeutic use in congestive heart failure due to left ventricular (LV) dysfunction. The possibility of directly stimulating the failing heart to contract more vigorously is intuitively appealing and there is widespread interest in the development of sympathomimetic agents which could supplement or in some instances replace cardiac glycosides. A large number of such compounds have been investigated, several of which are reviewed here.

Several major classes of nonparenteral sympathomimetic compounds exist: those with direct beta-agonist effects (for example, full agonists such as albuterol [salbutamol] or partial agonists such as corwin and prenalterol); agents with mixed alpha- and beta-agonist properties (such as ephedrine); and agents whose primary mechanism of action appears to be dopaminergic (such as levodopa and ibopamine). This chapter discusses the mechanism of action, pharmacologic properties, potential therapeutic effects, drug interactions, and intrinsic limitations of this class of inotropic agents. A representative list of sympathomimetic compounds with potential application as inotropic agents by nonparenteral administration is shown in Table 1.

Several of these compounds have been evaluated both parenterally and nonparenterally. This chapter will focus primarily on the effects of these drugs when administered orally.

151

TABLE 1 Representative Nonparenteral Sympathomimetic Cardiotonics

Name	References
Albuterol (salbutamol)	30, 33, 37, 39, 44-52, 128
Butopamine	53, 54
Corwin (ICI 118,587)	8, 55-59, 129-131
Ephedrine	4, 59a-61
Ibopamine (SB 7505)	24, 38, 69-77, 133, 134
Levodopa	25, 26, 68
Pirbuterol	24, 38, 69-77, 133-134
Prenalterol	9, 10, 12, 22, 23, 29, 32, 56, 77-101, 108, 115, 116, 135-147
Terbutaline	40, 41, 102-107, 109

II. MECHANISM OF ACTION AND PHARMACOLOGIC EFFECTS

A. Mechanism of Action

All sympathomimetic inotropic agents by definition either directly or indirectly stimulate myocardial adrenergic receptors to increase cardiac contractile force. These receptors appear to be predominantly of $beta_1$ type in humans. Alpha-adrenergic receptors affecting contractility may also be present in the myocardium (1), but are not discussed here because they appear to have a limited role in cardiac contraction. $Beta_2$-receptors are also present in the human heart (1a,2), and these could theoretically play a part in the contractile process. Buxton and Brunton, however, have reported that in the experimental animal, ventricular $beta_2$-receptors are located in nonmyocyte cell types (3). This finding supports the concept that $beta_1$-receptors are the primary adrenergic mediators of cardiac contractility. Extramyocardial receptor effects may in fact substantially enhance the therapeutic effects of these agents (such as vasodilation mediated by $beta_2$-receptor activation) or potentiate their adverse effects (such as alpha-receptor-mediated vasoconstriction or beta-receptor-mediated tachycardia). A diverse spectrum of compounds exists, ranging from almost pure $beta_1$-agonists to agents whose predominant effects are extracardiac.

Dopamine congeners may differ from other sympathomimetics by indirectly, as well as directly, stimulating cardiac $beta_1$-receptors. Storage pool release of myocardial catecholamines is thought to be responsible for this effect (4,5). This release appears to account for at least part of the inotropic effect of dopamine (4,5), and it has been speculated that arrhythmogenicity is increased because of this property (6).

The interaction between endogenous or exogenous sympathomimetics and myocardial beta-receptors mediating contractility has been reviewed elsewhere (7). This interaction is discussed briefly here and is presented schematically in Figure 1.

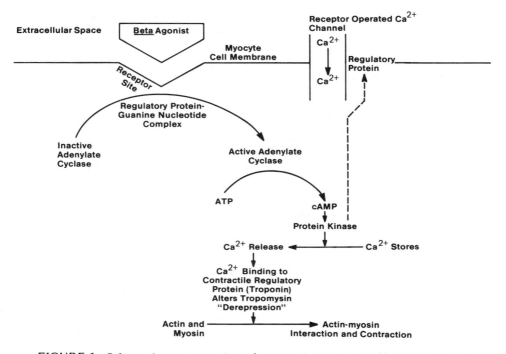

FIGURE 1 Schematic representation of proposed mechanism of myocardial cell membrane beta-receptor activation and subsequent intracellular events. Beta-agonists may directly stimulate myocyte contractile processes and enhance Ca^{2+} influx by recruitment of additional receptor-operated Ca^{2+} channels. The latter effect is illustrated by the broken line.

Beta-agonist-mediated receptor activation results in a sequence of biochemical events involving adenylate cyclase and guanine nucleotide regulatory protein in or near the cell membrane. These events ultimately produce increased intracellular calcium concentration in the region of troponin C, an inhibitory protein regulating actin-myosin interaction. Calcium-induced binding to troponin produces "derepression" of actin and myosin, thus enhancing myofibrillar shortening and global cardiac contraction. Additional recruitment of receptor-operated cell membrane calcium channels may also be induced by sympathomimetics. Relaxation of cardiac muscle is enhanced by beta-adrenergic stimulation; this property may contribute to a therapeutic effect in the failing ventricle (8,9).

It is evident that modulation of the $beta_1$-receptor agonist properties of these agents is possible. This may occur through alterations in $beta_1$-receptor density or affinity, administration of other agents which alter beta-receptor properties (such as beta-adrenergic blocking agents), or alterations in the chemical structure of the sympathomimetic (for example, production of a drug with both agonist and antagonist properties). In addition, a wide variety of interactions between beta agonists and other cardiovascular compounds is possible, as discussed in the section on drug interactions.

B. Hemodynamic Effects

The primary cardiovascular properties of oral sympathomimetics are due to the enhanced rate and force of cardiac contraction and the accompanying direct or reflex vasoactive properties. Specific responses are dependent on several factors, including the presence and severity of heart failure, the dose and duration of therapy, and the particular agent used. The pharmacologic properties associated with acute administration are discussed here. The problem of drug tolerance during chronic administration of these agents is referred to in the section on limitations.

In general, heart rate is increased due to stimulation of the sinoatrial (SA) node beta-receptors, although this effect is often attenuated in the presence of heart failure. Cardiac output is increased, predominantly by enhanced stroke volume and to a lesser extent by increased heart rate. Increased cardiac stroke volume reflects direct stimulation of contractile receptors and with some agents it reflects diminished arteriolar resistance ($\downarrow$ afterload) as well. It appears that the predominant contractile effect of sympathomimetics in the diseased ventricle may be on the residual normal myocardium rather than on abnormal tissue. In the case of ischemic ventricular dysfunction, normal tissue responsiveness to beta-agonists clearly exceeds that of the ischemic myocardium (10,11). In addition, the level of sympathetic activation prior to administration may be a major determinant of responsiveness. Hemodynamic response to the $beta_1$-agonist prenalterol, for example, appears to be diminished in subjects with increased heart rate or elevated plasma norepinephrine concentrations (12).

Systemic arterial pressure responds variably to sympathomimetics. Agents with prominent $beta_2$-agonist properties (such as terbutaline or albuterol) may increase pulse pressure and reduce mean pressure. Other compounds may elevate systemic arterial pressure by producing a cardiac output increase which more than offsets intrinsic vasodilating properties, or by directly stimulating vasoconstriction (such as agents with alpha agonist properties). Reflexly diminished vasoconstriction is also frequently elicited by a rising cardiac output. The overall effect is often a reduction in calculated systemic vascular resistance, particularly in the presence of heart failure. Because of direct or reflexly mediated vasodilation, there tends to be little or no change in systemic arterial pressure despite an increased cardiac output.

The LV filling pressure is decreased due to increased ventricular emptying in systole and enhanced diastolic compliance. Isovolumetric and ejection phase indices of LV function are enhanced by direct inotropic effect, arteriolar relaxation, or by both mechanisms. The LV peak rate of pressure development (dP/dt_{max}), LV ejection fraction and stroke work, and noninvasive systolic time interval indices of LV performance are all improved. In short-term treatment, the depressed ventricular function curve of the failing ventricle returns toward normal in response to the positive inotropic effect, and ventricular dilation diminishes.

Hemodynamic performance of the right ventricle (RV) and pulmonary circulation are also generally improved by sympathomimetic cardiotonics. Heart failure is associated with elevated pulmonary vascular resistance and increased RV filling pressure, both of which decline with administration of these agents. Direct or reflex relaxation of pulmonary resistance vessels and improved RV emptying are thought to occur in a manner analogous to systemic hemodynamic effects.

C. Myocardial Metabolic and Coronary Blood Flow Effects

Augmented myocardial oxygen consumption and myocardial blood flow frequently accompany the circulatory effects of sympathomimetic agents. Heart rate and contractile force, two major determinants of myocardial oxygen consumption, are increased by sympathetic stimulation. Increased systemic arterial pressure, if present, also contributes to the increased myocardial oxygen demand. Elevated cardiac oxygen requirements, however, are at least partly offset by a reduction in ventricular wall tension due to diminished ventricular size and pressure and increased myocardial blood flow. Reduced wall tension results from the inotropic and vasodilator properties of sympathomimetic cardiotonics. Increased myocardial blood flow may result from metabolically mediated or direct coronary vasodilation, increased coronary perfusion pressure, and possibly, enhanced collateral flow. The overall effect on oxygen balance in the ischemic ventricle is highly variable. Some sympathomimetic agents appear to worsen ischemic injury by diverting blood flow from underperfused tissue ("coronary steal" phenomenon) (11), whereas others may directly enhance oxygen delivery to ischemic myocardium. Because of this variability, assessment of the effect of each individual inotropic agent on myocardial metabolism is necessary.

D. Cardiac Electrophysiological Effects

Cardiac conduction system effects and arrhythmogenic potential frequently coexist with other cardiac effects of sympathomimetics. An increased rate of SA node discharge and enhanced atrioventricular (AV) conduction are present. In addition, increased automaticity from direct stimulation of ectopic ventricular or supraventricular foci may occur with resultant arrhythmias. Re-entrant dysrhythmias may also be provoked by direct effects on re-entry circuits or indirectly by aggravation of cardiac ischemia. Concurrent administration of other potentially arrhythmogenic agents (such as cardiac glycosides), hypotension, hypoxia, electrolyte abnormalities, and acid-base disturbances are frequently present in advanced

TABLE 2 Cardiovascular Properties of Nonparenteral Sympathomimetics

Parameter	Effect
Cardiac output	↑
Heart rate	↑
Stroke volume	↑
Systemic arterial pressure	Variable
LV filling pressure	↓ or →
LV stroke work	↑
RV filling pressure	Usually ↓
Systemic vascular resistance	Usually ↓
Pulmonary vascular resistance	Usually ↓
Coronary blood flow	Usually ↓
Myocardial oxygen consumption	Variable (usually ↑)
Cardiac electrophysiological effects	↑
SA node discharge	↑
AV conduction	↑
Automaticity	↑

Note: ↑ increased, ↓ decreased, → unchanged. LV = left ventricle; RV = right ventricle; SA = sinoatrial; AV = atrioventricular.

congestive heart failure; these factors may compound the arrhythmogenicity of sympathomimetic cardiotonics. Table 2 summarizes the cardiovascular effects of such agents.

E. Extracardiac Effects

Extracardiac effects of sympathomimetic agents are complex, and limited information is available for several compounds. Both circulatory and noncirculatory organ systems are affected.

1. Regional Blood Flow Alterations

The specific regional distribution of the increased cardiac output induced by sympathomimetics is incompletely understood. Heart failure itself produces marked alterations in regional blood flow distribution (13,14), with proportionately greater flow to the brain and heart and reduced flow to other vascular beds, including those of the skin and kidney. Blood flow distribution within a specific organ may also be altered by heart failure. This finding has been noted in the renal circulation (15,16), and it may occur in other organs. Studies of regional blood flow have been performed with the parenteral inotropic agents dobutamine and dopamine. Leier and colleagues (17) found no change in hepatic blood flow with either agent during sustained infusion in cardiomyopathic heart failure, although dobutamine increased forearm blood flow. Renal blood flow was not significantly altered by either drug during maintenance infusion. Vatner and colleagues noted similar results during acute dobutamine infusion in normal conscious dogs (18). In barbiturate anesthetized dogs, Robie and Goldberg (19) reported greater increases in renal and mesenteric blood flow with dopamine than with dobutamine. In normal conscious dogs, Liang and Hood (20) found that high-dose dobutamine infusions increased stomach blood flow as well as femoral and diaphragmatic skeletal muscle blood flow. The same group found similar regional blood flow changes with dobutamine administration following myocardial infarction (21).

Sustained (24 hr) intravenous prenalterol infusion in human subjects with heart failure has also been shown to improve forearm blood flow measured by plethysmography (22), and acute prenalterol infusion in the conscious dog enhances iliac blood flow (23). Pirbuterol has likewise been shown to enhance forearm blood flow and diminish forearm vascular resistance in heart failure (24). Whether the effects of these relatively short-term infusions are sustained during chronic oral sympathomimetic administration is uncertain.

2. Dopaminergic Effects

Parenterally administered dopamine selectively stimulates dopaminergic receptors, including renovascular receptors, producing increased urine flow. This property appears to be shared by its orally active precursor, levodopa (25,26) and by other dopaminelike oral inotropic agents (27,28). Postsynaptic dopamine-1 (DA_1) receptor stimulation is the likely mechanism.

3. Noncirculatory Effects

Because of the potential for prolonged use, noncardiovascular pharmacologic properties of sympathomimetic agents are also of theoretical and practical importance. Adrenergic regulation of skeletal muscle function, hormone and lipid metabolism, pulmonary function, and hematologic parameters is known to occur. However, only limited information regarding the effects of chronic sympathomimetic administration on these diverse functions is available. Several endocrine functions involve adrenergic receptors. Enhanced insulin release, enhanced glycogenolysis, and diminished serum potassium are potential adverse effects of prolonged sympathetic stimulation. Prenalterol has been reported to elevate plasma insulin levels (22,29), possibly by direct pancreatic $beta_1$-agonist activity. This effect is shared by other agents with $beta_1$-agonist activity (30,31). Plasma glucagon levels have been reported to rise with albuterol (30). Glycogenolysis is also enhanced by beta stimulation, and the net metabolic effect is often an increase in blood glucose concentration (29,30). This elevation in blood glucose may be more pronounced in diabetic subjects (29). However, there is substantial variability in these hormonal responses, and not all investigators have reported significant alterations in glucose, insulin, and glucagon levels (22,32). Reduced circulating potassium concentrations have been

reported with several beta-sympathomimetic agents, including albuterol, prenalterol, and isoproterenol (33-35). This effect is extrarenal, and appears to be due to
insulin-mediated potassium entry into cells or to activation of beta-dependent sodium-potassium ATPase (33-35). Beta$_2$-receptors appear to be the predominant
beta-adrenergic receptors responsible for this effect (34). Renin release is also
strongly influenced by beta-adrenergic stimulation, and increased plasma renin activity and elevations of plasma angiotensin II concentration can occur with administration of these inotropic agents (22,36,37). A diminished hemodynamic response
due to vasoconstriction and salt and fluid retention could result from this effect,
particularly if diuretics are not concurrently employed. Lipolysis depends largely
on beta-adrenergic regulation and increased levels of circulating free fatty acids
result from beta-agonist administration (30,38,39,40). Plasma triglyceride concentrations, however, do not appear to be altered acutely (29). Long-term effects on
plasma triglyceride, total serum cholesterol, and high-density lipoprotein cholesterol
levels are unknown. Beta-agonists may improve pulmonary function by bronchial
smooth muscle relaxation, diminished pulmonary vascular resistance, and increased
ventilation (41,42). Peripheral blood platelet count is also diminished by sympathomimetic cardiotonics, but the effect appears to be modest in subjects with initially normal platelet counts (42a). Skeletal muscle beta$_2$-receptor stimulation may
produce tremor, a relatively common side effect with terbutaline (41).

F. Pharmacologic Aspects of Oral Administration

Specific pharmacologic and pharmaceutical problems are inherent in the development of sympathetic stimulants intended for oral administration. An unmodified
catecholamine structure is unsuitable because of widespread catecholamine degra-
dative enzymes (catechol-O-methyltransferase and monoamine oxidase) present in
the digestive tract and liver (41). Sublingual administration does diminish the "first-
pass" effect of hepatic degradation; however, the generally short duration of action with this route of administration significantly limits its usefulness. Modification of the chemical structure of endogenous or synthetic catecholamines has been
the most widely used approach to improve oral bioavailability for this class of cardiotonics.

III. SPECIFIC AGENTS

This section discusses results reported with specific agents, presented alphabetically.
When available, studies pertinent to long-term oral administration are emphasized.

A. Albuterol (Salbutamol)

Albuterol (salbutamol) directly stimulates both beta$_1$ and beta$_2$-receptors; the latter effect appears predominant, particularly at lower doses (44). Arteriolar relaxa-

tion occurs, with a lesser inotropic effect. Albuterol has been widely used in bronchospastic disorders because of its relative beta$_2$-agonist specificity. Several intravenous trials have demonstrated its hemodynamic efficacy in acute LV dysfunction complicating myocardial infarction, including cardiogenic shock (45-49). In chronic heart failure, increased cardiac output, a reduction in elevated ventricular filling pressure and volume, and reduced systemic vascular resistance have also been reported after acute administration either intravenously or orally (50-52,44). These beneficial effects occur in both ischemic and nonischemic heart failure (50-52,44). Sharma and Goodwin reported improved hemodynamic performance during exercise as well as at rest (50). Enhanced cardiovascular effects are elicited when vasodilators (isosorbide dinitrate or sodium nitroprusside) are administered concurrently with albuterol (48,51). The results of long-term oral administration of this agent have not been reported.

B. Butopamine

Butopamine was synthesized in an attempt to develop an orally effective dobutamine derivative. A catechol ring hydrogen atom and a side chain beta-hydroxyl group were exchanged. Alteration of the parent compound to eliminate catechol-O-methyltransferase degradation in the digestive tract, however, produced an agent with reduced inotropic properties, but a significant retained chronotropic effect (53,54). Thompson and co-workers reported increased cardiac output and stroke work and reduced systemic and pulmonary vascular resistance after intravenous butopamine administration in congestive heart failure, but for equal increments in cardiac output, butopamine increased heart rate more than dobutamine (53). Two of eight patients developed substantial increases in ventricular ectopic activity during butopamine infusion. In normal human volunteers a prolonged butopamine infusion also produced pronounced chronotropic effects (54). In addition, it blunted isoproterenol and exercise-induced tachycardia for more than 48 hours after the infusion was discontinued. The latter effect may be due to beta-receptor "down regulation" after continuous sympathomimetic administration.

C. Corwin (ICI 118,587)

Corwin (ICI 118,587), like prenalterol, is a partial beta-agonist which appears to produce relatively selective beta$_1$-receptor stimulation (55,8,56). At low concentrations, or in states of diminished sympathetic drive, its agonist effects predominate; however, antagonist effects are more pronounced at higher doses or in states of heightened sympathetic activity (55,8,57). This property may have beneficial consequences in circumstances in which an excess inotropic response could be detrimental, as in ischemic heart disease. Rousseau et al. (58) demonstrated favorable hemodynamic and myocardial metabolic effects (unaltered myocardial oxygen consumption and lactate extraction) in patients with prior myocardial infarction.

The majority of these subjects, however, had well-preserved LV function. In moderate-to-severe cardiac failure due to idiopathic dilated cardiomyopathy, corwin has been reported to enhance indices of LV function (increased dP/dt_{max} and cardiac output with decreased ventricular filling pressure) without altering heart rate (59). Corwin possesses a relatively flat dose-response curve (55), an expected property of a partial beta-agonist. At present, there are insufficient data to assess the effects of long-term corwin administration in congestive heart failure.

D. Ephedrine

Ephedrine, a noncatecholamine, has pharmacologic properties similar to ephinephrine, producing both beta- and alpha-adrenergic stimulation. Unlike catecholamines, it is resistant to gastrointestinal degradation and it possesses a long duraction of action. Peripheral norepinephrine release may account for a significant portion of its cardiovascular effects (59a). Bronchodilation and nasal decongestion have been ephedrine's primary therapeutic applications. Franciosa and Cohn evaluated oral ephedrine as a single agent and combined ephedrine and intravenous sodium nitroprusside in 11 patients with severe congestive heart failure (60). Oral ephedrine alone enhanced cardiac output and diminished systemic vascular resistance. However, increases in heart rate, systemic arterial pressure, and pressure-rate product accompanied these effects. Combined nitroprusside and ephedrine administration produced a more pronounced favorable hemodynamic response than ephedrine alone. In addition, mean systemic arterial pressure declined and pressure-rate product was insignificantly altered from baseline when both agents were given together. There were no major adverse effects of ephedrine.

Chronic oral administration of ephedrine, however, has not been reported in congestive heart failure. As single-agent therapy, several disadvantages exist. First, an elevated pressure-rate product suggests increased myocardial oxygen consumption, with the attendant risk of myocardial ischemia. In addition, tolerance to ephedrine occurs rapidly. Also, ephedrine (as well as other sympathomimetic agents) has been reported to produce myocardial damage during prolonged administration (61).

E. Ibopamine (SB 7505)

The orally active dopamine derivative (diisobutyric ester of N-methyl-dopamine), ibopamine (SB 7505), possesses pharmacologic properties similar to its parent compound. Like dopamine, ibopamine appears to selectively activate renovascular and other dopaminergic receptors (27,28,62). Myocardial beta-receptor stimulation may occur through both direct and indirect effects. Longhini and co-workers (63) demonstrated increased arterial blood flow, decreased peripheral arterial resistance, and increased venous capacitance in the upper extremity of normal volunteers after a single oral dose of 150 mg of ibopamine. Systemic arterial pressure and heart rate were unaffected. Similar hemodynamic effects were sustained after 5-day oral administration. Peripheral vascular effects were counteracted by sulpiride, a specific vascular dopaminergic antagonist.

Several studies have assessed the hemodynamic effects of ibopamine in congestive heart failure. Reffo et al. demonstrated increased cardiac index and stroke work index, decreased mean pulmonary artery pressure, and decreased systemic and pulmonary vascular resistance after oral ibopamine administration in 10 subjects with refractory heart failure (64). Heart rate, mean systemic arterial pressure and pulmonary wedge pressure were insignificantly altered. Col and colleagues studied oral ibopamine in 8 patients with severe (New York Heart Association functional class IV) heart failure and found very similar results (65). Ren, Unverferth, and Leier compared the effects of oral ibopamine to intravenous dopamine in subjects with heart failure of various etiologies (66). Peripheral vascular effects were more prominent than improved inotropic parameters, with reduced peripheral and pulmonary arterial resistance and increased cardiac index and stroke volume index. Systemic and pulmonary artery pressure, heart rate, and ventricular filling pressures were unaltered. These results were comparable to those noted for 2-4 μg/kg per min of intravenous dopamine. Hemodynamic effects of oral ibopamine were relatively short-lived, with a duration of action of approximately 4 hours. Interestingly, a transient increase in central pressures occurred 30 minutes after oral ibopamine administration.

Dei Cas and co-workers noninvasively evaluated both acute and chronic (7-day) oral ibopamine therapy in heart failure subjects (28). Systolic time interval indices of LV function (pre-ejection period and electromechanical systole) improved significantly, without changes in heart rate or blood pressure. Hemodynamic effects were sustained over 7 days, and were associated with increased urine flow and increased urinary sodium and potassium excretion. The same group reported the effects of oral ibopamine on invasive hemodynamic parameters in idiopathic dilated cardiomyopathy subjects (67) with results very similar to those previously described. Hemodynamic effects were sustained for 5-7 hr. Trials examining the effects of chronic oral ibopamine therapy in cardiac failure are currently underway.

F. Levodopa

Dopa (dihydroxyphenylalanine) is the immediate biochemical precursor of dopamine. Aromatic acid decarboxylase enzymatically catalyzes this conversion. As previously discussed, dopamine can both directly and indirectly stimulate cardiac beta-receptors. Oral levodopa has been extensively used in the treatment of Parkinson's disease; in 1971 Finlay and co-workers reported that oral levodopa increased renal plasma flow, glomerular filtration rate, and sodium and potassium excretion in subjects with Parkinson's disease. Similar data were obtained in three additional subjects with heart failure. Systolic time interval indices of LV function improved acutely in both groups of patients (25). These studies were extended to assess chronic oral therapy in Parkinson's disease (68). It was demonstrated that acute hemodynamic effects were attenuated by 3 months. Inotropic responsiveness to intravenous dopamine and epinephrine, however, were unaltered by chronic levodopa administration, suggesting that altered myocardial beta-receptor responsiveness was not the cause of tolerance. Acute beta-adrenergic blockade abolished the inotropic effect of levodopa. Heart rate did not significantly change during acute or chronic administration, but systemic arterial pressure declined with acute levodopa administration.

Rajfer and colleagues reported both acute and chronic beneficial hemodynamic effects in a subsequent assessment of oral levodopa in chronic severe heart failure (26). A dose of 1.5-2.0 g increased depressed stroke volume index and cardiac index while decreasing systemic vascular resistance in 10 subjects with New York Heart Association functional class III-IV cardiac failure. Mean arterial pressure, heart rate, and ventricular filling pressures were unaltered. Hemodynamic effects were temporally associated with peak plasma levodopa and dopamine concentrations. Six chronically treated patients experienced sustained hemodynamic benefit from oral levodopa administered for several months. A similar pattern of hemodynamic response occurred during long-term treatment with the additional effect of a reduced heart rate.

G. Pirbuterol

Pirbuterol, like terbutaline and albuterol, predominantly stimulates $beta_2$-adrenergic receptors, with some direct $beta_1$-effect. $Beta_2$-receptor activation enhances vasodilation, including venodilation. Pirbuterol possesses greater $beta_2$-receptor specificity and a longer duration of action than albuterol (69,24).

Several investigators have assessed both acute and chronic pirbuterol administration in heart failure. Awan and associates (24) evaluated the acute circulatory effects of oral pirbuterol (0.4 mg/kg) in patients with heart failure refractory to digitalis and diuretics. Sustained (6 hr) hemodynamic benefit occurred with both increased cardiac output and reduced LV filling pressure. Systemic vascular resistance declined, as did forearm venous tone. Forearm blood flow increased. Systemic arterial pressure was diminished, presumably due to pronounced arteriolar relaxation. Heart rate increases were modest, with no significant change in pressure-rate product, suggesting unaltered myocardial oxygen consumption. Other investigators have measured myocardial oxygen consumption and have supported this finding (70), as well as pirbuterol's acute beneficial hemodynamic effects. The addition of oral isosorbide dinitrate to pirbuterol further reduced the LV filling pressure, reduced the right atrial pressure, and reduced the heart rate (71). Variable effects of pirbuterol on coronary sinus flow have been reported (70,38). None of these investigations indicate clinical or biochemical parameters of worsened myocardial ischemia in the presence of coronary artery disease. Fowler and co-workers, however, reported increased myocardial oxygen consumption and decreased myocardial lactate extraction after high-dose intravenous pirbuterol in six patients with heart failure due to ischemic heart disease (72). One of six developed angina pectoris.

Long-term trials of oral pirbuterol have resulted in conflicting results. Pamelia et al. (73) documented acute hemodynamic benefit, with subsequent chronic oral therapy in the 20 subjects investigated. Of the 20 subjects, 6 failed to respond by 3 weeks. The 14 responders received oral pirbuterol therapy for an additional 3 weeks. After 6 weeks, responsive patients had a significantly improved heart failure symptom score as well as increased treadmill exercise duration. In responders, the investigators also noted increased LV ejection fraction, cardiac index, and LV stroke work, with reduced LV filling pressure and systemic vascular resistance. Subjects with nonischemic LV dysfunction and those with higher baseline LV ejection fractions responded more favorably than other subjects. Awan and co-workers also reported symptomatic improvement, increased exercise duration, and improved LV ejection fraction after 6 weeks of oral pirbuterol treatment of cardiac failure due to ischemic heart disease (74). A large British trial (75) of 63 patients treated with oral pirbuterol for 3 months also reported improved exercise capacity and symptoms status in the 35 subjects who completed the study. Chronic hemodynamic improvement was also demonstrated in these 35 subjects. The favorable hemodynamic responses, however, had no apparent relationship to increased exercise duration and symptomatic benefit. Of the 63 patients, 12 (19%) had pirbuterol withdrawn because of adverse effects or a poor response; 20 subjects (32%) died during therapy, 16 of whom were taking pirbuterol at the time of death. Because the trial was uncontrolled, it is unknown whether this high mortality was excessive compared to alternative modes of therapy.

In a smaller trial of New York Heart Association functional class III-IV heart failure, Colucci and collaborators found largely negative effects of long-term (1 month) oral pirbuterol therapy despite an initial beneficial effect (76). The LV ejection fraction and cardiac index returned to baseline after chronic drug administration. This attenuated hemodynamic effect was associated with decreased peripheral blood lymphocyte beta-receptor density. Drug tolerance due to cardiac or vascular beta-receptor "down regulation" appears to be the mechanism for this effect. This phenomenon is discussed further in the section on limitations of nonparenteral sympathomimetic agents.

In summary, oral pirbuterol clearly produces favorable acute hemodynamic effects in congestive heart failure. Several investigators have reported continued long-term clinical and hemodynamic improvement. However, a significant portion of patients are intolerant of long-term pirbuterol or experience no beneficial effect. Pharmacologic tolerance attributable to beta-receptor "down regulation" is a significant concern with long-term administration of this agent.

H. Prenalterol

The beta-agonist prenalterol is among the most well-studied nonparenteral sympathomimetic cardiotonics. Prenalterol is a relatively cardioselective drug with mixed beta-agonist and beta-antagonist properties. There are similarities to isoproterenol in its chemical structure, although prenalterol is not a true catecholamine. Whether prenalterol is truly $beta_1$-selective is controversial. Kenakin and coworkers (77,78,79) have suggested that this agent may lack $beta_1$-selectivity, but still possesses relative cardiac selectivity by virtue of organ-specific differences in receptor-tissue coupling responses. Some radioligand binding studies, however, have supported $beta_1$-receptor selectivity with prenalterol (56). Because it is effective both parenterally and orally, it possesses the advantage of interchangeable administration by either route. As do other sympathomimetics, prenalterol produces acute beneficial hemodynamic effects in congestive heart failure. Increased cardiac output (mediated by increased stroke volume and heart rate), reduced LV filling pressure, increased LV ejection fraction, and diminished pulmonary and systemic vascular resistance have been reported (80-86). Enhanced diastolic emptying is also present (9). Dose-dependent increases in cardiac cyclic adenosine monophosphate (cyclic AMP) concentrations are mediated by myocardial $beta_1$-receptor activation (43). In ischemic LV dysfunction, prenalterol improves hemodynamic performance at the cost of increased myocardial oxygen consumption, although coronary blood flow increases proportionately (87,88). The latter effect may be due in part to direct coronary vasodilation (89). The majority of subjects have no adverse cardiac metabolic response (87,88). Stimulation of residual nonischemic myocardium appears to be prenalterol's primary inotropic mechanism in the regionally ischemic ventricle (10). In the presence of acute myocardial infarction, prenalterol has also been shown to improve hemodynamic performance and to reverse unwanted side effects of beta-adrenergic blockade. Because of its residual antagonist characteristics, prenalterol does not produce the full inotropic effect of a pure beta-agonist such as dobutamine (90). Heart failure subjects with markers of high basal sympathetic activity (elevated resting heart rate or elevated resting plasma norepinephrine level) appear to respond less favorably to prenalterol (12). This may reflect a general tendency for patients with high sympathetic tone to be relatively unresponsive to further sympathetic stimulation.

After acute oral administration, prenalterol causes sustained hemodynamic effects for approximately 4-6 hr. It is well absorbed from the gastrointestinal tract, although significant hepatic metabolism occurs after oral administration (91). Approximately 13% of an oral dose and approximately 60% of an intravenous dose appear in the urine as unchanged drug (91). An elimination phase half-life ($t_{1/2}$) of approximately 2-3 hr has been reported for both normal subjects and heart failure patients (91-93). The systemic metabolic effects of prenalterol administration reflect beta adrenergic activation. Lipolysis occurs, elevating plasma free fatty acid concentrations. Modest increases in circulating insulin and glucose have been reported (29). Plasma catecholamine, cortisol, and glucagon concentrations are unaltered during intravenous infusion in heart failure subjects, while plasma renin activity and plasma angiotension II levels rise (22). Renal effects in heart failure subjects reported during prenalterol administration include increasing urinary potassium and aldosterone excretion and unaltered sodium excretion (22). In normal volunteers, however, plasma renin activity and urinary potassium excretion were unaltered, while transient decreases in urinary volume and free water clearance were noted (94).

Cardiac electrophysiological effects of prenalterol include an increased rate of SA node discharge and accelerated AV conduction. The functional refractory period of the atrium, AV node, and ventricle are decreased. His-Purkinje conduction is unaltered, but ventricular automaticity is enhanced (95). Knauss and co-workers (96) found an increased rate of sinus arrhythmias in normal volunteers. Significant ventricular arrhythmias have been noted in some reports, particularly in the presence of cardiac inschemia (97,80,98). Concurrent administration of cardiac glycosides may increase prenalterol's arrhythmogenic potential (80).

Several long-term clinical trials of oral prenalterol in congestive heart failure have been performed. Despite the short-term hemodynamic benefit obtainable with this cardiotonic, long-term studies generally have been less encouraging. Roubin and co-workers (99) performed a double-blind cross-over trial of 11 patients with moderately severe LV dysfunction (mean LV ejection fraction of 24%). Each subject received 2 weeks of placebo or prenalterol. With the exception of a reduced heart rate during exercise, prenalterol produced no significant hemodynamic effect. Similarly, exercise duration and exercise oxygen consumption were unaltered. Lambertz et al. performed a double-blind trial of oral prenalterol versus placebo in severe (New York Heart Association functional class III or IV) congestive heart failure (98). While receiving maintenance digitalis and diuretic therapy, 16 subjects were randomized (8 in each group) to double-blind therapy for 3 months followed by open-label prenalterol for 3 additional months. Short-term improvement in echocardiographic ejection fraction and circumferential fiber shortening and in LV filling pressure and stroke work were demonstrated, but these effects were no longer present at 3 and 6 months. Maximum exercise workload was similarly improved short-term, but returned to baseline by 6 months. Symptom status also failed to improve during long-term therapy.

In an uncontrolled trial, Strauer and collaborators (100) also noted attenuation of prenalterol's beneficial acute hemodynamic effects after 4-7 months of therapy. Currie and co-workers in fact observed hemodynamic deterioration during sustained oral prenalterol administration in patients with New York Heart Association functional class II-III heart failure (101). Sharpe and Coxon, however, reported improved cardiac output and exercise capacity during long-term (4 weeks) treatment with this cardiotonic in an uncontrolled trial (86). These studies suggest that the majority of subjects receiving chronic oral prenalterol therapy are unlikely to respond despite unequivocal acute beneficial hemodynamic effects.

I. Terbutaline

Terbutaline, a beta-agonist, possesses pharmacologic properties similar to albuterol (salbutamol) and pirbuterol. Beta$_2$-receptor stimulation predominates, with significant residual beta$_1$ activity. Terbutaline was initially employed as a bronchodilator, but was noted to enhance contractile function in the normal ventricle (102). Several groups have subsequently evaluated its acute hemodynamic effects in congestive heart failure. Slutsky (103) noted improved cardiac output, stroke volume, LV filling pressure, and LV and RV ejection fraction after inhalation of 0.5 mg of nebulized terbutaline by 13 subjects with ischemic or cardiomyopathic heart failure. In addition, systemic vascular resistance and ventricular volumes declines. Systemic arterial pO$_2$ declined, however, and the hemodynamic response was brief. Intravenous terbutaline produced similar acute hemodynamic improvement in 8 subjects with severe heart failure from a variety of causes (mean cardiac index of 1.79 liters/min/m^2) in a study reported by Wang and co-workers (104). Potential adverse effects included increased heart rate and decreased plasma potassium concentration. In patients with heart failure due to coronary artery disease, the same group reported similar favorable systemic circulatory effects (increased cardiac index and stroke volume with reduced LV filling pressure and reduced vascular resistance) after acute intravenous terbutaline administration (105). Coronary sinus oxygen content and myocardial lactate extraction were unaltered. No clinical or electrocardiographic evidence of myocardial ischemia was noted. Slutsky et al. (105) demonstrated increased LV ejection fraction and stroke volume following terbutaline administration in ischemic heart disease patients with prior myocardial infarction. The maximal response occurred in subjects with significantly decreased LV contractile function. In chronic obstructive lung disease with RV dysfunction, terbutaline offers the advantage of a cardiac inotropic effect coupled with pulmonary vascular and bronchial relaxation. One group has reported improved RV performance, enhanced systemic oxygen delivery, and diminished pulmonary vascular resistance in such patients following acute terbutaline administration (107).

These observations support the short-term use of terbutaline as a cardiotonic with favorable vasodilating properties. The availability of oral terbutaline offers the possibility of long-term nonparenteral therapy with this agent. However, insufficient data are available to support chronic oral terbutaline therapy in congestive heart failure.

IV. DRUG INTERACTIONS

Multiple interactions between nonparenteral sympathomimetic cardiotonics and other pharmacologic agents may occur. Three major types of drug interactions are discussed here: (1) interactions involving other agents with beta-adrenergic activity, (2) interactions with other cardiovascular drugs which enhance the hemodynamic effects of oral sympathomimetics, and (3) interactions with other cardiovascular agents which may produce a deleterious effect.

A. Interactions with Other Beta-Receptor Active Agents

Both beta-adrenergic blocking agents and beta-adrenergic stimulants may modify the outcome of administering sympathomimetic cardiotonics. Prior administration of beta-receptor blocking agents substantially diminishes the hemodynamic response of beta-agonists (92). An increased dose of the agonist may be necessary to overcome this effect. Beta-stimulants of the type discussed in this chapter may be of use in reversing unwanted hemodynamic effects of beta-blockade in patients with reduced contractile function (108).

Complex drug interactions may result from the administration of more than one beta-adrenergic inotropic agent at or nearly at the same time. Although different agents in this class of cardiotonics are ordinarily not employed simultaneously, sequential administration of these agents is not unlikely in the clinical setting. Prior treatment with a partial beta-agonist (such as corwin or prenalterol) or a dopaminergic agent may lead to significant reductions in the hemodynamic response to subsequently administered full beta-agonists (54,55). Prior administration of full agonists may produce the same effect (78). "Down regulation" of beta-adrenergic receptors appears to be the most likely cause for this phenomenon. Markedly diminished inotropic responsiveness should be anticipated during sequential administration of sympathetic stimulants. In addition, the cardiovascular response to other sympathetic stimuli (such as exercise) is also blunted (54). It is not known how long this homologous beta-receptor "down regulation" persists after discontinuation of all the beta-adrenergic stimulants discussed in this chapter. One week after discontinuation of chronic oral pirbuterol therapy for congestive heart failure, Colucci et al. noted a return to pretreatment lymphocyte beta-receptor density in a small number of patients (76).

B. Favorable Interactions with Other Cardiovascular Agents

The major beneficial interaction with other cardiovascular drugs is the hemodynamic improvement obtained with the combined administration of a vasodilator and inotropic agent. The complementary effects of these agents optimize reductions in elevated ventricular filling pressure and vascular resistance while providing maximal cardiac output. Agents with predominant venodilating properties (such as isosorbide dinitrate), arteriolar dilating properties (such as hydralazine) or mixed vasorelaxant effects (such as captopril or nitroprusside) enhance the response to nonparenteral sympathomimetics (48,51,60,71,82,109). Concurrent parenteral use of both dopaminergic and pure beta-agonists has been employed in cardiogenic shock in an attempt to maximize both renal blood flow and overall cardiovascular performance (110). Combined use of these agents in chronic heart failure has not been investigated.

C. Deleterious Drug Interactions

Potentially adverse drug interactions may occur with the use of these agents. The most serious interaction is enhanced arrhythmogenicity, which may occur by a direct effect, or because of reduced blood potassium concentrations caused by concurrent diuretic use coupled with beta-receptor-mediated entry of plasma potassium into cells. Cardiac glycoside administration may also enhance the arrhythmogenic potential of sympathetic stimulants. There is evidence that serious ventricular arrhythmias inducible by digitalis are in part due to enhanced sympathetic drive (111). The combination of sympathomimetic cardiotonics and digitalis may excessively increase sympathetic tone and precipitate significant rhythm disturbances (80). Other inotropic agents, including the bipyridine derivative amrinone, may also predispose to cardiac arrhythmias (112). Whether an adverse proarrhythmic interaction between bipyridine inotropic agents and sympathomimetics exists is uncertain.

V. LIMITATIONS

Several major potential limitations of chronic administration of sympathetic stimulants in congestive heart failure are discussed here—drug tolerance, aggravated myocardial ischemia, arrhythmogenicity, and myocardial structural damage. Adverse metabolic effects of long-term administration of these agents (such as altered glucose, lipid, or potassium homeostasis) is another limitation. The latter possibility is discussed in the section on pharmacologic effects.

A. Drug Tolerance

Diminished pharmacologic effectiveness despite sustained administration may be a major limitation of sympathetic stimulants. A reduced inotropic response has been reported after chronic pirbuterol and prenalteral therapy (76,98,99,101). Tolerance during prolonged administration of beta-adrenergic stimulants in reversible airways disease has also been recognized. The primary mechanism by which cardiovascular tolerance may develop appears to be homologous "down regulation" of beta-receptors to further stimulation after repetitive or sustained beta-adrenergic receptor activation. A reduced number of receptors or altered receptor affinity or both may play a role. Reduced numbers of beta-receptors may result from "internalization" of exposed receptors on the cell surface to unexposed sites within the cell membrane or intracellular space (7,113). Heart failure itself causes diminished cardiac beta-receptor density (114), probably in part due to elevated circulating catecholamine levels. A further reduction in receptor number due to superimposed sympathetic stimulation may be deleterious if the failing ventricle is dependent on these receptors for inotropic support. Altered receptor affinity may represent a shift from a high affinity state to a lower affinity state, or a reduction in affinity in the presence of only one affinity state (7). Precisely which mechanisms play a role in possible beta-receptor "down regulation" during prolonged sympathetic inotropic stimulation in congestive heart failure is uncertain. After 1 month of pirbuterol administration, Colucci and co-workers reported a decrease in beta-receptor number on peripheral blood lymphocytes associated with a diminished LV ejection fraction response (76). Upon withdrawal of pirbuterol, lymphocyte beta-receptor number returned to prior levels in the small number of subjects in which this effect was evaluated.

The effect of partial beta-agonists (for example, corwin or prenalterol) on cardiac beta-receptor density during chronic administration is unknown. Because these agents possess both agonist and antagonist properties, receptor interactions are complex. Diminished hemodynamic responsiveness during sustained prenalterol therapy (98,99,101) raises the possibility that beta-receptor desensitization may occur with these agents.

Intermittent drug administration or progressively increased dosage may be effective in diminishing receptor "down regulation" or the effects of this phenomenon. Use of these techniques, however, has not been adequately evaluated with this class of agents. Limas and Limas have shown that isoproterenol induced beta-receptor "down regulation" occurs rapidly and is short-lived after withdrawal (113). Therefore, intermittent administration with interruptions of as little as 1 or 2 days could theoretically restore receptor responsiveness.

A second mechanism by which prolonged sympathetic stimulation may result in a diminished therapeutic response is activation of the renin-angiotensin-aldosterone system or other counteractive neuroendocrine axes. Stimulation of the renin-angiotensin-aldosterone system has been reported with nonparenteral sympathomimetic cardiotonics (115,22,36,37), and resultant vasoconstriction and salt and water retention could diminish their hemodynamic effects. This phenomenon has been labeled "pseudotolerance" because tissue responsiveness to the inotropic agent is not necessarily altered. Concurrent diuretic use, however, is frequently employed and ordinarily offsets any fluid retention that may occur.

B. Aggravation of Myocardial Ischemia

As previously noted, myocardial ischemia may be worsened by elevated oxygen demand out of proportion to increases in ischemic zone blood flow. This appears to occur infrequently with the agents discussed here. However, instances of aggravated cardiac ischemia have been reported in several patients receiving beta-adrenergic stimulants (72,88,116). This adverse outcome appears to be more frequent at higher doses (72). Agents with partial antagonist properties may partially protect against this effect by producing only limited inotropic stimulation.

C. Arrhythmogenicity

Arrhythmogenicity is a potentially serious limitation of all inotropic agents which activate beta-receptors. The frequent coexistence of LV dysfunction and serious rhythm disturbances is a major clinical concern even in the absence of exogenous sympathetic stimulants. As previously discussed, cardiac electrophysiological effects of these agents include enhanced automaticity. In addition, re-entrant or afterdepolarization dysrhythmias may also be precipitated. Published reports of the cardiotonics discussed in this chapter suggest that the majority of patients do not develop serious arrhythmias during long-term administration. However, isolated instances of serious rhythm disturbances have been recorded (80,97,98). As previously noted, cardiac glycosides appear to enhance sympathetic stimulation of the heart, and their arrhythmogenic effect may be potentiated by concurrent beta-agonist administration.

D. Possible Adverse Cardiac Morphological Effects

Structural cardiac pathology is an additional adverse effect that may be associated with prolonged administration of beta-agonists. Animal studies have demonstrated cardiac enzyme release, myocardial degeneration, cardiac fibrosis, and and inflammation with pharmacologic doses of catecholamines (117-121). Pheochromocytomas and high doses of exogenous catecholamines in human patients can also produce significant structural abnormalities and cardiac dysfunction (117,122,123). Diminished contractile function accompanies prolonged norepinephrine infusions in experimental animals (124). Hemodynamic dysfunction in this setting may be due not only to diminished beta-receptor density but also in part to structural abnormalities, since myocardial responsiveness to nonadrenergic stimuli (such as exogenous calcium) is also depressed (124). Extrapolation of these data to chronic human heart failure is conjectural, but it is possible that high levels of endogenous sympathetic drive induced by heart failure coupled with chronic exogenous sympathomimetic cardiotonic use may be detrimental to cardiac structure and function. Favorable myocyte ultrastructural changes after sustained intravenous dobutamine infusion however, suggest that this effect does not occur during short-term use (125).

Reports that chronic beta-adrenoceptor blockade is beneficial in congestive heart failure are of interest in light of the potential adverse effects of prolonged sympathomimetic use (126). It is somewhat paradoxical that both beta-agonists and beta-blocking agents have been proposed for chronic heart failure therapy. Both could have a useful role if patients were prospectively selected for the appropriate therapy. At present this is not possible, but future studies may delineate this issue more clearly. Some patients with advanced heart failure do appear to be dependent on sustained sympathetic drive (127). One hypothesis which may reconcile these conflicting reports is that heart failure subjects with low sympathetic tone may benefit from further beta-adrenergic stimulation, while those with higher sympathetic drive may benefit from beta-adrenergic inhibition as long as they are not critically dependent on sympathetic support.

VI. SUMMARY

The pharmacologic rationale, mechanism of action, clinical effects, limitations, and drug interactions of nonparenteral sympathomimetic cardiotonics intended for chronic oral use in congestive heart failure have been discussed in this chapter. This heterogeneous class of agents, which either directly or indirectly stimulate myocardial beta-receptors, may ultimately prove to be of long-term benefit in drug treatment of the failing ventricle. However, at present the use of these inotropic agents is largely investigational. Significant unanswered questions remain regarding their long-term effects on hemodynamic performance, cardiac arrhythmias, endocrine function, and cardiac structure. Whether these agents alter the adverse prognosis associated with heart failure is unknown. Preliminary data from the few long-term trials undertaken with this class of cardiotonics are conflicting, although they suggest that the pharmacologic response to these drugs diminishes with time.

ACKNOWLEDGMENTS

The author gratefully acknowledges the manuscript preparation skills and support of Donna McEwen, Sylvia Leonard, Pat Moore, Jackie Jennings, and Susan Clifford.

REFERENCES

1. H. Aass, T. Skomedal, and J. Osnes. Demonstration of an *alpha* adrenoceptor-mediated inotropic effect of norepinephrine in rabbit papillary muscle. *J. Pharmacol. Exper. Ther. 226*: 572 (1983).
1a. P. Robberecht, M. Delhaye, G. Taton, P. De Neef, M. Waelbroeck, J. M. De Smet, J. L. Leclerc, P. Chatelain, and J. Christophe. The human heart beta-adrenergic receptors. *Mol. Pharmacol. 24*: 169 (1983).
2. G. L. Stiles, S. Taylor, and R. J. Lefkowitz. Human cardiac beta-adrenergic receptors: Subtype heterogeneity delineated by direct radioligand binding. *Life Sci. 33*: 467 (1983).
3. I. L. O. Buxton, and L. L. Brunton. Direct analysis of β-adrenergic receptor subtypes on intact adult ventricular myocytes of the rat. *Circ. Res. 56*: 126 (1985).
4. L. I. Goldberg. Cardiovascular and renal actions of dopamine: Potential clinical applications. *Pharmacol. Rev. 24*: 1 (1972).
5. L. I. Goldberg, Y.-Y. Hsieh, and L. Resnekov. Newer catecholamines for treatment of heart failure and shock: an update on dopamine and a first look at dobutamine. *Prog. Cardiovasc. Dis. 19*: 317 (1977).
6. R. R. Tuttle, and J. Mills. Development of a new catecholamine to selectively increase cardiac contractility. *Circ. Res. 36*: 185 (1975).

7. R. J. Lefkowitz. Direct binding studies of adrenergic receptors: Biochemical, physiological, and clinical implications. *Ann. Intern. Med. 91*: 450 (1979).

8. H. Pouleur, H. Van Mechelen, H. Balasim, M. F. Rousseau, and A. A. Charlier. Comparisons of the inotropic effects of the *beta*-1-adrenoceptor partial agonists SL 75.177.10 and ICI 118,587 with digoxin on the intact canine heart. *J. Cardiovasc. Pharmacol. 6*: 720 (1984).

9. F. Cucchini, G. Baldi, R. Bolognesi, R. Farrari, and O. Visioli. Effect of prenalterol on contractility, relaxation, and filling phase in coronary artery disease patients with previous myocardial infarction. *J. Cardiovasc. Pharmacol. 6*: 822 (1984).

10. P. C. Kirlin, J. L. Romson, B. Pitt, and B. Lucchesi. Regional myocardial contractile response to the *beta*-adrenergic stimulant prenalterol in the conscious dog following myocardial infarction. *Pharmacol. 28*: 51 (1984).

11. S. F. Vatner, and H. Baig. The effects of inotropic stimulation on ischemic myocardium in conscious dogs. *Trans. Assoc. Am. Physicians 91*: 282 (1978).

12. H. Leinberger, W. Maurer, H. Haneisen, G. Schuler, and W. Kubler. Dose-dependent hemodynamic response to prenalterol in patients with congestive heart failure. *Acta Med. Scand. (suppl.) 659*: 299 (1982).

13. R. Zelis, S. H. Nellis, J. Longhurst, G. Lee, and D. T. Mason. Abnormalities in the regional circulations accompanying congestive heart failure. *Prog. Cardiovasc. Dis. 18*: 181 (1975).

14. C. B. Higgins, S. F. Vatner, D. Franklin, and E. Braunwald. Effects of experimentally produced heart failure on the peripheral vascular response to severe exercise in conscious dogs. *Circ. Res. 31*: 186 (1972).

15. M. M. Kilcoyne, D. H. Schmidt, and P. J. Cannon. Intrarenal blood flow in congestive heart failure. *Circulation 47*: 786 (1973).

16. H. V. Sparks, H. H. Kopald, S. Carriere, J. E. Chimoskey, M. Kinoshita, and A. C. Barger. Intrarenal distribution of blood flow with chronic congestive heart failure. *Am. J. Physiol. 223*: 840 (1972).

17. C. V. Leier, P. T. Heban, P. Huss, C. A. Bush, and R. P. Lewis. Comparative systemic and regional hemodynamic effects of dopamine and dobutamine in patients with cardiomyopathic heart failure. *Circulation 58*: 466 (1978).

18. S. F. Vatner, R. J. McRitchie, and E. Braunwald. Effects of dobutamine on left ventricular performance, coronary dynamics, and distribution of cardiac output in conscious dogs. *J. Clin. Invest. 53*: 1265 (1974).

19. N. W. Robie, and L. I. Goldberg. Comparative systemic and regional hemodynamic effects of dopamine and dobutamine. *Am. Heart J. 90*: 340 (1975).

20. C.-S. Liang, and W. B. Hood, Jr. Dobutamine infusion in conscious dogs with and without autonomic nervous system inhibition: Effects on systemic hemodynamics, regional blood flows and cardiac metabolism. *J. Pharmacol. Exp. Ther. 211*: 698 (1979).

21. C.-S. Liang, J. M. Yi, L. G. Sherman, J. Black, H. Gavras, and W. B. Hood, Jr. Dobutamine infusion in conscious dogs with and without acute myocardial infarction. *Circ. Res. 49*: 170 (1981).

22. D. Fitzpatrick, H. Ikram, M. G. Nicholls, and E. A. Espiner. Hemodynamic, hormonal and electrolyte responses to prenalterol infusion in heart failure. *Circulation 67*: 613 (1983).

23. W. T. Manders, S. F. Vatner, and E. Braunwald. Cardio-selective beta adrenergic stimulation with prenalterol in the conscious dog. *J. Pharmacol. Exp. Ther. 215*: 266 (1980).
24. N. A. Awan, M. K. Evenson, K. E. Needham, T. O. Evans, J. Hermanovich, C. R. Taylor, E. Amsterdam, and D. T. Mason. Hemodynamic effects of oral pirbuterol in chronic severe congestive heart failure. *Circulation 63*: 96 (1981).
25. G. D. Finlay, T. L. Whitsett, E. A. Cucinell, and L. I. Goldberg. Augmentation of sodium and potassium excretion, glomerular filtration rate and renal plasma flow by levodopa. *N. Engl. J. Med. 284*: 865 (1971).
26. S. I. Rajfer, A. H. Anton, J. D. Rossen, and L. I. Goldberg. Beneficial hemodynamic effects of oral levodopa in heart failure. *N. Engl. J. Med. 310*: 1357 (1984).
27. G. F. Melloni, G. M. Minoja, G. Scorazzati, R. Bauer, B. Brusoni, and P. Ghiradi. Renal effects of SB 7505: A double-blind study. *Eur. J. Clin. Pharmacol. 19*: 177 (1981).
28. L. Dei Cas, C. Manca, B. Bernardini, G. Vasini, and O. Visioli. Noninvasive evaluation of the effects of oral ibopamine (SB 7505) on cardiac and renal function in patients with congestive heart failure. *J. Cardiovasc. Pharmacol. 4*: 436 (1982).
29. D. Oltmans. Metabolic effects of prenalterol in diabetic patients. *Acta Med. Scand. (suppl.) 659*: 147 (1982).
30. D. E. Potter, L. C. Woodson, R. R. Kempen, and S. Ellis. Comparative metabolic and cardiovascular effects of carbuterol, isoproterenol, metaproterenol and salbutamol in the baboon. *Horm. Metab. Res. 12*: 323 (1980).
31. G. Holm. Adrenergic regulation of insulin release. *Acta Med. Scand. (suppl.) 672*: 21 (1983).
32. G. Klein, A. Wirtzfeld, G. Schmidt, and T. Eilker. Metabolic effects of prenalterol in healthy volunteers. *Acta Med. Scand. (suppl.) 659*: 137 (1982).
33. M. L. Wahlqvist, E. A. Shanahan, P. M. Dennis, P. T. Pullan, and E. G. Wilmshurst. Cardiac effects of salbutamol-induced hypokalaemia in the conscious dog. *Clin. Exp. Pharmacol. Physiol. 5*: 617 (1978).
34. H. H. Vincent, F. Boomsma, A. J. Man in 't Veld, F. H. M. Derkx, G. J. Wenting, and M. A. D. H. Schalekamp. Effects of selective and nonselective β-agonists on plasma potassium and norepinephrine. *J. Cardiovasc. Pharmacol. 6*: 107 (1984).
35. T. Clausen. Adrenergic control of Na^+-K^+-homeostasis. *Acta Med. Scand. (suppl.) 672*: 111 (1983).
36. B. E. Karlberg. Adrenergic regulation of renin release and effects on angiotensin and aldosterone. *Acta Med. Scand. (suppl.) 672*: 33 (1983).
37. E. J. Johns, H. K. Richards, and B. Singer. Effects of adrenaline, noradrenaline, isoprenaline and salbutamol on the production and release of renin by isolated renal cortical cells of the cat. *Br. J. Pharmacol. 53*: 67 (1975).
38. A. D. Timmis, G. Bergman, L. Walker, M. J. Monaghan, and D. E. Jewitt. Potential value of oral *beta*-2-adrenoceptor agonists in congestive heart failure: a haemodynamic and metabolic study. *Int. J. Cardiol. 5*: 327 (1984).
39. J. G. Kelly, and R. G. Shanks. Metabolic and cardiovascular effects of isoprenaline and salbutamol in the dog. *Br. J. Pharmacol. 53*: 157 (1975).

40. S. Carlstrom, and H. Westling. Metabolic, circulatory and respiratory effects of a new sympathomimetic *beta*-receptor-stimulating agent, terbutaline, compared with those of orciprenaline. *Acta Med. Scand. (suppl.) 512*: 33 (1970).

41. N. Weiner. Norepinephrine, epinephrine and the sympathomimetic amines. In *The Pharmacologic Basis of Therapeutics*. A. G. Gilman, L. S. Goodman, and A. Gilman (eds.). Macmillan, New York, 1980.

42. D. D. Heistad, R. C. Wheeler, A. L. Mark, P. G. Schmid, and F. M. Abboud. Effects of adrenergic stimulation on ventilation in man. *J. Clin. Invest. 51*: 1469 (1972).

42a. K. Freden, P. Lundborg, L. Vilen, and J. Kutti. The peripheral platelet count in response to adrenergic alpha and beta-1-receptor stimulation. *Scand. J. Haematol. 21*: 427 (1978).

43. H. Mattson, A. Hedberg, and E. Carlsson. Basic pharmacologic properties of prenalterol. *Acta Med. Scand. (suppl.) 659*: 9 (1982).

44. P. D. V. Bourdillon, J. R. Dawson, R. A. Foale, A. D. Timmis, P. A. Poole-Wilson, and G. C. Sutton. Salbutamol in treatment of heart failure. *Br. Heart J. 43*: 206 (1980).

45. J. R. Dawson, P. A. Poole-Wilson, and G. C. Sutton. Salbutamol in cardiogenic shock-complicating acute myocardial infarctions. *Br. Heart J. 43*: 523 (1980).

46. A. D. Timmis, M. B. Fowler, and D. A. Chamberlain. Comparison of haemodynamic responses to dopamine and salbutamol in severe cardiogenic shock complicating acute myocardial infarction. *Br. Med. J. 282*: 7 (1981).

47. A. D. Timmis, S. K. Strak, and D. A. Chamberlain. Haemodynamic effects of salbutamol in patients with acute myocardial infarction and severe left ventricular dysfunction. *Br. Med. J. 2*: 1101 (1979).

48. M. B. Fowler, A. D. Timmis, and D. A. Chamberlain. Synergistic effects of a combined salbutamol-nitroprusside regimen in acute myocardial infarction and severe left ventricular failure. *Br. Med. J. 280*: 435 (1980).

49. M. B. Fowler, A. D. Timmis, J. P. Crick, R. Vincent, and D. A. Chamberlain. Comparison of haemodynamic responses to dobutamine and salbutamol in cardiogenic shock after acute myocardial infarction. *Br. Med. J. 284*: 73 (1982).

50. B. Sharma, and J. F. Goodwin. Beneficial effect of salbutamol on cardiac function in severe congestive cardiomyopathy. *Circulation 58*: 449 (1978).

51. J. D. Stephens, S. O. Banim, and R. A. J. Spurrell. Haemodynamic effects of oral salbutamol alone and in combination with sublingual isosorbide dinitrate in patients with severe congestive cardiac failure. *Br. Heart J. 43*: 220 (1980).

52. J. Mifune, K. Kuramoto, K. Ueda, S. Matsushita, I. Kuwajima, M. Sakai, T. Iwasaki, N. Moroki, and M. Murakami. Hemodynamic effects of salbutamol, and oral long-acting beta-stimulant, in patients with congestive heart failure. *Am. Heart J. 104*: 1011 (1982).

53. M. J. Thompson, P. Huss, D. V. Unverferth, A. Fasola, and C. V. Leier. Hemodynamic effects of intravenous butopamine in congestive heart failure. *Clin. Pharmacol. Ther. 28*: 324 (1980).

54. C. V. Leier, S. Nelson, R. D. Magorien, H. Boudoulas, L. Gibb, and D. V. Unverferth. Heart rate responsiveness after sustained chronotopic stimulation with a *beta*-1-adrenergic receptor agonist. *J. Lab. Clin. Med. 101*: 955 (1983).

55. A. Nuttall, and H. M. Snow. The cardiovascular effects of ICI 118,587: A *beta*-1-adrenoceptor partial agonist. *Br. J. Pharmacol. 77*: 381 (1982).

56. N. Cook, A. Richardson, and D. B. Barnett. Comparison of the *beta*-1 selective affinity of prenalterol and corwin demonstrated by radioligand binding. *Eur. J. Pharmacol. 98*: 407 (1984).

57. M. Fukushima, H. Sato, T. Matsuyama, H. Ozaki, M. Matsumoto, M. Inoue, and H. Abe. Hemodynamic effects of new *beta*-1 partial agonist (ICI 118-587) in association with sympathetic nervous activity. *J. Am. Coll. Cardiol. (abstr.) 5*: 517 (1985).

58. M. F. Rousseau, H. Pouleur, and M. F. Vincent. Effects of a cardioselective *beta*-1 partial agonist (corwin) on left ventricular function and myocardial metabolism in patients with previous myocardial infarction. *Am. J. Cardiol. 51*: 1267 (1983).

59. S. Simonsen. Haemodynamic effects of ICI 118,587 in cardiomyopathy. *Br. Heart J. 51*: 654 (1984).

59a. J. N. Cohn. Comparative cardiovascular effects of tyramine, ephedrine, and norepinephrine in man. *Circ. Res. 16*: 174 (1965).

60. J. A. Franciosa, and J. N. Cohn. Hemodynamic effects of oral ephedrine given alone or combined with nitroprusside infusion in patients with severe left ventricular failure. *Am. J. Cardiol. 43*: 79 (1979).

61. L. B. To, J. F. Sangster, D. Rampling, and I. Cammens. Ephedrine-induced cardiomyopathy. *Med. J. Aust. 2*: 35 (1980).

62. S. Stefoni, L. Coli, G. Masconi, and R. Prandini. Ibopamine (SB 7505) in normal subjects and in chronic renal failure: A preliminary report. *Br. J. Clin. Pharmac. 1*: 69 (1981).

63. C. Longhini, G. F. Musacci, L. Ansani, T. Toselli, M. Artioli, L. Bianco, and P. Ghirardi. Effect of ibopamine on peripheral haemodynamics. *Eur. J. Clin. Pharmacol. 24*: 585 (1983).

64. G. C. Reffo, M. Turrin, A. Gabellini, and C. Forattini. Haemodynamic evaluation of ibopamine in severe congestive heart failure. *Eur. J. Clin. Pharmacol. 26*: 19 (1984).

65. J. Col, E. Mievis, and M. Reynaert. Ibopamine in very severe congestive heart failure: Pilot haemodynamic invasive assessment. *Eur. J. Clin. Pharmacol. 24*: 297 (1983).

66. J. H. Ren, D. V. Unverferth, and C. V. Leier. The dopamine congener, ibopamine, in congestive heart failure. *J. Cardiovasc. Pharmacol. 6*: 748 (1984).

67. L. Dei Cas, R. Bolognesi, F. Cucchini, A. Fappani, S. Riva, and O. Visioli. Hemodynamic effects of ibopamine in patients with idiopathic congestive cardiomyopathy. *J. Cardiovasc. Pharmac. 5*: 249 (1983).

68. T. L. Whitsett, and L. I. Goldberg. Effects of levodopa on systolic preejection period, blood pressure, and heart rate during acute and chronic treatment of Parkinson's disease. *Circulation 45*: 97 (1972).

69. B. Sharma, J. Hoback, G. Francis, M. Hodges, R. W. Asinger, J. N. Cohn, and C. R. Taylor. Pirbuterol: An oral beta agonist for therapy of congestive heart failure. *Circulation (abstr.) 59-60*: II-229 (1979).

70. R. E. Rude, Z. Turi, E. J. Brown, B. H. Lorell, W. S. Colucci, G. H. Mudge, Jr., C. R. Taylor, and W. Grossman. Acute effects of oral pirbuterol on myo-

cardial oxygen metabolism and systemic hemodynamics in chronic congestive heart failure. *Circulation 64*: 139 (1981).

71. J. Balyliss, M. Norell, R. Canepa-Anson, S. R. Reuben, P. A. Poole-Wilson, and G. C. Sutton. Acute haemodynamic comparison of amrinone and pirbuterol in chronic heart failure. *Br. Heart J. 49*: 214 (1983).

72. M. B. Fowler, G. Bergman, A. D. Timmis, L. Atkinson, L. Howell, and D. E. Jewitt. Pirbuterol therapy in left ventricular failure associated with a positive inotropic action and what is its metabolic cost? *Circulation (abstr.) 66*: II-137 (1982).

73. F. X. Pamelia, M. Georghiade, G. A. Beller, H. L. Bishop, A. Y. Olukotun, C. R. Taylor, D. D. Watson, A. M. Grunwald, J. Sirowatka, and B. A. Carabello. Acute and long-term hemodynamic effects of oral pirbuterol in patients with chronic severe congestive heart failure: Randomized double-blind trial. *Am. Heart J. 106*: 1369 (1983).

74. N. A. Awan, K. Needham, M. K. Evenson, J. Hermanovich, J. A. Joye, A. N. DeMaria, and D. T. Mason. Therapeutic efficacy of oral pirbuterol in severe chronic congestive heart failure: Acute hemodynamic and long-term ambulatory evaluation. *Am. Heart J. 102*: 555 (1981).

75. J. R. Dawson, R. Canepa-Anson, P. Kuan, S. R. Reuben, P. A. Poole-Wilson, and G. C. Sutton. Symptoms, haemodynamics, and exercise capacity during long term treatment of chronic heart failure: Experience with pirbuterol. *Br. Heart J. 50*: 282 (1983).

76. W. S. Colucci, R. W. Alexander, G. H. Williams, R. E. Rude, B. L. Holman, M. A. Konstam, J. Wynne, G. H. Mudge, Jr., and E. Braunwald. Decreased lymphocyte *beta*-adrenergic-receptor density in patients with heart failure and tolerance to the beta-adrenergic agonist pirbuterol. *N. Engl. J. Med. 305*: 185 (1981).

77. T. P. Kenakin, and R. M. Ferris. Effects of *in vivo-beta* adrenoceptor down-regulation on cardiac responses to prenalterol and pirbuterol. *J. Cardiovasc. Pharmacol. 5*: 90 (1983).

78. T. P. Kenakin, and D. Beek. In vitro studies on the cardiac activity of prenalterol with reference to use in congestive heart failure. *J. Pharmacol. Exp. Ther. 220*: 77 (1982).

79. T. P. Kenakin. Prenalterol as a selective cardiostimulant: Differences between organ and receptor selectivity. *J. Cardiovasc. Pharmacol. 7*: 208 (1985).

80. P. C. Kirlin, and B. Pitt. Hemodynamic effects of intravenous prenalterol in severe heart failure. *Am. J. Cardiol. 670* (1981).

81. N. A. Awan, K. E. Needham, M. K. Evenson, A. Win, and D. T. Mason. Hemodynamic actions of prenalterol in severe congestive heart failure due to chronic coronary disease. *Am. Heart J. 101*: 158 (1981).

82. H. Drexler, H. Lollgen, and H. Just. Short- and long-term effects of hydralazine and combined hydralazine-prenalterol therapy in severe chronic congestive heart failure. *Klin. Wochenschr. 59*: 647 (1981).

83. W. Klein, D. Brandt, and E. Maurer. Hemodynamic assessment of prenalterol: A cardioselective beta agonist in patients with impaired left ventricular function. *Clin. Cardiol. 4*: 325 (1981).

84. F. Waagstein, S. Reiz, R. Ariniego, and A. Hjalmarson. Clinical results with prenalterol in patients with heart failure. *Am. Heart J. 102*: 548 (1981).
85. A. C. Tweddel, R. G. Murray, D. Pearson, W. Martin, and I. Hutton. Cardiovascular effects of prenalterol on rest and exercise haemodynamics in patients with chronic congestive cardiac failure. *Br. Heart J. 47*: 375 (1982).
86. D. N. Sharp, and R. Coxon. Prenalterol, an oral *beta*-1 adrenoceptor agonist, in the treatment of chronic heart failure. *Eur. J. Clin. Pharmacol. 25*: 539 (1983).
87. W. Kupper, K. H. Kuck, F. Sonntag, and W. Bleifeld. Effects of the new *beta*-1-agonist prenalterol on myocardial metabolism and left ventricular function in patients with chronic heart failure. *Circulation (abstr.) 62*: III-298 (1980).
88. P. C. Kirlin, J. A. Walton, Jr., J. F. Brymer, G. Beauman, and B. Pitt. Hemodynamic and myocardial metabolic effects of the *beta*-agonist prenalterol in ischemic left ventricular dysfunction. *J. Cardiovasc. Pharmacol. 6*: 825 (1984).
89. S. F. Vatner, T. H. Hintze, and P. Macho. Regulation of large coronary arteries by *beta*-adrenergic mechanisms in the conscious dog. *Circ. Res. 51*: 56 (1982).
90. P. C. Kirlin, B. Pitt, and B. R. Lucchesi. Comparative effects of prenalterol and dobutamine in a canine model of acute ischemic heart failure. *J. Cardiovasc. Pharmacol. 3*: 896 (1981).
91. C. Graffner, K.-J. Hoffmann, G. Johnsson, P. Lundborg, and O. Ronn. Pharmacokinetic studies in man of the selective *beta*-1-adrenoceptor agonist, prenalterol. *Eur. J. Clin. Pharmacol. 20*: 91 (1981).
92. O. Ronn, C. Graffner, G. Johnsson, L. Jordo, P. Lundborg, and J. Wikstrand. Haemodynamic effects and pharmacokinetics of a new selective *beta*-1 adrenoceptor agonist, prenalterol, and its interaction with metoprolol in man. *Eur. J. Clin. Pharmacol. 15*: 9 (1979).
93. O. Ronn. Pharmacokinetics of prenalterol in healthy subjects and patients with congestive heart failure. *Acta Med. Scand. (suppl.) 659*: 89 (1982).
94. K. A. Meurer, R. Lang, V. Hombach, and A. Helber. Effects of a *beta*-1-selective adrenergic agonist in normal human volunteers. *Klin. Wochenschr. 58*: 425 (1980).
95. E. Moore, G. Aberg, J. F. Spear, A. B. Hodess, I. Herrman, and G. Adler. Inotropic, chronotropic and dromotropic effects of prenalterol, a new cardiostimulant drug. *Acta Med. Scand. (suppl.) 659*: 53 (1982).
96. M. Knaus, B. Pfister, U. C. Dubach, and P. R. Imhof. Human pharmacology studies with a new, orally active stimulant of cardiac adrenergic beta-receptors. *Am. Heart J. 95*: 602 (1978).
97. W. Doering, B. Waner, and J. Isbary. Effects of I.V. prenalterol in patients with severe cardiac failure at rest and during exercise. *Acta Med. Scand. (suppl.) 659*: 307 (1982).
98. H. Lambertz, J. Meyer, and R. Erbel. Long-term hemodynamic effects of prenalterol in patients with severe congestive heart failure. *Circulation 69*: 298 (1984).
99. G. S. Roubin, M. B. Christopher, Y. P. Choong, S. Devenish-Meares, N. N. Sadick, P. J. Fletcher, D. T. Kelly, and P. J. Harris. *Beta*-adrenergic stimula-

tion of the failing ventricle: A double-blind, randomized trial of sustained oral therapy with prenalterol. *Circulation 69*: 955 (1984).

100. B. E. Strauer, I. Bohn, B. Hahn, A. Kment, and U. Motz. Contractile, coronary, and metabolic effects of the acute and long-term treatment of cardiac failure with prenalterol. *J. Cardiovasc. Pharmacol. 6*: 491 (1984).

101. P. J. Currie, M. J. Kelly, K. Middlebrook, J. Federman, E. Sainsbury, J. Ashley, and A. Pitt. Acute intravenous and sustained oral treatment with the *beta*-1 agonist prenalterol in patients with chronic severe cardiac failure. *Br. Heart J. 51*: 530 (1984).

102. B. Arner, A. Bertler, T. Karlefors, and H. Westling. Circulatory effects of orciprenaline, adrenaline and a new sympathomimetic *beta*-receptor-stimulating agent, terbutaline, in normal human subjects. *Acta Med. Scand. (suppl.) 512*: 25 (1970).

103. R. Slutsky. Hemodynamic effects of inhaled terbutaline in congestive heart failure patients without lung disease: Beneficial cardiotonic and vasodilator beta-agonist properties evaluated by radionuclide angiography. *Am. Heart J. 101*: 556 (1981).

104. R. Y. C. Wang, T. F. Tse, D. Y. C. Yu, P. K. Lee, and M. S. S. Chow. Beneficial hemodynamic effects of intravenous terbutaline in patients with severe heart failure. *Am. Heart J. 104*: 1016 (1982).

105. R. Y. C. Wang, P. K. Lee, D. Y. C. Yu, T. F. Tse, and M. S. S. Chow. Myocardial metabolic effects of intravenous terbutaline in patients with severe heart failure due to coronary artery disease. *J. Clin. Pharmacol. 23*: 362 (1983).

106. R. Slutsky, W. Hooper, K. Gerber, W. Ashburn, G. Curtis, and J. Karliner. Left ventricular size and function after subcutaneous administration of terbutaline. *Chest 79*: 501 (1981).

107. B. N. Brent, D. Mahler, H. J. Berger, R. A. Matthay, L. Pytlik, and B. L. Zaret. Augmentation of right ventricular performance in chronic obstructive pulmonary disease by terbutaline: A combined radionuclide and hemodynamic study. *Am. J. Cardiol. 50*: 313 (1982).

108. R. Ariniego, F. Waagstein, B. Mombay, and A. Hjalmarson. Haemodynamic effects of a new *beta*-1-receptor agonist in acute myocardial infarction. *Br. Heart J. 42*: 139 (1979).

109. N. A. Awan, K. E. Needham, B. S. H. Lui, J. Rutledge, E. A. Amsterdam, and D. T. Mason. Complementary combined captopril and terbutaline therapy in severe chronic congestive heart failure. *Am. Heart J. 104*: 1224 (1982).

110. C. Richard, J. L. Ricome, A. Rimailho, G. Bottineau, and P. Auzepy. Combined hemodynamic effects of dopamine and dobutamine in cardiogenic shock. *Circulation 67*: 620 (1983).

111. R. A. Gillis, A. Raines, Y. J. Sohn, B. Levitt, and F. G. Standaert. Neuroexcitatory effects of digitalis and their role in the development of cardiac arrhythmias. *J. Pharmacol. Exper. Ther. 183*: 154 (1972).

112. C. V. Leier, K. Dalpiaz, P. Huss, J. B. Hermiller, R. D. Magorien, T. M. Bashore, and D. V. Unverferth. Amrinone therapy for congestive heart failure

in outpatients with idiopathic dilated cardiomyopathy. *Am. J. Cardiol. 52*: 304 (1983).

113. C. J. Limas, and C. Limas. Rapid recovery of cardiac β-adrenergic receptors after isoproterenol-induced "down"-regulation. *Circ. Res. 55*: 524 (1984).

114. M. R. Bristow, R. Ginsburg, W. Minobe, R. S. Cubicciotti, W. S. Sageman, K. Lurie, M. E. Billingham, D. C. Harrison, and E. B. Stinson. Decreased catecholamine sensitivity and B-adrenergic-receptor density in failing human hearts. *N. Engl. J. Med. 307*: 205 (1982).

115. U. Kopp, M. Aurell, L. Svensson, and B. Ablad. Effects of prenalterol, a *beta*-1 adrenoceptor agonist, on renal function in anaesthetized dogs. *Acta Physiol. Scand. (abstr.) Suppl. 473*: 49 (1979).

116. A. L. Muir, W. J. Hannan, N. G. Dewhurst, and I. M. Slessor. The effects of intravenous prenalterol on ventricular performance, as assessed by radionuclide ventriculography, in patients with ischaemic heart disease. *Br. J. Clin. Pharmacol. 12*: 475 (1981).

117. J. E. Szakacs, and A. Cannon. 1-Norepinephrine myocarditis. *Am. J. Clin. Pathol. 30*: 425 (1958).

118. R. S. Eliot, G. L. Todd, F. C. Clayton, and G. M. Pieper. Experimental catecholamine-induced acute myocardial necrosis. *Adv. Cardiol. 25*: 107 (1978).

119. A. J. Moss, I. Vittands, and E. A. Schenk. Cardiovascular effects of sustained norepinephrine infusions. I. Hemodynamics. *Circ. Res. 18*: 596 (1966).

120. E. A. Schenk, and A. J. Moss, Cardiovascular effects of sustained norepinephrine infusions. II. Morphology. *Circ. Res. 18*: 605 (1966).

121. E. A. Shenk, R. Galbreath, and A. J. Moss. Cardiovascular effects of sustained norepinephrine infusions. III. Lactic dehydrogenase isoenzyme release. *Circ. Res. 18*: 616 (1966).

122. I. K. Kline. Myocardial alterations associated with pheochromocytomas. *Am. J. Pathol. 38*: 539 (1961).

123. R. Garcia, and J. M. Jennings. Pheochromocytoma masquerading as a cardiomyopathy. *Am. J. Cardiol. 29*: 568 (1972).

124. R. R. Fripp, J. C. Lee, and S. E. Downing. Inotropic responsiveness of the heart in catecholamine cardiomyopathy. *Am. Heart J. 101*: 17 (1981).

125. D. V. Unververth, C. V. Leier, R. D. Magorien, R. Croskery, J. R. Svirbely, A. J. Kolibash, M. R. Dick, J. A. Mecham, and N. Baba. Improvement of human myocardial mitochondria after dobutamine: A quantitative ultrastructural study. *J. Pharmacol. Exp. Ther. 215*: 527 (1980).

126. K. Swedberg, A. Hjalmarson, F. Waagstein, and I. Wallentin. Beneficial effects of long-term *beta*-blockade in congestive cardiomyopathy. *Br. Heart J. 44*: 117 (1980).

127. B. I. Hoffbrand. Letter. *Lancet 1*: 1031 (1980).

128. M. H. Chamales, R. D. Gourley, and B. J. Williams. Effect of acetylcholine on changes in contractility, heart rate and phosphorylase activity produced by isoprenaline, salbutamol and aminophylline in the perfused guinea-pig heart. *Br. J. Pharmacol. 53*: 531 (1975).

129. I. Amende, R. Simon, and P. Lichtlen. Effects of a new cardioselective *beta*-1 partial agonist on left ventricular function in patients with dilative cardiomyopathy. *Circulation (abstr.) 68*: III-374 (1983).

130. G. Svensson, N. Rehnqvist, A. Sjogren, and L. Erhardt. Hemodynamic effects of ICI 118.587 (corwin) in patients with mild cardiac failure after myocardial infarction. *J. Cardiovasc. Pharmacol.* 7: 97 (1985).

131. A. Ohyagi, S. Sasayama, Y. Nakamura, J. D. Lee, Y. Kihara, and C. Kawai. Effect of ICI 118,587 on left ventricular function during graded treadmill exercise in conscious dogs. *Am. J. Cardiol.* 54: 1108 (1984).

132. K. Kawahara, and J. Inui. Analysis of the positive inotropic effect of ibopamine in the blood-perfused canin papillary muscle. *J. Cardiovasc. Pharmacol.* 7: 316 (1985).

133. R. Canepa-Anson, C. Ilsley, J. Bayliss, S. Reuben, G. Sutton, and P. Poole-Wilson. Effects of oral pirbuterol on haemodynamics, distribution of blood flow and lactate production during treadill exercise in patients with chronic heart failure. *Am. J. Cardiol. (abstr.)* 49: 1001 (1982).

134. K. P. Kunze, K. H. Kuck, A. Costard, and W. Bleifield. Acute and long term effects of oral pirbuterol in patients with chronic congestive heart failure. *Circulation (abstr.)* 68: III-374 (1983).

135. E. Carlsson, C. G. Dahlof, A. Hedberg, H. Persson, and B. Tangstrand. Differentiation of cardiac chronotropic and inotropic effects of *beta*-adrenoceptor agonists. *Neunyn-Schmiedeberg's Arch. Pharmacol.* 300: 101 (1977).

136. U. Johansson, and B. Waldeck. On the stereospecificity of the *beta*-2-adrenoceptor blocking properties of prenalterol. *J. Pharm. Pharmacol.* 32: 659 (1980).

137. T. P. Kenakin, and D. Beek. Is prenalterol (H133/80) really a selective beta 1 adrenoceptor agonist? Tissue selectivity resulting from differences in stimulus-response relationships. *J. Pharmacol. Exp. Ther. 213*: 406 (1980).

138. A. Weiss, B. Pfister, P. Imhof, P. H. Degen, D. Burckhardt, and U. C. Dubach. Haemodynamic effects, plasma concentrations and tolerance of orally administered prenalterol in man. *Eur. J. Clin. Pharmacol.* 18: 383 (1980).

139. T. Svendsen, O. J. Hartling, and J. Trap-Jensen. Immediate haemodynamic effects of prenalterol, a new adrenergic *beta*-1-receptor agonist, in healthy volunteers. *Eur. J. Clin. Pharmacol.* 18: 219 (1980).

140. N. Rohm, J. Wagner, and H. J. Schumann. The lack of a pronounced preference of prenalterol for the beta-1-adrenoceptor subtype. *Naunyn-Schmiedeberg's Arch. Pharmacol.* 315: 85 (1980).

141. G. Jennings, C. Oddie, M. Hargreaves, and A. Bobik. Cardioselectivity of prenalterol. *Circulation (abstr.)* 66: II-20 (1982).

142. D. W. Wahr, K. Swedberg, M. Rabbino, M. J. Hoyle, D. Curran, W. W. Parmley, and K. Chatterjee. Intravenous and oral prenalterol in congestive heart failure. *Am. J. Med.* 76: 999 (1984).

143. W. G. Hendry, M. B. Comerford, and E. M. M. Besterman. A dose response study with oral prenalterol in patients with chronic congestive cardiac failure. *Clin. Cardiol.* 7: 23 (1984).

144. M. C. Petch, C. Wisbey, O. Ormerod, C. Scott, and R. M. Goodfellow. Acute haemodynamic effects of oral prenalterol in severe heart failure. *Br. Heart J.* 52: 49 (1984).

145. I. Hutton, R. G. Murray, R. N. Boyes, A. P. Rae, and W. S. Hillis. Haemo-dynamic effects of prenalterol in patients with coronary heart disease. *Br. Heart J. 43*: 134 (1980).
146. M. F. Shiu, M. A. Ireland, and W. A. Littler. Hemodynamic effects of atrial pacing and prenalterol infusion in patients taking beta-adrenergic blocking drugs. *Circulation 64*: 1135 (1981).
147. G. I. C. Nelson, B. Silke, R. C. Ahuja, C. Walker, D. R. Forsyth, S. P. Ver-ma, and S. H. Taylor. Hemodynamic trial of sequential treatment with diur-etic, vasodilator, and positive inotropic drugs in left ventricular failure fol-lowing acute myocardial infarction. *Am. Heart J. 107*: 1202 (1984).

6

Phosphodiesterase Inhibition
Enoximone (MDL-17043) in the Acute and Chronic Therapy of Congestive Heart Failure

BARRY F. URETSKY
University of Pittsburgh School of Medicine, Presbyterian-University Hospital, Pittsburgh, Pennsylvania

Digitalis is the most powerful remedy we possess in restoring and maintaining [cardiac] compensation.

William Osler, 1885

This form of treatment is exactly the same as the driver gives his horse when he is greatly overloaded and the going is too heavy for him, merely a stimulation with a gad, which is just what drugs are in failure of the heart. . . .

William Hay, 1922

I. INTRODUCTION

Debate continues over the value of positive inotropic therapy in the acute and chronic treatment of congestive heart failure (1-3). This controversy has centered mainly around the digitalis compounds, the major clinically utilized inotropic agents in heart failure (4-12). The development of the intravenously active sympathomimetic inotropic agents, isoproterenol, dopamine, and dobutamine, have added a large body of data, either supporting (13-16) or opposing (17-23) the use of positive inotropic agents in the acute treatment of heart failure. Most recently, orally active agents with both positive inotropic and vasodilator properties, including the bipyridine derivatives, amrinone and milrinone, and the imidazolone derivatives, enoximone (MDL 17043) and piroximone (MDL 19205) (24), have been investigated to determine their long-term efficacy in chronic heart failure. This chapter reviews studies that concern the potential of enoximone as a clinically useful therapeutic agent, in both acute and chronic therapy for congestive heart failure.

II. PHOSPHODIESTERASE INHIBITION AND CYCLIC ADENOSINE MONOPHOSPHATE GENERATION

Enoximone is a cyclic AMP-dependent phosphodiesterase (PDE) inhibitor (25). Its proposed mechanism of action of inotropy is the generation of increased levels of intracellular cyclic AMP by inhibition of its breakdown by the enzyme phosphodiesterase. A large body of data for a number of compounds correlates increases in intracellular myocardial cyclic AMP levels and increases in contractile state (26-31). In myocardial tissue, cyclic AMP performs several actions that would facilitate both contraction and relaxation. It phosphorylates a sarcolemmal protein kinase which increases calcium conductance through the slow channel, thus enhancing the concentration of intracellular calcium (26). It also phosphorylates

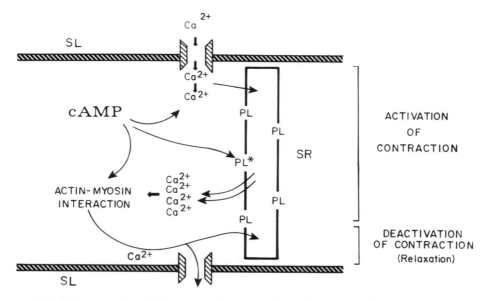

FIGURE 1 Cyclic AMP has several important functions in cardiac muscle contraction and relaxation. The strength of contraction is directly related to the concentration of intracellular calcium (Ca^{2+}). Cyclic AMP increases intracellular calcium by phosphorylating a protein kinase in the sarcolemma (SL), which increases calcium conductance through the slow channel. Cyclic AMP also phosphorylates a protein, phospholamban (PL), in the sarcoplasmic reticulum (SR). Activated phospholamban (PL*) increases calcium uptake into the SR, thus increasing the total amount of calcium which may be released into the cytoplasm on subsequent cardiac contractions. Thus, intracellular calcium concentration and the force of contraction are affected by the effects of the cyclic AMP on both the SL and SR.

a constituent of the sarcoplasmic reticulum (SR), phospholamban (32-34). Activated phospholamban enhances intracellular calcium uptake into the SR. Thus, the addition of these two actions culminates in larger SR stores of calcium available for release in future cardiac cycles (See Fig. 1).

Myocardial contractile force is directly related to the concentration of intracellular calcium (35). Intracellular calcium is raised both by calcium traversing the slow channel during depolarization and by calcium-triggered release of larger stores of calcium from the SR (35). Thus, the two actions of cyclic AMP summate in increasing contractile force by providing more intracellular calcium through the slow channel, increasing the size of the calcium signal for release of SR-stored calcium, and providing larger stores of SR calcium to be released. Cyclic AMP also decreases the affinity of calcium during active contraction for the regulatory protein troponin subunit TnI (36). This action has the effect of decreasing the cross-bridging

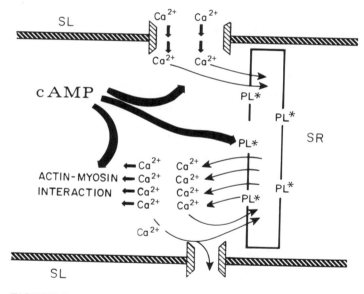

FIGURE 2 Cyclic AMP also promotes cardiac relaxation by allowing intracellular calcium to be taken up more quickly by the SR through activated phospholamban. Furthermore, the phosphorylation of the troponin subunit TnI by cyclic AMP decreases the affinity for calcium for the actin-myosin complex, thus promoting the more rapid decrease in actin-myosin cross-bridging, or more rapid cardiac relaxation. Increases in cyclic AMP, such as by beta-agonist stimulation or phosphodiesterase inhibition, will allow for greater stimulation of the related cyclic AMP effects, with consequent improvement in cardiac contraction and relaxation.

period of actin and myosin; stated conversely, this effect increases the speed of myocardial relaxation (See Fig. 2).

The methylxanthine PDE inhibitors, caffeine and theophylline, produce a lengthening rather than an abbreviation of the contractile state. This effect has been attributed to an additional action of these drugs on the SR to inhibit calcium uptake (37). If this is the case, then certain PDE inhibitors have actions other than those related to cyclic AMP generation.

It should also be pointed out that it is not certain that increased cyclic AMP levels are the basis for the inotropic effects of PDE inhibitors, or of beta-agonists. As vanBelle (38) has noted, several enzymological and stoichiometric criteria for cyclic AMP as the "second messenger" have not been fulfilled. That cyclic AMP is a major hormone for inotropic control in this regard should be accepted with caution.

III. PHOSPHODIESTERASE INHIBITION AS A MECHANISM OF SMOOTH MUSCLE RELAXATION

Vasodilation from smooth muscle relaxation results from lowering of intracellular calcium (37). Increases in cyclic AMP from PDE inhibition may decrease intracellular calcium concentration by phosphorylation of a Ca^{2+}-dependent ATPase in the SR (37). This phosphorylation increases SR calcium uptake, thereby decreasing intracellular calcium and promoting vasodilation. This SR-sequestered calcium must, in turn, be extruded extracellularly; the mechanism of this movement is unknown. Cyclic AMP also phosphorylates myosin kinase, making it less active in its combination with intracellular calcium and the regulatory protein calmodulin. The myosin kinase-calmodulin-calcium complex is required to activate myosin in order for it to cross-link with actin and produce muscular contraction (26,39).

It should be noted that the methylxanthine PDE inhibitors, caffeine and theophylline, may actually produce vasoconstriction (40). This effect has been related to inhibition of calcium uptake by the smooth muscle SR, an effect considered independent of its PDE inhibitory action.

IV. ENOXIMONE: EXPERIMENTAL STUDIES

In vitro effects of enoximone have been studied in cat papillary muscle, guinea pig left atrium, and spontaneously beating cat right atrium (41). In all three preparations, contractile force increased in a dose-dependent manner and was not blocked by alpha-, beta-, or histamine-receptor antagonists. Under constant loading conditions, the normal canine left ventricle responded to enoximone with increases in contractile force, again in a dose-dependent manner and unaffected by alpha- or beta-adrenergic blockade, reserpine-induced catecholamine depletion, bilateral vagotomy, or bilateral carotid sinus denervation (42). In the working canine heart, enoximone produced marked increases in contractile force (approximately +75%) with a smaller increase in heart rate (approximately +10%), particularly at larger doses (42). A moderate (– 35%) decrease in pulmonary artery wedge pressure and smaller decrease in systemic arterial pressure (– 10%) were reported. In a canine model of propranolol-induced heart failure, enoximone reversed abnormalities in cardiac function (42). Myocardial oxygen consumption after enoximone does not change significantly (43).

Enoximone has also produced direct arterial vasodilation in the isolated hind limb of the dog. Vasodilation was not blocked by bilateral sympathectomy, alpha- or beta-adrenergic receptor blockade, cholinergic or histaminergic receptor blockade, or prostaglandin synthesis inhibition. These findings are compatible with, but clearly not proof of, a cyclic AMP-mediated mechanism of vasodilation.

V. INTRAVENOUS ENOXIMONE IN ACUTE THERAPY FOR HEART FAILURE

Intravenous positive inotropic agents are frequently used to treat potentially reversible or to stabilize cardiac dysfunction. Such conditions include postcardiac surgery myocardial dysfunction, acute myocardial infarction, or an acute exacerbation of chronic heart failure. Intravenous positive inotropic agents have also been used in selected cases to support the failing circulation until surgical intervention, that is, until cardiac transplantation is performed (44,45). Enoximone may have a therapeutic role in all of these settings.

In patients with severe heart failure, enoximone produces dose-related changes in most central hemodynamic parameters. Using relatively large doses (an average cumulative dose of 5.8 mg/kg), we demonstrated an average 76% increase in cardiac output (46). Other studies have demonstrated the expected improvement in cardiac output related to the overall cumulative dose (47,48). This improvement is primarily the result of an increase in stroke volume, but small increases in heart rate also occur. In our initial study, which used the largest mean dose, heart rate increases were also greatest (46). These data are in accord with animal studies that demonstrate cardioacceleration with enoximone, predominantly at high doses (41). Among the effects that accompany improvement in cardiac performance have been a decrease of 30-50% in both right atrial and pulmonary artery wedge pressure. A smaller decrease in mean pulmonary artery pressures (approximately 20-25%) and systemic arterial pressure (5-20%) also have been reported. The greatest decrease in systemic arterial pressure was noted in our initial study, when the largest doses were employed; this finding emphasizes the dose-dependence of hemodynamic changes. Both systemic vascular (27-52%) and pulmonary arteriolar (21-49%) resistance fell in these initial studies.

We have demonstrated that after intravenous dosages, enoximone is hemody-
namically effective for at least 6 hours. Individual patients have shown improvement in 8-24 hr. In a preliminary study, Ferry et al. (49) have suggested that enoximone may be given as an infusion for as long as 48 hours without attenuation
of hemodynamic effect.

All studies have demonstrated that this agent may be given intravenously with
minimal side effects. An occasional episode of gastrointestinal distress has been reported, and the subjective observation of increased ventricular ectopy in individual
patients has been reported (46,47,48,50).

Improvement in cardiac performance has not been associated with large increases
in myocardial oxygen consumption. In a study by Amin et al. (47) myocardial
oxygen consumption fell by 18% (p<0.01), whereas in a study by Martin et al.
(51), myocardial oxygen consumption increased slightly (+7%) but significantly
(p<0.01). Although these results are somewhat contradictory, neither study
demonstrated large changes in myocardial oxygen consumption. Four patients
(18% of the overall population) did, however, have a positive lactate balance, suggesting the development of myocardial ischemia. Thus, although in general it may
be said that enoximone does not have a major effect on myocardial oxygen consumption and does not produce adverse myocardial effects (that is, lactate production), such adverse effects may occur in individual cases. For this reason we
suggest minimizing the dose to the lowest effective hemodynamic dose possible.
In this context, it should be emphasized that such a conclusion may also be drawn
regarding the use of the bipyridine derivatives, amrinone (52) and milrinone (53),
and the sympathomimetic agent, dobutamine (54,55).

Changes in organ blood flow other than to the heart have not been reported to
date with enoximone.

Comparative studies of enoximone with dobutamine have been reported (56,
57). We found that at a comparable improvement in cardiac output, pulmonary
artery and pulmonary artery wedge pressures tended to drop to a greater extent
with enoximone than dobutamine, whereas heart rate rose to a greater extent with
dobutamine than enoximone (57). Similar findings have been reported by others,
except that the change in heart rate was similar with both drugs, and the decrease
in mean arterial pressure was somewhat greater with enoximone than dobutamine
(58). The comparative effects of intravenous nitroprusside and enoximone have
also been examined (56). The hemodynamic effects of the two agents were similar.
When hemodynamics were compared at the same level of pulmonary arterial wedge
pressure, Amin et al. found a greater increase in cardiac output and stroke work
index and a lesser decrease in mean arterial pressure with enoximone. These findings raised the possibility that the additional improvement in the former parameters were related to the inotropic property of enoximone.

That enoximone can increase the contractile state of the myocardium in man
has been clearly demonstrated (50). The relative contributions of inotropy and

vasodilation toward the efficacy of this agent have not been fully clarified, however.

We have also reported that intravenous enoximone produces a significant rise in plasma renin activity (59). In a subsequent study, we demonstrated that dobutamine at a comparable improvement in cardiac output produced a significantly greater increase in plasma renin activity than did enoximone (57). It is not clear whether further drug-induced increases in plasma renin activity are deleterious, although inhibition of the renin-angiotensin system has been clearly demonstrated to be efficacious in patients with severe heart failure (60). Thus, further stimulation of plasma renin activity would not appear to be beneficial in this setting. We have also demonstrated a heterogeneous response to enoximone of both plasma norepinephrine and arginine vasopressin with a tendency of the former to decrease and no significant directional change in the latter (59,61).

Do the present data satisfy the requirements to recommend intravenous enoximone in the short-term treatment of heart failure? In an extremely practical sense they do, in that intravenous enoximone has presumably fulfilled a set of Food and Drug Administration criteria for acceptance as a marketable inotropic drug similar to the criteria applied to intravenous amrinone. There are, however, several important considerations which required further clinical studies and experience. For example, does the improvement in cardiac output translate to improvement in specific organ function? Is there an improvement in renal function that can be measured by increases in urine volume and sodium excretion? What is the relative arrhythmogenicity of enoximone when compared to other available inotropic agents, including dobutamine, dopamine, and most recently, amrinone? Is an agent with a relatively long half-life, such as enoximone or amrinone, appropriate in the short-term management of heart failure? Because of the nature of the patient population, it may be difficult to answer these questions in controlled studies. However, with demonstration of the safety of the intravenous preparation and its salutary effects on hemodynamics it may be propitious at present to consider its use in clinical practice.

VI. LONG-TERM TREATMENT OF CONGESTIVE HEART FAILURE WITH ENOXIMONE

The end point in evaluating the efficacy of an agent in the chronic treatment of heart failure has remained difficult to determine (62). Chronic hemodynamic improvement would appear to signal clinical improvement, but unfortunately this is not always the case (61,63). On the other hand, it seems unlikely that agents that develop hemodynamic attenuation over time, such as the oral beta-agonists, would produce clinical improvement (64,65). Functional improvement and clinical status have been utilized to determine the efficacy of a drug in this setting (60).

Using such criteria, no inotropic agent has demonstrated clinical efficacy, and at least one, amrinone, has failed the test (66,67).

What data are currently available on the efficacy of *oral* enoximone? We have reported on the acute hemodynamic response to a single oral dose of enoximone (3,68). Hemodynamics were quite similar to the intravenous agent, except that cardiac output peaked at only 28% above baseline. An oral dose of 3 mg/kg was as effective as 6 mg/kg in producing this effect. These data contrast with two studies in which oral enoximone was given every 1 or 2 hours until peak hemodynamic effect was reached (48,69). In these latter two studies, the improvement in cardiac output with oral enoximone equaled that of the intravenous agent. The difference between our findings and the data from these studies may be explained by a limitation of absorption at or below 3 mg/kg. Thus, multiple dosages may allow for repeated periods of absorption, and due to the long half-life of the drug and its metabolically active metabolite, MDL 19438, higher plasma drug levels may be available to produce a greater improvement in cardiac output (68).

We have reported (61) continued hemodynamic efficacy in eight patients studied at between 4 weeks (six patients, each clinically improved) and several months (two patients, neither clinically improved). All patients demonstrated continued hemodynamic improvement with enoximone. Rubin and Tabak (70) have suggested that attenuation may occur with chronic use of enoximone. Of their seven patients, four demonstrated continued hemodynamic efficacy, and three had lost hemodynamic responsiveness. These data overall suggest that enoximone probably maintains hemodynamic efficacy in the majority of patients. Clearly, however, more studies with larger numbers will be required to substantiate this viewpoint.

Oral enoximone, like its intravenous counterpart, has been shown to produce a small rise in plasma renin activity with a tendency toward lower norepinephrine levels and no change in arginine vasopressin (3).

Enoximone is metabolized in the liver primarily by conversion to a sulfoxide metabolite, MDL 19438, which has approximately 20% of the hemodynamic efficacy of the parent compound (68). This metabolite, as well as other quantitatively less important compounds, are excreted by the kidneys. Thus, it is not unexpected that patients who have severe congestive heart failure with relatively poor renal and hepatic blood flow would metabolize this agent at rates that differ from those of normal subjects. In a study of normal males, the time to reach peak plasma level of enoximone was 0.17 hours (10 min) and 0.67 hours (40 min) for MDL 19438 (71). In contrast, time to reach peak plasma level for enoximone in patients with severe heart failure was 1.6 hours, or ten times as long as in normal subjects. These data suggest a sluggish absorption of this agent in patients with severe heart failure. In normal subjects, the elimination half-life was 1.3 hours for enoximone and 2.3 hours for MDL 19438. These data contrast with findings for the half-life of enoximone and MDL 19438 in patients with severe heart failure and a serum creatinine level of less than 2 mg%. The half-life of enoximone was 20±5.8 hours, and the half-life of MDL 19438 was 25.6 ± 25 hours (3). The large standard deviations attest to the wide variation in drug disposition of enoximone seen in heart failure patients.

Dose schedules depend on the plasma level of enoximone desired. The long half-life would suggest infrequent dosages, but the limitation in absorption suggests that more frequent dosages would allow for higher drug levels.

Little functional data is available for patients receiving enoximone. Rubin and Tabak (70) reported a small, nonsignificant increase in peak oxygen uptake, in acute therapy and after 4 weeks of chronic therapy in a small group of patients, but they concluded that enoximone was ineffective in improving exercise tolerance. It is obvious that more studies will be required to determine whether improvement in functional capacity, short-term and long-term, does occur.

Several investigators have reported long-term clinical follow-up studies of patients with severe heart failure who received enoximone (48,61,69). Most patients have been characterized as having "refractory heart failure." Of the 95 cases reported in two studies (48,61), 79% had had an inadequate response to previous vasodilator therapy. Of the 95, 72% were classified as New York Heart Association (NYHA) functional class IV. These patients as a group probably have had more advanced heart failure than those studied in natural history studies and controlled trials with vasodilators. In our own series of 57 patients, in NYHA class III patients (n = 14) we found an improvement rate of 79% in 1 month, 69% in 6 months and 54% in 1 year. In contrast, we found an improvement in 49% of NYHA class IV patients (n = 39) at 1 month, 11% at 6 months and only 3% (1 patient) at 1 year. Survival at 1 month was 93% in NYHA class III, 69% at 6 months, and 54% in 1 year. For NYHA class IV patients, 1 month survival was 72%, 6 months survival was 11% and 1 year survival was 3%. Deaths were approximately equally divided between sudden deaths (n = 20) and heart failure deaths (n = 17) as well as two noncardiac deaths.

Adverse effects required drug termination in 7% of our patients. Major side effects were related to gastrointestinal symptoms, such as nausea or vomiting, loose stools, and abdominal cramps. Although they occurred frequently in our study (75% of patients), most symptoms were mild and could be controlled by reducing the dosage. Similar improvement, mortality, and adverse reaction rates have been reported in a study of 37 patients undertaken by Kereiakes et al. (48). In a smaller study of 13 bedridden NYHA class IV patients reported by Shah et al. (64), all but 1 patient was dead by 21 weeks.

Based on these studies, we can conclude that enoximone does not fall into that special group of drugs, which includes penicillin for pneumococcal pneumonia, in which clinical efficacy is "obvious" and controlled trials are either unnecessary or may actually be unethical. The relatively poor survival rates in uncontrolled studies may be more a function of the extreme severity of the patient's illness than a function of the drug effect. Whether enoximone is efficacious, has no advantage over placebo, or is actually deleterious cannot be discerned from available data. We believe, however, that the existing data are promising enough to proceed with a randomized trial similar to that applied to captopril (60) to determine whether enoximone is an efficacious agent in chronic heart failure.

If a randomized, placebo-controlled trial with enoximone demonstrates a lack of clinical efficacy, should these data, along with the negative results in similar studies with amrinone, lead us to conclude that positive inotropic therapy is an ineffective approach in chronically treating heart failure? Such a conclusion is probably too broad. If one reviews studies evaluating the clinical efficacy of vasodilator therapy, it is difficult to conclude, with the exception of angiotensin-converting enzyme inhibition (CEI) (60,72) and possibly the nitrate preparation isosorbide dinitrate (73), that vasodilator therapy is an effective mode of treatment for chronic heart failure. Hydralazine, prazosin, other nitrate preparations, and minoxidil all have demonstrated limitations in long-term use (63,74,75-79). Is this lack of efficacy a negative summation between a salutary vasodilation on the plus side and an adverse effect, such as sodium retention, on the negative side? Or is the vasodilation in the group of drugs just mentioned ineffective in producing a salutary effect chronically—and might it provoke, depending on the agent, other unwanted side effects? CEI on the other hand, has been demonstrated to be clinically efficacious, which may in part be related to its vasodilatory property. If investigators had concluded that vasodilators were ineffective based on experience with vasodilators other than CEI, the only clearly effective therapy (other than diuretics) in the treatment of heart failure would not have been developed. It should be added in this context, however, that it is possible that the clinical efficacy of CEI in the setting of chronic heart failure may be independent of its vasodilator effect (80). The same investigative sequence may be occurring with the positive inotropic agents. It may be that enoximone, as well as amrinone, may not be effective in chronic heart failure. The reasons for failure may include the possibility that the particular activating mechanism, namely phosphodiesterase inhibition, has an overall negative vector on the cardiovascular system. In other words, the advantage of positive inotropy may be outweighed by an unwanted side effect such as production of serious arrhythmia or cell "burnout," although neither of these possibilities has actually been documented. Another possibility is that the vasodilator aspect of enoximone (or amrinone), rather than the inotropic aspect, is a negative factor, acting to shunt blood to metabolically inactive tissues and to provoke salt retention. Finally, the unwanted effect of renin stimulation by enoximone may adversely affect long-term results; the addition of a converting enzyme inhibitor may counteract this effect and allow the potentially salutary effects of positive inotropy to be realized. Other agents, with different mechanisms of action, may indeed be effective in the long-term treatment of congestive heart failure. Efforts at promoting improved function with inotropic therapy, whether studies with enoximone prove fruitful or fruitless, should not yet be abandoned.

ACKNOWLEDGMENTS

I would like to acknowledge the short-term but invaluable assistance of Elsie F. Eberman in typing and preparing this chapter. Additionally, I would like to acknowledge the long-term, unselfish, and loving support of my wife Sybil, and my parents Jack and Lillian Uretsky.

REFERENCES

1. A. M. Katz. A new inotropic drug: Its promise and a caution. *N. Engl. J. Med. 299*: 1409-1410 (1978).
2. T. H. LeJemtel, and E. H. Sonnenblick. Should the failing heart be stimulated? *N. Engl. J. Med. 310*: 1384-1385 (1984).
3. B. F. Uretsky, T. Generalovich, J. G. Verbalis, A. M. Valdes, and P. S. Reddy. MDL 17,043 therapy in severe congestive heart failure: Characterization of the acute and chronic hemodynamic, pharmacokinetic, hormonal, and clinical response. *J. Am. Coll. Cardiol. 5*: 1414-1421 (1985).
4. S. B. Arnold, C. B. Randolph, W. Meister, K. Melmon, M. D. Cheitlin, D. Bristow, W. W. Parmley, and K. Chatterjee. Long-term digitalis therapy improves left ventricular function in heart failure. *N. Engl. J. Med. 303*: 1443-1448 (1980).
5. E. Braunwald. Effects of digitalis on the normal and the failing heart. *J. Am. Coll. Cardiol. 5*: 51A-59A (1985).
6. J. L. Fleg, S. H. Gottlieb, and E. G. Lakatta. Is digoxin really important in treatment of compensated heart failure? *Am. J. Med. 73*: 244-250 (1982).
7. M. Gheorghiade, and G. A. Beller. Effects of discontinuing maintenance digoxin therapy in patients with ischemic heart disease and congestive heart failure in sinus rhythm. *Am. J. Cardiol. 51*: 1243-1250 (1983).
8. J. Hamer. The paradox of the lack of the efficacy of digitalis in congestive heart failure with sinus rhythm. *Br. J. Clin. Pharmacol. 8*: 109-113 (1979).
9. D. C. Lee, R. A. Johnson, J. B. Bingham, M. Leahy, R. E. Dinsmore, A. H. Goröll, J. B. Newell, H. W. Strauss, and E. Haber. Heart failure in outpatients: A randomized trial of digoxin versus placebo. *N. Engl. J. Med. 306*: 699-705 (1982).
10. A. J. Moss, H. T. Davis, D. L. Conrad, J. J. DeCamilla, C. L. Odoroff. Digitalis-associated cardiac mortality after myocardial infarction. *Circulation 64*: 1150-1156 (1981).
11. C. D. Mulrow, J. R. Feussner, and R. Velez. *Ann. Intern. Med. 101*: 113-117 (1984).
12. T. J. Ryan, K. R. Bailey, C. H. McCabe, S. Luk, L. D. Fisher, M. B. Mock, and T. Killip. The effects of digitalis on survival in high-risk patients with coronary artery disease: The coronary artery surgery study (CASS). *Circulation 67*: 735-742 (1983).
13. C. Liang, J. M. Ui, L. G. Sherman, J. Black, H. Gavras, and W. B. Hood, Jr. Dobutamine infusion in conscious dogs with and without acute myocardial infarction. *Circ. Res. 49*: 170-180 (1981).

14. D. V. Unverferth, R. D. Magorien, R. Altschuld, A. J. Kolibash, R. P. Lewis, and C. V. Leier. The hemodynamic and metabolic advantages gained by a three-day infusion of dobutamine in patients with congestive cardiomyopathy. *Am. Heart J. 106*: 29-34 (1983).

15. R. E. Rude, L. R. Bush, C. Izquierdo, L. M. Buja, J. T. Willerson. Effects of inotropic and chronotropic stimuli on acute myocardial ischemic injury. III. Influence of basal heart rate. *Am. J. Cardiol. 53*: 1688-1694 (1984).

16. R. E. Rude, C. Izquierdo, L. M. Buja, and J. T. Willerson. Effects of inotropic and chronotropic stimuli on acute myocardial ischemic injury. I. Studies with dobutamine in the anesthetized dog. *Circulation 65*: 1321-1328 (1982).

17. S. Davidson, P. R. Maroko, and E. Braunwald. Effects of isoproterenol on contractile function of the ischemic and anoxic heart. *Am. J. Physiol. 227*: 439-443 (1974).

18. J. C. Lee, and S. E. Downing. Ventricular function in norepinephrine-induced cardiomyopathic rabbits. *Am. J. Physiol. 242*: H191-H196 (1982).

19. P. R. Maroko, J. K. Kjekshus, B. E. Sobel, T. Watanabe, J. W. Covell, J. Ross, Jr., and E. Braunwald. Factors influencing infarct size following experimental coronary artery occlusions. *Circulation 43*: 67-82 (1971).

20. P. R. Maroko, P. Libby, and E. Braunwald. Effect of pharmacologic agents on the function of the ischemic heart. *Am. J. Cardiol. 32*: 930-936 (1973).

21. S. F. Vatner, R. J. McRitchie, P. R. Maroko, T. A. Patrick, and E. Braunwald. Effects of catecholamines, exercise, and nitroglycerin on the normal and ischemic myocardium in conscious dogs. *J. Clin. Invest. 54*: 563-575 (1974).

22. S. F. Vatner, R. W. Millard, T. A. Patrick, and G. R. Heyndrickx. Effects of isoproterenol on regional myocardial function, electrogram, and blood flow in conscious dogs with myocardial ischemia. *J. Clin. Invest. 57*: 1261-1271 (1976).

23. J. C. Yates, R. E. Beamish, and N. S. Dhalla. Ventricular dysfunction and necrosis produced by adrenochrome metabolite of epinephrine: Relation to pathogenesis of catecholamine cardiomyopathy. *Am. Heart J. 102*: 210-221 (1981).

24. M. Petein, B. Levine, and J. Cohn. Hemodynamic effects of a new inotropic agent, piroximone (MDL 19,205), in patients with chronic heart failure. *J. Am. Coll. Cardiol. 4*: 364-371 (1984).

25. T. Kariya, L. J. Wille, and R. C. Dage. Biochemical studies on the mechanism of cardiotonic activity of MDL 17,043. *J. Cardiovasc. Pharmacol. 4*: 509-514 (1982).

26. R. S. Adelstein, M. D. Pato, and M. A. Conti. The role of phosphorylation in regulating contractile proteins. In *Advances in Cyclic Nucleotide Research*, vol. 14. J. E. Dumont, P. Greengard, and G. A. Robinson (eds.). Raven Press, New York, 1981, pp. 361-373.

27. G. I. Drummond, and D. L. Severson. Cyclic nucleotides and cardiac function. In *Brief Reviews from Circulation Research 1980*, monograph 69. Dallas, American Heart Association, 1980, pp. 8-16.

28. M. Endoh, S. Yamashita, and N. Taira. Positive inotropic effect of amrinone in relation to cyclic nucleotide metabolism in the canine ventricular muscle. *J. Pharmacol. Exp. Ther. 221*: 775-783 (1982).

29. P. Honerjager, M. Schafer-Korting, and M. Reiter. Involvement of cyclic AMP in the direct inotropic action of amrinone. *Arch. Pharmacol. 318*: 112-120 (1981).

30. W. R. Kukovetz, G. Poch, and A. Wurm. Quantitative relations between cyclic AMP and contraction as affected by stimulators of adenylate cyclase and inhibitors of phosphodiesterase. In *Advances in Cyclic Nucleotide Research*, vol. 5. G. I. Drummond, P. Greengard, and G. A. Robinson (eds.). Raven Press, New York, 1975, pp. 395-414.

31. R. W. Tsien. Cyclic AMP and contractile activity in heart. In *Advances in Cyclic Nucleotide Research*, vol. 8. P. Greengard, and G. A. Robinson (eds.). Raven Press, New York, 1977, pp. 363-420.

32. A. M. Katz. Cyclic adenosine monophosphate effects on the myocardium: A man who blows hot and cold with one breath. *J. Am. Coll. Cardiol. 2*: 143-149 (1983).

33. A. M. Katz. Role of the contractile proteins and sarcoplasmic reticulum in the response of the heart to calecholamines: An historical review. In *Advances in Cyclic Nucleotide Research*. P. Greengard, and G. A. Robinson (eds.). Raven Press, New York, 1979, pp. 303-349.

34. A. M. Katz, M. Tada, and M. A. Kirchberger. Control of calcium transport in the myocardium by the cyclic-AMP-protein kinase system. In *Advances in Cyclic Nucleotide Research*, vol. 5. G. I. Drummond, P. Greengard, and G. A. Robinson (eds.). Raven Press, New York, 1975, pp. 453-472.

35. H. Scholz. Inotropic drugs and their mechanisms of action. *J. Am. Coll. Cardiol. 4*: 389-397 (1984).

36. P. J. England, H. T. Pask, and D. Mulls. Cyclic-AMP-dependent phosphorylation of cardiac contractile proteins. In *Advances in Cyclic Nucleotide and Protein Phosphorylation Research*, vol. 17. P. Greengard (ed.). Raven Press, New York, 1984, pp. 383-391.

37. M. A. Movsesian. Calcium-physiology in smooth muscle. *Prog. Cardiovasc. Dis. 25*: 211-224 (1982).

38. H. vanBelle. A critical review of cyclic AMP and its role in cellular metabolism and heart muscle contractility. In *Cardiac Metabolism*. A. J. Drake-Holland, and M. I. M. Noble (eds.). John Wiley & Sons, New York, 1983, pp. 417-444.

39. J. C. Ruegg, M. P. Sparrow, and U. Mrwa. Cyclic-AMP mediated relaxation of chemically skinned fibres of smooth muscle. *Pflugers Arch. 390*: 198-201 (1981).

40. A. W. Jones, D. B. Bylund, and L. R. Forte. cAMP-dependent reduction in membrane fluxes during relaxation of arterial smooth muscles. *Am. J. Physiol. 246 (Heart Circ. Physiol. 15)*: H306-H311 (1984).

41. L. E. Roebel, R. C. Dage, H. C. Cheng, and J. K. Woodward. Characterization of the cardiovascular activities of a new cardiotonic agent MDL 17,043 (1,3-dihydro-4-methyl-5-[4-(methylthio)-benzoyl]-2H-imidazol-2-one). *J. Cardiovasc. Pharmacol. 4*: 721-729 (1982).

42. R. C. Dage, L. E. Roebel, C. P. Hsieh, D. L. Weiner, and J. K. Woodward. Cardiovascular properties of a new cardiotonic agent: MDL 17,043, (1,3-dihydro-4-methyl-5-[4-(methylthio)-benzoyl]-2H-imidazol-2-one). *J. Cardiovasc. Pharmacol. 4*: 500-508 (1982).

43. L. E. Roebel, R. J. Hodgeman, N. L. Velayo, R. C. Dage, and J. K. Woodward. Effect of MDL 17,043, a new cardiotonic agent, on myocardial oxygen consumption. *J. Pharm. Pharmacol. 17*: 247-249 (1983).

44. R. L. Hardesty, B. P. Griffith, A. Trento, M. E. Thompson, P. S. Ferson, and H. T. Bahnson. Morbidly ill patients and excellent survival following cardiac transplantation. *J. Am. Coll. Cardiol. 3*: 562 (1984).

45. R. L. Hardesty, B. P. Griffith, A. Trento, M. E. Thompson, P. F. Ferson, and H. T. Bahnson. Mortally ill patients and excellent survival following transplantation. *Ann. Thorac. Surg. 41*: 126-129 (1986).

46. B. F. Uretsky, T. Generalovich, P. S. Reddy, R. B. Spangenberg, and W. P. Follansbee. The acute hemodynamic effects of a new agent, MDL 17,043, in the treatment of congestive heart failure. *Circulation 67*: 823-828 (1983).

47. D. K. Amin, P. K. Shah, S. Hulse, F. G. Shellock, and H. J. C. Swan. Myocardial metabolic and hemodynamic effects of intravenous MDL-17,043, a new cardiotonic drug, in patients with chronic severe heart failure. *Am. Heart J. 108*: 1285-1292 (1984).

48. D. Kereiakes, K. Chatterjee, W. W. Parmley, B. Atherton, D. Curran, A. Kereiakes, and R. Spangenberg. Intravenous and oral MDL 17.043 (a new inotropic-vasodilator agent) in congestive heart failure: Hemodynamic and clinical evaluation in 38 patients. *J. Am. Coll. Cardiol. 4*: 884-889 (1984).

49. D. R. Ferry, G. T. Kennedy, R. A. O'Rourke, and M. H. Crawford. Prolonged effectiveness of intravenous MDL 17,043 for treating severe congestive heart failure. *J. Am. Coll. Cardiol. 5*: 514 (1985).

50. M. H. Crawford, K. L. Richards, M. T. Sodums, and G. T. Kennedy. Positive inotropic and vasodilator effects of MDL 17,043 in patients with reduced left ventricular performance. *Am. J. Cardiol. 53*: 1051-1053 (1984).

51. J. L. Martin, M. J. Likoff, J. S. Janicki, W. K. Laskey, J. W. Hirshfeld, Jr., and K. T. Weber. Myocardial energetics and clinical response to the cardiotonic agent MDL 17,043 in advanced heart failure. *J. Am. Coll. Cardiol. 4*: 875-830 (1984).

52. J. R. Benotti, W. Grossman, E. Braunwald, and B. A. Carabello. Effects of amrinone on myocardial energy metabolism and hemodynamics in patients with severe congestive heart failure due to coronary artery disease. *Circulation 62*: 28-34 (1980).

53. E. S. Monrad, D. S. Baim, H. S. Smith, A. Lanoue, E. Braunwald, W. Grossman. Effects of milrinone on coronary hemodynamics and myocardial energetics in patients with congestive heart failure. *Circulation 71*: 972-979 (1985).

54. P. Coté, M. G. Bourassa, J. F. Tubau, M. Enjalbert, and M. Vandormael. Effects of dobutamine on left ventricular performance and myocardial metabolic demands in patients with ischemic heart disease. *Clin. Cardiol. 7*: 14-22 (1984).

55. R. G. Pozen, R. Dibianco, R. J. Katz, R. Bortz, R. J. Myerburg, and R. D. Fletcher. Myocardial metabolic and hemodynamic effects of dobutamine in heart failure complicating coronary artery disease. *Circulation 63*: 1279-1285 (1981).

56. D. K. Amin, P. K. Shah, S. Hulse, and F. Shellock. Comparative acute hemo-dynamic effects of intravenous sodium nitroprusside and MDL-17,043, a new inotropic drug with vasodilator effects in refractory congestive heart failure. *Am. Heart J. 109*: 1006-1012 (1985).

57. B. F. Uretsky, J. G. Verbalis, T. Generalovich, A. M. Valdes, and P. S. Reddy. Comparative hormonal and hemodynamic responses to intravenous MDL 17, 043 and dobutamine. *J. Am. Coll. Cardiol. 5*: 515 (1985).

58. D. K. Amin, F. G. Shellock, S. Hulse, G. Brandon, R. Spangenberg, and H. J. C. Swan. Comparative hemodynamic effects of intravenous dobutamine and MDL-17,043, a new cardioactive drug, in severe congestive heart failure. *Am. Heart J. 109*: 91-98 (1985).

59. B. F. Uretsky, T. Generalovich, and P. S. Reddy. The relationship of catecho-lamine and plasma renin activity levels to improved hemodynamics with MDL 17,043 in patients with congestive heart failure. *J. Am. Coll. Cardiol. 1*: 676 (1983).

60. Captopril Multicenter Research Group. A placebo-controlled trial of captopril in refractory chronic congestive heart failure. *J. Am. Coll. Cardiol. 2*: 755-763 (1983).

61. B. F. Uretsky, A. M. Valdes, and P. S. Reddy. Positive inotropic therapy for short-term support and long-term management of congestive heart failure: The hemodynamic and clinical efficacy of MDL 17,043. *Circulation 73* (Suppl. 3): III-219-III-229 (1986).

62. E. Braunwald, and W. S. Colucci. Evaluating the efficacy of new inotropic agents. *J. Am. Coll. Cardiol. 3*: 1570-1574 (1984).

63. J. A. Franciosa, R. A. Jordan, M. M. Wilen, and C. L. Leddy. Minoxidil in patients with chronic left heart failure: Contrasting hemodynamic and clini-cal effects in a controlled trial. *Circulation 70*: 33-38 (1984).

64. W. S. Colucci, R. W. Alexander, G. H. Williams, R. E. Rude, B. L. Holman, M. A. Konstam, J. Wynne, Jr., G. H. Mudge, and E. Braunwald. Decreased lym-phocyte beta-adrenergic-receptor density in patients with heart failure and tolerance to the beta-adrenergic agonist pirbuterol. *N. Engl. J. Med. 305*: 185-190 (1981).

65. H. Lambertz, M. Jurgen, and R. Erbel. Long-term hemodynamic effects of prenalterol in patients with severe congestive heart failure. *Circulation 69*: 298-305 (1984).

66. R. DiBianco, R. Shabetai, B. D. Silverman, C. V. Leier, J. R. Benotti, with the Amrinone Multicenter Study Investigators. Oral amrinone for the treatment of chronic congestive heart failure: Results of a multicenter randomized dou-ble-blind and placebo-controlled withdrawal study. *J. Am. Coll. Cardiol. 4*: 855-866 (1984).

67. B. Massie, M. Bourassa, R. DiBianco, M. Hess, M. Konstam, M. Likoff, and M. Packer, for the Amrinone Multicenter Trial Group. Long-term oral administra-tion of amrinone for congestive heart failure: Lack of efficacy in a multicen-ter controlled trial. *Circulation 71*: 963-971 (1985).

68. B. F. Uretsky, T. Generalovich, P. S. Reddy, R. Salerni, A. M. Valdes, J. F. Lang, and R. A. Okerholm. Acute hemodynamic effect of oral MDL 17,043 in severe congestive heart failure. *Am. J. Cardiol. 54*: 357-362 (1984).

69. P. K. Shah, D. K. Amin, S. Hulse, F. Shellock, and H. J. C. Swan. Inotropic therapy for refractory congestive heart failure with oral fenoximone (MDL 17,043): Poor long-term results despite early hemodynamic and clinical improvement. *Circulation 71*: 326-331 (1985).

70. S. A. Rubin, and L. Tabak. MDL 17,043: Short- and long-term cardiopulmonary and clinical effects in patients with heart failure. *J. Am. Coll. Cardiol. 5*: 1422-1427 (1985).

71. R. G. Alken, G. G. Belz, K. D. Haegele, T. Meinicke, and P. J. Schechter. Kinetics of fenoximone, a new cardiotonic in healthy subjects. *Clin. Pharmacol. Ther. 36*: 209-216 (1984).

72. B. L. Kramer, B. M. Massie, and N. S. Topic. Controlled trial of captopril in chronic heart failure: a rest and exercise hemodynamic study. *Circulation 67*: 807-816 (1983).

73. C. V. Leier, P. Huss, R. D. Magorien, and D. V. Unverferth. Improved exercise capacity and differing arterial and venous tolerance during chronic isosorbide dinitrate therapy for congestive heart failure. *Circulation 67*: 817-822 (1983).

74. S. B. Arnold, R. L. Williams, T. A. Ports, R. A. Baughman, L. Z. Benet, W. W. Parmley, and K. Chatterjee. Attenuation of prazosin effect on cardiac output in chronic heart failure. *Ann. Intern. Med. 91*: 345-349 (1979).

75. J. A. Franciosa, K. T. Weber, T. B. Levine, G. T. Kinasewitz, J. S. Janicki, J. West, M. M. Hennis, and J. N. Cohn. Hydralazine in the long-term treatment of chronic heart failure: Lack of difference from placebo. *Am. Heart J. 104*: 587-594 (1982).

76. M. Packer. Conceptual dilemmas in the classification of vasodilator drugs for severe chronic heart failure. *Am. J. Med. 76*: 3-13 (1984).

77. P. Packer, J. Meller, R. Gorlin, and M. V. Herman. Hemodynamic and clinical tachyphylaxis to prazosin-mediated afterload reduction in severe chronic congestive heart failure. *Circulation 59*: 531-539 (1979).

78. M. Packer, J. Meller, N. Medina, M. Yushak, and R. Gorlin. Hemodynamic characterization of tolerance to long-term hydralazine therapy in severe chronic heart failure. *N. Engl. J. Med. 306*: 57-62 (1982).

79. M. Packer, J. Meller, N. Medina, M. Yushak, and R. Gorlin. Serial hemodynamic studies indicate that early tolerance to prazosin in heart failure is not reversible. *Circulation (suppl. 2) 66*: 210 (1982).

80. R. C. Tarazi, P. M. Fouad, J. K. Ceimo, and E. L. Bravo. Renin, aldosterone and cardiac decompensation: Studies with an oral converting enzyme inhibitor in heart failure. *Am. J. Cardiol. 44*: 1013-1018 (1979).

81. P. J. Silver, C. Schmidt-Silver, and J. DiSalvo. Beta-adrenergic relaxation and cAMP kinase activation in coronary arterial smooth muscle. *Am. J. Physiol. 242 (Heart Circ. Physiol. 11)*: H177-H184 (1982).

82. B. F. Uretsky. Is inotropic therapy appropriate for treatment of chronic congestive heart failure? *Postgrad. Med.* (1986).

7

The Bipyridine Derivatives
Amrinone and Milrinone

ROBERT DiBIANCO
Georgetown University, Veterans Administration Medical Center, Washington, D.C., and Washington Adventist Hospital, Takoma Park, Maryland

I. INTRODUCTION

Amrinone, and its more recently discovered analog, milrinone, are bipyridine derivatives which have been demonstrated to possess positive inotropic and vasodilator activity when administered either intravenously or orally in a variety of research evaluations. The discussion that follows will attempt to summarize the substantial body of information available about these new agents.

Formal investigation of amrinone or WIN 40680 [5-amino-3,4'-bipyridin-6(1H)-one] began with the IND submission to the Food and Drug Administration (FDA) in October 1977, by the Sterling-Winthrop Research Institute, Rensselaer, New York (Fig. 1). Amrinone was synthesized by Lesher and Opalka and first reported as a cardioactive compound in 1978 by Farah and Alousi (1-4). These investigators confirmed that amrinone possessed positive inotropic and peripheral vasodilating action. Using several experimental models to determine amrinone's effects, including initial studies in isolated cat atria and papillary muscles, and intact anesthetized and unanesthetized dogs, these investigators characterized amrinone to have inotropic activity that was not mediated through the autonomic nervous system, adrenergic receptor, or Na^+,K^+-activated ATPase inhibition (1-3,5). They described amrinone as a noncatechol, nonglycoside inotropic agent and showed that pretreatment with reserpine, dl-propranolol, metiamide (an H_2 receptor blocker), atropine, phenoxybenzamine, or chlorisondamine (a ganglionic blocker) was not associated with reductions in the inotropic activity of amrinone. Amrinone improved the disturbed hemodynamics of pentabarbital-induced heart failure (see Table 1). These early investigators could not confirm meaningful phosphodiesterase activity for amrinone or an increase in myocardial cyclic AMP (3,6). This latter finding has

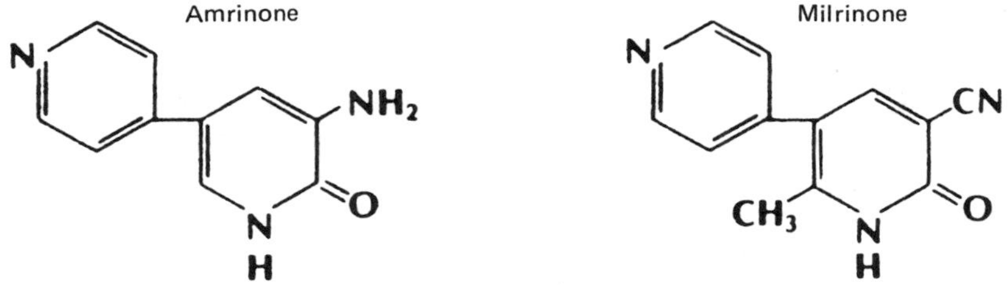

Amrinone

NH_2

N
H

5-Amino [3,4'-Bipyridine]
-6(1H)-one

Milrinone

CN

CH_3 N
H

1,6-Dihydro-2-methyl-6-oxo-
[3,4'-bipyridine] -5-carbonitrile

FIGURE 1   Structural formulas of amrinone and milrinone. (From E. Braunwald, E. H. Sonnenblick, L. W. Chakrin, and R. P. Schwartz, eds., *Milrinone—Investigation of a New Inotropic Therapy for Congestive Heart Failure*, Raven Press, New York, 1984, p. 22.)

TABLE 1   Effect of Amrinone on Pentobarbital-Induced Heart Failure in Dogs

	Cardiac output (liters/min)	Contractile force (g)	Central venous pressure (mm Hg)	Heart rate (beats/min)	Blood pressure Systolic	Diastolic
Control	4.07	27	0.7	168	180	150
Pentobarbital failure induced						
	2.54	15	3.8	126	105	55
Amrinone, 1 mg/kg, and infusion of 100 µg/kg per min						
After infusion						
2 min	3.78	20	1.3	132	130	70
10 min	3.46	25	0.7	132	125	60
15 min	4.01	33	0.4	150	130	60
60 min	3.69	36	0.2	138	125	50
Stop amrinone infusion						
After 90 min	3.28	22	1.5	120	110	50

Note: Anesthesia: 15.2 kg pentobarbital (30 mg/kg, intravenous); heart failure induced by bolus injections of 45 mg/kg, followed by constant infusion of pentobarbital (0.25 mg/kg/ min).
Source: From Ref. 3.

been a topic of extensive study and has been disputed by others (6-10). It is now recognized that amrinone is a phosphodiesterase inhibitor, although this classification may not explain all of its actions (6,7,11-14). In some species, other mechanisms may play a role in producing positive inotropy (that is, beta-adrenergic receptor and slow entry calcium channels) (14,15,17-20).

The increase in developed tension produced by amrinone in the isolated cat atrium and papillary muscle was shown to be dose dependent and not associated with changes in the duration of the contractile cycle, right atrial rate, or the time-to-peak tension (1-4,16,21). Some studies have found a slight but definite positive chronotropic effect (21-23), but few other electrophysiological actions (24-30). Increases in peak developed tension, peak rate of tension development, and rate of relaxation of electrically stimulated or potassium-contracted cells after treatment with amrinone have been confirmed in most species tested (1-4,7,15,16,31-38).

In the intact dog, intravenous amrinone in dosages of 0.3-10 mg/kg produced increases in the rate of left ventricular pressure development (dP/dt_{max}) which were attended by minimal increases in heart rate and slight reductions in blood pressure (1-5,39). There is controversy over the effect on myocardial oxygen consumption; some studies report favorable reductions (40,41) and others report increases (21,34). At higher dosages, significant reductions in systolic pressure become manifest (1,3,4,13,21,23,41) (see Fig. 2). In addition to systemic vasodilator activity, pulmonary and coronary activities have been shown (36,42-47). In December 1977, the first human subject was treated with intravenous amrinone

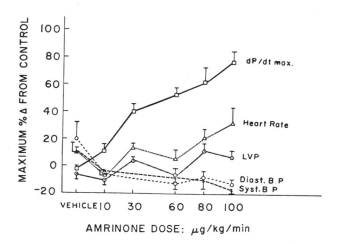

FIGURE 2   Dose-response curve of the cardiovascular effects of intravenously infused amrinone in the anesthetized dog. (From Ref. 3.)

and in August 1978, the first subject received oral drug. Short-term clinical studies in patients with heart failure then commenced (22,48-63).

These short-term studies of the intravenous administration of amrinone found the drug to be a safe and well-tolerated agent effective in the treatment of heart failure. It was approved by the FDA for use in the United States in 1984. Unlike short-term intravenous use which showed limited side effects, chronic use of oral amrinone has been attended by a high incidence of both major and minor side effects that have significantly compromised the patient group capable of tolerating treatment and the maximum daily dose that can be given (64-70). Questions have also been raised (and to date left unanswered) regarding the risks of chronic oral amrinone treatment for producing adverse effects on left ventricular function (71-75) and provoking arrhythmia (74-78). In addition, oral amrinone has not been found to be effective for reducing symptoms or enhancing exercise capacity in well-controlled, single- and double-blind studies of patients with chronic heart failure (79-82). As a result, the Sterling-Winthrop Research Institute has withdrawn oral amrinone from use and further development worldwide (letter to U.S. physicians, January 18, 1984). These findings will be discussed in greater detail in the section on human studies.

Milrinone, WIN 47203, 1,6-dihydro-2-methyl-6-oxo-[3,4'bipyridine] -5-carbonitrile (Fig. 1), is an analog of amrinone, synthesized by Lesher and Philion, and introduced by Alousi et al. in 1981 (31,83-86). As is evident from Figure 1, milrinone results from a combined carbonitrile substitution for the C5 amino group and methyl substitution at the C2 position of amrinone. Developed for its increased potency and enhanced safety, which have been observed in preliminary studies, the preclinical testing of milrinone has been very similar to that of amrinone. Milrinone is confirmed to be a noncatechol, nonglycoside inotropic agent and vasodilator which has demonstrated positive inotropic activity in in vitro and in vivo systems in several species, including guinea pig, rabbit, cat, and hamster, as well as direct and indirect vasodilator activity (6,32,84-88). Like amrinone, milrinone may be given intravenously or orally. Blockade of the adrenergic system (reserpine or d1-propranolol) and the H_1 and H_2 receptors does not alter milrinone's effect on contractility, nor does pretreatment with a prostaglandin synthetase inhibitor. As with amrinone, milrinone's parent compound, pretreatment with beta-adrenergic agonist (dopamine) or digitalis glycoside (ouabain) does not reduce the inotropic action of milrinone (Fig. 3). Milrinone has been shown to inhibit cardiac adenosine 3' 5' monophosphate (cyclic AMP) phosphodiesterase and to increase myocardial cyclic AMP levels (6,32,85), although it is controversial whether this finding completely explains its inotropic activity (6,32,85). Since the time course of the increase in cyclic AMP does not correlate with the increase in developed tension, other mechanisms probably play a role in initiation of the inotropic response (32).

In isolated guinea pig atria and papillary muscle, milrinone produced increases in rate and level of developed tension that were concentration dependent (6,85).

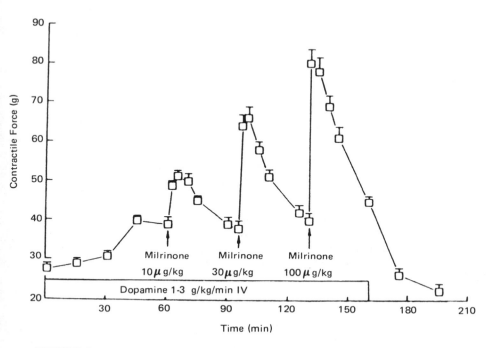

FIGURE 3 Effect of intravenously administered milrinone on cardiac contractile force during dopamine infusion in anesthetized dogs (n = 5, X ± SEM). (From Ref. 100, permission granted.)

An approximate rise of developed tension of 25%, which required 3.0 μg/ml of amrinone, was accomplished by a concentration of 0.1 μg/ml of milrinone, thereby confirming a 30-fold per weight increase in inotropic potency using this model (32,85) (see Figure 4).

In the anesthetized dog, bolus injections of intravenous milrinone in dosages of 0.01-0.1 mg/kg are associated with significant increases in left ventricular dP/dt (24 ± 6 to 119 ± 16%) and cardiac output (16 ± 5 to 33 ± 9%) (32). Dosages in excess of 0.3 mg/kg (up to 10 mg/kg) are associated with significant vasodilator action and increases in heart rate (Fig. 5). Milrinone has been effective in the treatment of heart failure induced by halothane, pentobarbital, propranolol, and verapamil in dogs (Table 2) (6).

The use of intravenous and oral milrinone in normal human subjects and patients with congestive heart failure has been limited. Preliminary data suggests that the high incidence of adverse effects associated with chronic oral amrinone (including gastrointestinal distress, fever, flulike illness, and laboratory abnormalities such as thrombocytopenia and elevation of hepatic enzymes) are lacking with milrinone

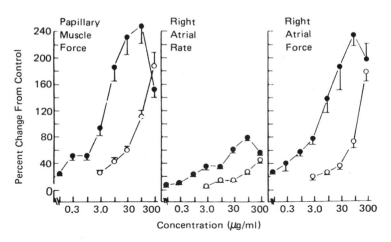

FIGURE 4 Inotropic responses to amrinone (o) and milrinone (•). (From E. Braunwald, E. H. Sonnenblick, L. W. Chakrin, and R. P. Schwartz, eds., *Milrinone—Investigation of a New Inotropic Therapy for Congestive Heart Failure*, Raven Press, New York, 1984, p. 29.)

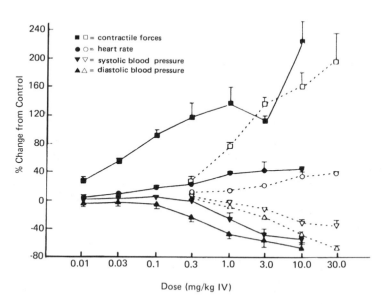

FIGURE 5 Bolus injections of amrinone (open symbols) and milrinone (closed symbols). (From E. Braunwald, E. H. Sonnenblick, L. W. Chakrin, and R. P. Schwartz, eds., *Milrinone—Investigation of a New Inotropic Therapy for Congestive Heart Failure*, Raven Press, New York, 1984, p. 29.)

204

TABLE 2 Effect of Milrinone on Verapamil-Induced Heart Failure in Anesthetized Dogs

Parameter	Baseline values	Absolute values	
		Verapamil failure	Verapamil plus milrinone
Contractile force (g)	63.8 ± 6.6	18.6 ± 4.6	65.2 ± 11.6[a]
Cardiac output (liters/min)	1.5 ± 0.14	0.9 ± 0.06	1.8 ± 0.29[a]
Mean right atrial pressure (mmHg)	−3.0 ± 1.04	2.6 ± 0.59	−1.0 ± 1.14[b]
Total peripheral resistance (Dyne/sec/cm^5) $\times$ 10^{-3}	6.42 ± 0.717	4.97 ± 0.341	2.85 ± 0.402[b]
Heart rate (beats/min)	145 ± 13.8	60 ± 7.6	53 ± 8.1
Blood pressure (mmHg)			
Systolic	156 ± 5.5	98 ± 7.0	126 ± 7.6[b]
Diastolic	101 ± 2.9	36 ± 4.8	24 ± 4.0[c]
Pulmonary artery systolic	21 ± 3.4	18 ± 3.0	21 ± 1.6
Pulmonary artery diastolic	16 ± 3.8	9 ± 1.9	12 ± 2.6[a]

Note: Values are means ± SEM (n = 4-5)
[a]$P < 0.05$.
[b]$P < 0.01$.
[c]$P < 0.001$; significance determined by t test for paired data.
Source: From Ref. 32.

(86). Significant hypotension may be produced by increased dosages of milrinone and represents a dose-related relaxant action on the peripheral vasculature. Two large-scale, placebo-controlled and randomized double-blind trials are now in progress to evaluate the chronic safety and efficacy of milrinone in the treatment of moderately severe heart failure. These trials have the further purpose of evaluating the progression of heart failure and should help determine whether treatment with milrinone is associated with an acceleration of left ventricular dysfunction—a hypothesis raised by several amrinone investigators (56,63,71,73-75,89) and incompletely answered by prior small and uncontrolled trials of the bipyridine derivatives (55, 89). The hypothesis as stated by Katz suggests that an especially delicate balance exists between energy production and utilization in the myocardial cells and that there is a possibility that under the influence of a powerful inotrope, the lack of chemical energy might lead to cell death and patchy fibrosis. Substantiation of this theory is still awaited (71).

II. PHARMACOKINETICS

Amrinone for intravenous use (amrinone lactate solution preserved with sodium metabisulfite) is light sensitive and has a pH adjusted to 3.2-4.0 units, because at increased pH, amrinone becomes less soluble (falling from 25 g/ml solubility at pH 4.1 to 0.7 g/ml solubility at pH 8.0) (78). Amrinone is detectable in plasma using a liquid chromatographic technique (90). In one study, the plasma elimination half-life ($t_{1/2}$) was 2.6 ± 1.4 hours and a direct relationship of $t_{1/2}$ to dose was suggested (91). Plasma protein binding is reported to be in the range of 10-49%, depending on the methodology employed (78). In the dog, rat, and monkey, the biotransformation of amrinone has been evaluated and found to be similar using ^{14}C-labeled amrinone (92). The primary route of excretion of amrinone and several metabolites (including N-glycolyl, N-acetate, O-glucuronide, and N-glucuronide) is via the kidney. Each of these metabolic pathways is conjugative and saturable; hence, increased dosages of amrinone are associated with increases in free amrinone in the urine, without large changes in metabolite excretion (92). At 96 hours after an oral dose of radioactive ^{14}C-labeled amrinone, 63% of the label was present in the urine and 18% in the feces. At 8 hours after oral administration, 51% of the

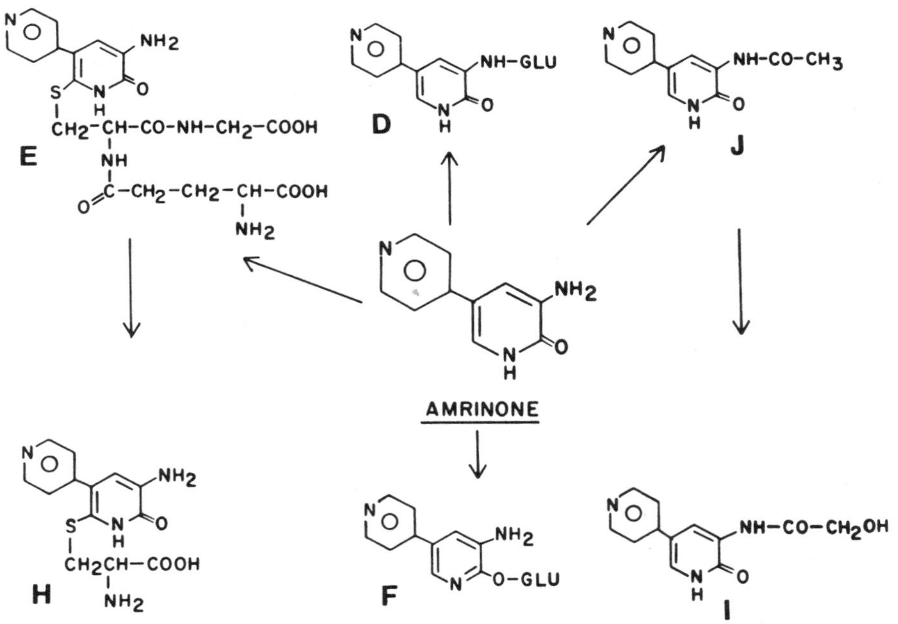

FIGURE 6   Scheme for the metabolism of amrinone. From Ref. 92.

radioactivity was amrinone, 5% was N-acetate, 8% was N-glycolate, and less than 8% of each glucuronide metabolite was present. These biotransformations are illustrated in Figure 6. In human volunteers, 0.8-2.2 mg/kg given intravenously had a volume of distribution of 1.2 liters/kg and an elimination half-life of approximately 2.6 ± 1.4 hours. The maximum plasma concentration was found to be correlated to the oral dosage between 25 and 250 mg (0.3-3.5 mg/kg) (91). Heart failure is associated with prolongations of the plasma elimination half-life of amrinone to variable degrees (range 3-15 hr), which probably result from reductions in hepatic and renal blood flow and depend on the severity of the hemodynamic disturbances (78,93).

In most reported studies, intravenous amrinone was given as a 0.5 mg/kg bolus followed by 0.5 mg/kg repeat boluses or a continuous infusion of approximately 40 µg/kg/min until an optimal hemodynamic response or an adverse effect occurred. In heart failure patients, the plasma level of amrinone was shown to correlate with the improvement in cardiac index in 13 of 14 patients after initial treatment (r = 0.81; P < 0.001); however, this improvement in cardiac index was not sustained at the initial high value after 4-5 hr despite continuous and constant plasma levels of amrinone (58,93,94).

Oral amrinone was usually given at 100 mg three times daily with increases of 50 mg per dose (that is, 150 mg daily) up to total daily dosages of 600 mg per day. Oral administration is associated with rapid absorption; peak blood levels appear at 1 hour (51,94). Maximal hemodynamic effects occur within 1-4 hr and the onset of action may vary from 0.5-2 hr. Almost all effects are dissipated by 6 hours (range 4-7 hr) after an initial dose (50). On chronic dosing, effects last ≥ 8 hours (50,51). Oral administration requires a two- or threefold increment in dose in order to obtain the same plasma level and hemodynamic response as that obtained with intravenous administration (49,51,91,93,94).

Milrinone is a nonhygroscopic compound of high solubility in acid media. An intravenous bolus injection of milrinone in doses of 0.01-0.1 mg/kg produces hemodynamic changes similar to those produced by amrinone within the first minute which reach a peak effect within 2-5 min (95). This finding has been demonstrated in anesthetized dog preparations in which the duration of activity ranged from 0.5 to 2 hours as measured by changes in cardiac contractile force, heart rate, and left ventricular dP/dt (Fig. 7). The time course of hemodynamic changes after milrinone administration are similar to those occurring after amrinone administration (95). As with amrinone, there is a good correlation between the plasma concentration of milrinone and the hemodynamic alterations (95). Milrinone can be measured in plasma using a liquid chromatographic technique (96). In the anesthetized dog preparation, milrinone shows 10 to 30 times greater potency per weight than does amrinone (6,31). The metabolic fate of milrinone discerned from studies of the rat, dog, and monkey show unchanged milrinone in the urine to be the major excretion product (97). There are two metabolic pathways identified; each plays a

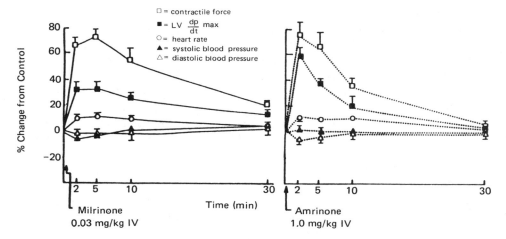

FIGURE 7   Effect of a single bolus of milrinone (0.03 mg/kg intravenously and amrinone 1.0 mg/kg intravenously) on the cardiovascular system of the anesthetized dog. (From E. Braunwald, E. H. Sonnenblick, L. W. Chakrin, and R. P. Schwartz, eds., *Milrinone—Investigation of a New Inotropic Therapy for Congestive Heart Failure*, Raven Press, New York, 1984, p. 29.)

minor role with oxidative end products of pyridyl-N-oxide and carboxamide; in the rat 98% of excreted drug is the parent compound (see Fig. 8) (97). Animal studies have suggested that the bioavailability of oral milrinone is high (>90%) and that absorption shows some dependence on gastric emptying (97).

Milrinone has a bioavailability of 92% in normal subjects and is eliminated with a mean apparent first-order elimination rate constant of 0.86 ± 0.23/hr corresponding to a half-life of 0.8 hours. Approximately 80% is recoverable from the urine by 24 hours (98). In patients with heart failure, intravenous doses of 12.5 µg/kg of milrinone produced a significant rise in cardiac output and an accompanying fall in pulmonary capillary wedge pressure without systemic hypotension (99). Dosages in excess of 12.5 µg (that is, 25-75 mg) also showed prompt and short-lived increases in cardiac index and reductions in left and right ventricular filling pressures; however, these were not proportional to the dose given and seemed to represent a plateau response (see Fig. 9) (99,100). In contrast, another study of 12.5-75.0 µg/kg of milrinone (given as sequential 10 mg boluses) intravenously in 11 patients with moderate-to-severe heart failure, found the hemodynamic effects to be serum concentration dependent (101). At higher dosages of 50-75 µg/kg, a significant reduction in mean arterial pressure was observed. The plasma half-life of intravenous milrinone was measured at 1.7 hours (99). The duration of action of intravenous milrinone did not exceed 1 hour. The volume of distribution was 0.35 ± 0.02 liters/kg with a plasma

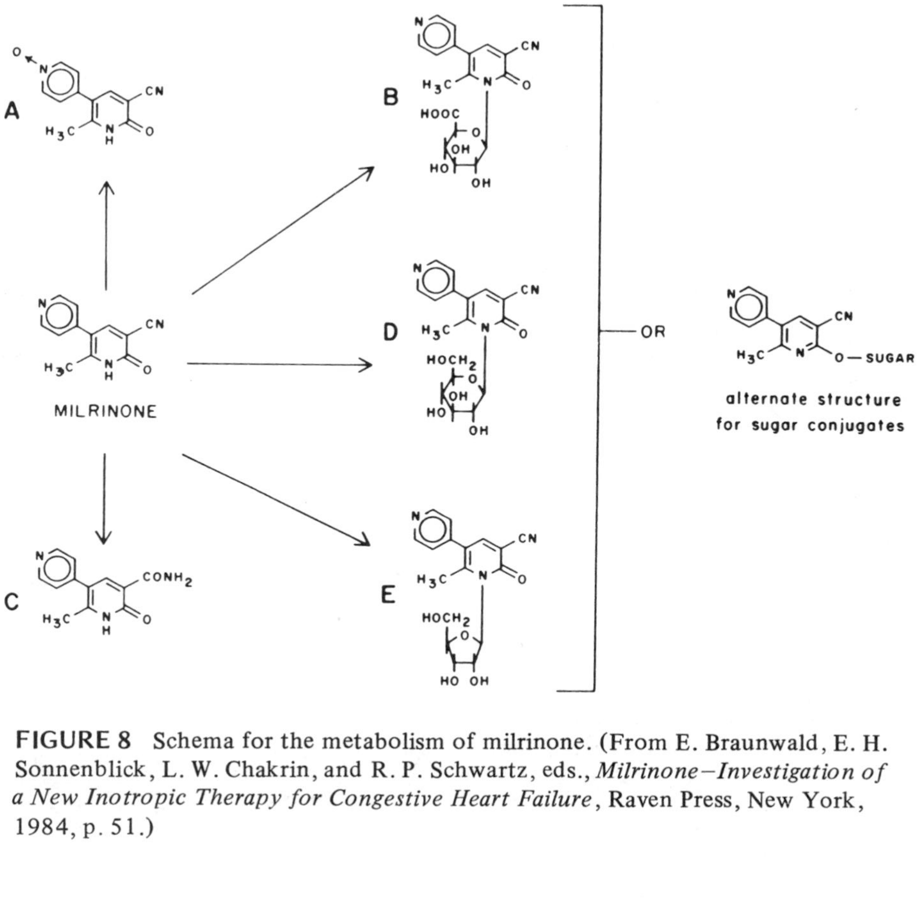

FIGURE 8   Schema for the metabolism of milrinone. (From E. Braunwald, E. H. Sonnenblick, L. W. Chakrin, and R. P. Schwartz, eds., *Milrinone—Investigation of a New Inotropic Therapy for Congestive Heart Failure*, Raven Press, New York, 1984, p. 51.)

clearance of 0.15 ± 0.03 liters/min per kg. For sustained action with intravenous use a continuous infusion is needed (99).

Oral milrinone was given to 21 patients as part of a dose-ranging study (102-103). At single doses of 5 mg or less there were no hemodynamic changes, whereas 7.5 mg and 10 mg doses consistently produced increases in cardiac index (mean improvement approximately 26%), reductions in left ventricular filling pressures (approximately 25%), and systemic vascular resistance (approximately 20%). A dose-response relationship was evident (see Fig. 10) and the largest increases in cardiac index occurred at the highest dose tested (15 mg); however, at this dose there was a significant reduction in mean arterial pressure. In 4 patients, mean arterial pressure was reduced from 18 to 36% and, although asymptomatic, was associated with a reflex sinus tachycardia. As the effect on peripheral resistance

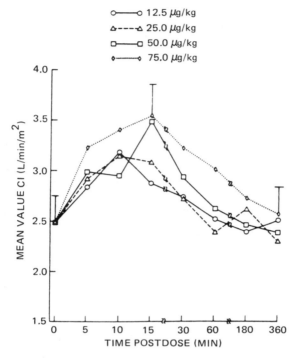

FIGURE 9 Effects of increasing milrinone dose on group mean cardiac index (CI) as a function of time (single bolus milrinone). (From E. Braunwald, E. H. Sonnenblick, L. W. Chakrin, and R. P. Schwartz, eds., *Milrinone—Investigation of a New Inotropic Therapy for Congestive Heart Failure*, Raven Press, New York, 1984.)

may be variable, it is suggested that initial dosages be observed and individualized (102).

III. MECHANISMS OF ACTION

The biochemical mechanism of amrinone's action is incompletely understood; although speculation continues to be centered about an augmentation of transcellular calcium delivery, increased calcium entry (mediated by Na-dependent and slow channel mechanisms) into the myocardial cell, and elevations of cyclic AMP that are mediated by phosphodiesterase inhibition activity of the drug (6,7,11,14,24, 33,104,105) (see Fig. 3).

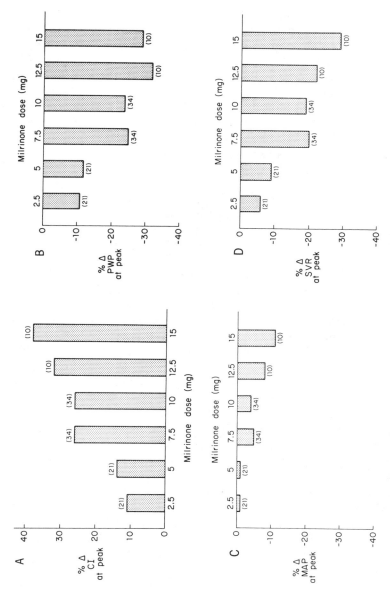

FIGURE 10 A-D. Dose-response relation of oral milrinone showing the peak changes in cardiac index (CI), pulmonary wedge pressure (PWP), mean arterial pressure (MAP), and systemic vascular resistance (SVR) for the six doses of milrinone. (From Ref. 49.)

The original studies of Alousi and Farah demonstrated quite clearly that amrinone does not manifest its inotropic action through mechanisms similar to those of cardiac glycosides or beta-adrenergic agonists (3). Amrinone does not show alterations of its activity as a result of pretreatment with reserpine designed to deplete endogenous catecholamine stores, nor does pretreatment with dl-propranolol or beta-agonists, such as dopamine or dobutamine, affect its activity, confirming a lack of participation through the beta-adrenergic receptor (3). Amrinone does not cause the release of endogenous catecholamines (3,104,105). Pretreatment with digitalis glycoside also fails to alter the hemodynamic response, suggesting that Na^+,K^+-ATPase inhibition does not play a direct role in mediating amrinone's activity—although one study suggests a nonadditive effect of amrinone and ouabain on cat papillary muscle (38). Other types of blockade, including H_1 and H_2 receptor blockade (with metiamide), ganglionic blockade (with chlorisondamine), cholinergic blockade (with atropine), and alpha-receptor blockade (with phentolamine or phenoxybenzamine), have similarly not blocked amrinone's inotropic activity (3,10,13). One study supported a minor histaminergic effect of amrinone (15). Amrinone produces an increase in calcium influx in cardiac myocytes and has shown a partial reduction in inotropic action after pretreatment with calcium channel blockers. This finding lends additional support for amrinone's calcium-mediated action (12,18,20,39,106). Amrinone may act to release calcium intracellularly by increasing intracellular levels of cyclic AMP, or possibly other modulators, as well as by enhancing calcium entry into the cell (6,12,18,20,106). Amrinone increases intracellular calcium in dog erythrocytes, but it is unclear whether calcium moves through myocardial membranes in similar fashion (11, 14). Furthermore, the accumulation of cellular Ca^{2+}, although increasing with time and with the concentration of amrinone in the dog erythrocytes, was apparent later than increases in developed tension and did not occur at inotropic drug concentrations. This suggests other mechanisms for the positive inotropic action (14). It has been suggested that myocardial cell levels of cyclic AMP rise after treatment with amrinone secondary to amrinone's inhibition of the cyclic nucleotide phosphodiesterase F-III (7,9,13,30,33,107). To determine whether or not cyclic AMP is involved in the actions of amrinone, studies of cat and canine ventricular muscle contraction were done in the presence of carbachol, a muscarinic agonist which specifically antagonizes cyclic AMP-mediated events without altering Ca^{2+} or alpha-receptor-mediated events. The inotropic responses were depressed markedly, confirming the relationship to increases in cyclic AMP (7,30). At high concentrations, amrinone produces a prolongation of contraction similar to that produced by theophylline (105,108). In a preliminary report, an antibiotic ionophore (R02-2985) produced similar changes in open-chested dogs as did amrinone, but did not appear to involve increases in calcium transport or adenyl cyclase activity (107). Another study suggested that amrinone's activity was mediated by nonspecific effects on vascular smooth muscle or by potentiation of the vasodilator action of adenosine (109).

Intravenous bolus injection of amrinone produces an increase in left ventricle dP/dt and peripheral vasodilatation in almost all mammalian species tested including humans (3,4,6,7,15-18,21,33,36,39,76,110-122). Most studies have shown amrinone to have vasodilator activity which in some investigations has been substantial and exceeded its effects on contractility (33,48,49,51-55,72,89,113,123). It is likely that a combination of inotropic and vasodilator activity is produced by amrinone and that improvements in left ventricular function result from direct drug-mediated positive inotropy and reductions in peripheral vascular resistance. The indirect withdrawal of augmented sympathetic nerve activity which occurs with improved hemodynamics in the setting of congestive heart failure (CHF) would further serve to lower peripheral vascular resistance (73,124-126). The regional circulatory effects of amrinone reveal an increase in coronary blood flow (21,114) that appears to be secondary to a nonspecific smooth muscle relaxant effect (17). An increase in myocardial oxygen consumption has been seen in the two different animal models (21,37), which may be associated with a relative decline in subendocardial perfusion in the dog (114).

Electrophysiological actions of amrinone were studied in Purkinje fibers from the dog (25-27). No significant changes were observed in resting membrane potential, action potential amplitude, maximum upstroke, or conduction velocity (3). In cat papillary muscle and guinea pig ventricular muscle, the increased contractile force also was not attended by changes in standard electrophysiological values and action potential characteristics (3,6). Unlike many positive inotropic drugs and interventions which induce oscillatory afterpotentials and aftercontractions in Purkinje tissue or myocardium, amrinone did not, despite tests using high concentrations and using depolarized Purkinje cells (24). In combination with acetylstrophantidin, amrinone increased the amplitude of the oscillatory afterpotentials (24). The significance of this finding is unclear; when amrinone was given to anesthetized dogs treated with arrhythmogenic doses of ouabain, no significant worsening of arrhythmia occurred (5).

In the intact animal, electrophysiological actions may be indirectly mediated, through the autonomic nervous system, through effects on electrolyte concentrations, or through interactions with other drugs or mechanisms. Amrinone may facilitate atrioventricular nodal conduction, leading to an enhanced response to supraventricular arrhythmia (28,77). Some investigators have suggested that amrinone may be proarrhythmic, that is, it may have the potential for arrhythmia generation or aggravation (30,50,54,69,75); this was not observed in a large controlled trial of oral amrinone, however (80).

Preliminary work has demonstrated that amrinone (and milrinone) relax pulmonary vascular smooth muscle in conscious newborn lambs at dosages beginning at 0.3 mg/kg, which are lower than those required to produce an increase in cardiac index (usually greater than 1.0 mg/kg). This effect is not dependent on muscarinic or beta-adrenergic receptors or on the formation of cyclo-oxygenase products (42, 44-46). One group found that amrinone produced a transient stimulation of ileal smooth muscle from the guinea pig, probably resulting from suspected postgang-lionic release of acetylcholine from cholinergic nerve terminals (49). One report suggested that amrinone blocked doxorubicin cardiotoxicity, although there was no investigation of the possible mechanism (111).

Milrinone, like amrinone, does not act through inhibition of the myocardial Na^+,K^+-ATPase or activation of adrenergic or cholinergic receptors and is there-fore unaffected by pretreatment with ouabain, reserpine, d1-propranolol, phenoxy-benzamine, dopamine, or atropine (31,32). Milrinone has been shown to be a phos-phodiesterase inhibitor and to increase myocardial levels of cyclic AMP; however, the onset of developed tension precedes the accumulation of cyclic AMP, which suggests other mechanisms for initiation of the inotropic response (6,32). Milrinone does not act via the release of endogenous norepinephrine. Its action is not altered by pretreatment with H_1 and H_2 receptor blockers (mepyramine and metiamide, respectively) or prostaglandin synthetase inhibitor (indomethacin). Milrinone pro-duces favorable increases in contractile force despite toxic doses of ouabain; in the presence of propranolol-, pentabarbital-, or verapamil-induced heart failure; and despite autonomic denervation (32). As with amrinone, the exact biochemical mechanism of action for milrinone remains unknown. It is highly likely that milri-none induces its positive inotropic action by modifying the availability of Ca^{2+} to the contractile elements; the lack of correlation of developed tension with cyclic AMP-phosphodiesterase and cyclic AMP levels is confounding (32).

Milrinone has proven vasodilator activity (87,101,127). When given intra-arter-ially, milrinone increased forearm blood flow in seven patients with chronic heart failure. Its action was concluded not to be solely the result of vasodilatation after a comparison with sodium nitroprusside (101); in this study, equipotent dosages of milrinone and nitroprusside for reducing arterial pressure had differing effects on stroke work, stroke volume, cardiac indices, and dP/dt. Milrinone increased the cardiac index 20% greater than did nitroprusside ($P<0.02$). Although stroke volume increased comparably for both drugs, the left ventricular end-diastolic pressure was lower with milrinone; that is, the stroke work index was higher with milrinone. The peak dP/dt was unchanged by nitroprusside and was increased by 32% with milri-none (101). A comparison of milrinone and dobutamine revealed that the vaso-dilator action of milrinone may mask the positive inotropic effect through a reduc-tion in preload and consequent reduction in measured dP/dt at the lowered pre-load (127).

Milrinone (7.5 mg orally), was compared to captopril (12.5 mg orally) in a study of 11 patients with heart failure (128). Cardiac output and arterial pressures were higher with milrinone, whereas systemic arterial pressure was less with captopril. Milrinone showed favorable increases in skeletal muscle blood flow as estimated by femoral vein oxygen content; femoral vein oxygen content remained unaltered after captopril administration. Renal blood flows were comparable with both treat-ments (128).

The electrophysiological effects of milrinone are similar to those of amrinone. Action potential characteristics of Purkinje cells are undisturbed at concentrations of 0.2-20 μg/ml of milrinone (129). These same investigators revealed that at therapeutic concentrations of 0.1-0.4 μg/ml milrinone enhanced conduction across areas of depressed conductivity and ischemic cells, which suggests that electrophysiological effects with clinical relevance in arrhythmia generation or prevention are yet to be determined (127). Milrinone restored electrical activity to K^+-inactivated tissues, a finding also seen with amrinone (15).

IV. CLINICAL STUDIES

Studies of amrinone effects in healthy subjects were performed for the purposes of determining dose-ranging intravenous and oral administration and elucidation of pharmacology (see above) and safety (see below). These studies have been limited with respect to the number of individuals studied and duration of treatment (23). Adverse effects during short-term administration have been few, consisting largely of excessive dose-related hypotension and reflex tachycardia.

Studies of intravenous and oral amrinone in patients with heart failure have been numerous (22,48-54,56,58-63,75,94,115,130,131); unfortunately only a limited number have had adequate placebo-controlled and double-blind designs (79-81).

Intravenous amrinone has been studied in patients with New York Heart Association functional class III-IV heart failure. Amrinone has been confirmed to act within 2-5 min of bolus injection, improving cardiac performance through reductions in preload and afterload and through enhanced contractility. At dosages of 1.5-3.6 mg/kg per day given as intermittent boluses or a continuous intravenous infusion, amrinone has been shown to reduce systemic vascular resistance and to decrease left and right ventricular filling pressures (22,44,49,59); its ability to improve cardiac contractility has been observed, though the validity and mechanism of this observation is controversial (48,53,60). Some have suggested that an indirect activation of catecholamines may account for discrepant observations (48). In uncontrolled patient studies, the hemodynamic changes after intravenous amrinone dosages have been associated with improvements in symptomatology, oftentimes described as dramatic, without a rise in heart rate or fall in mean arterial pressure (54). Studies of exercise capacity after intravenous amrinone administration in patients with heart failure have found improvement (52,54); however, conflicting hypotheses have been expressed and the mechanism has been debated (48,74).

Short-term comparisons of intravenous amrinone with beta-agonists (including isoproterenol, dopamine, dobutamine, and pirbuterol) and the vasodilators, sodium nitroprusside and prazosin, have found amrinone to be generally comparable in effectiveness to each of these agents with respect to magnitudes of cardiac index augmentation and reduction in left ventricular filling pressures. In 10 patients with a range of global left ventricular function (ejection fractions of 0.24-0.77, mean 0.47 ± 0.23), a maximum dose of 30 μg/kg per min of intravenous amrinone produced a significant reduction in left ventricular end-diastolic pressure without a change in cardiac rate, output, systemic resistance, or blood pressure (60). A maximum dose of 4 μg/min of isoproterenol lowered end-diastolic pressure comparably; however, it was associated with significant increases in heart rate, cardiac output, and maximum left ventricular dP/dt. Isoproterenol also lowered arterial mean pressure and total systemic vascular resistance (60). With amrinone treat-

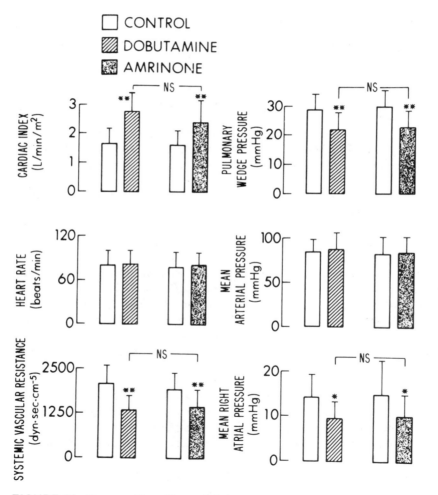

FIGURE 11   Comparative effects of dobutamine and amrinone on hemodynamic status. The initial responses relative to control values are shown (* = P<0.01; ** = P<0.001). (From Ref. 24.)

ment, a rise in cardiac output was correlated closely with a reduction in systemic vascular resistance (r = 0.90; P<0.001) in patients with a pre-existing elevation in left ventricular filling pressure. With isoproterenol, increases in left ventricular dP/dt and cardiac output occurred in all patients (after correction for increases of heart rate alone).

In 8 patients with heart failure, dobutamine and amrinone produced similar hemodynamic changes (see Fig. 11) (58). Both drugs showed a slightly better immediate than delayed response obtained using a continued infusion of 8 hours. Each was free of adverse effects at 11.8 μg/kg/min of dobutamine and 40 μg/kg per min for 1 hour followed by 10 μg/kg per min thereafter (58). Another comparison of 13 patients with heart failure given amrinone and the beta$_2$-agonist pirbuterol found the hemodynamic changes with amrinone to be indistinguishable from those with pirbuterol (see Figs. 12 and 13) (59). Both of these agents lowered systemic vascular resistance by approximately 32-33%, left ventricular end-diastolic pressure by 19-27%, and right atrial pressures by 16-21%; they increased the cardiac index by 55-65%. The addition of isosorbide dinitrate further reduced left ventricular end-diastolic pressure and right atrial pressure by 30%; the response to 20 mg of oral isosorbide dinitrate was similar after both amrinone and pirbuterol. Comparison of amrinone (1.5-3.5 mg/kg) to sodium nitroprusside (55-110 μg/min) revealed similarities of a dose relationship to reductions in left ventricular end-diastolic pressure and aortocoronary sinus oxygen difference and elevations of cardiac index (53). Systemic blood pressure was significantly reduced with nitroprusside and did not fall significantly with amrinone. In patients with cardiac failure

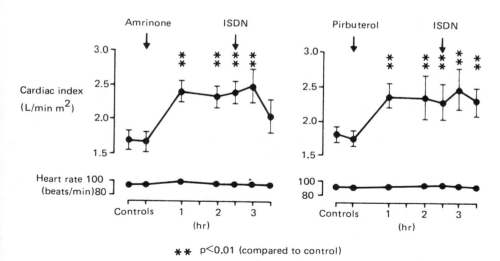

** p<0.01 (compared to control)

FIGURE 12 Changes with time in cardiac index and heart rate in 13 patients given oral amrinone and oral pirbuterol, and in 10 patients after the addition of 20 mg of isosorbide dinitrate (ISDN). (From Ref. 59.)

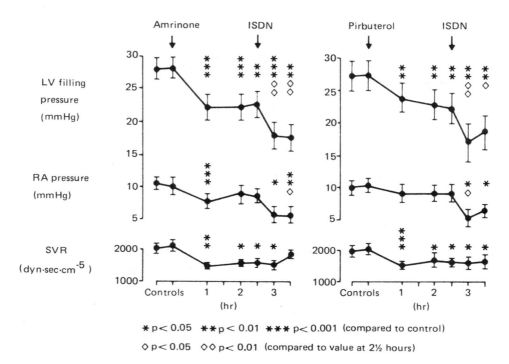

FIGURE 13 Changes with time in left ventricular filling pressure, right atrial pressure, and systemic vascular resistance in 13 patients given oral amrinone and pirbuterol, and in 10 patients after the addition of 20 mg of oral isosorbide dinitrate (ISDN). (From Ref. 59.)

secondary to coronary artery disease, amrinone (unlike nitroprusside) produced an increased heart rate ($+5\%$; $P = NS$). Left ventricular work increased with both drugs, reaching statistical significance for amrinone only. The maximum rate of pressure development (dP/dt), which tended to fall with nitroprusside, remained unchanged with amrinone (neither effect was statistically significant). Increases in peripheral and coronary sinus metabolite concentrations (including free fatty acid, glycerol, and glucose) were present after amrinone but not nitroprusside administration. In 4 of 14 patients, maximum dP/dt increased greater than 20% after amrinone treatment and was associated with a significant rise in free fatty acid concentration (43-129%), suggesting that catecholamine release had occurred; no direct correlation of contractility indices was found with either amrinone or sodium nitroprusside (53). A comparison of amrinone (2.5 mg/kg intravenously), pirbuterol (20-30 mg orally), and prazosin (3.5 mg average dose orally) supported similar directional changes with different magnitudes for each drug; cardiac index and stroke work index were increased and left ventricular filling pressures, systemic vascular resistance, and mean blood pressures were reduced (11).

Oral amrinone on initial administration has produced the same short-term hemodynamic changes as does intravenous amrinone (50,51,56,57,122). Investigations have confirmed that oral amrinone produces short-term hemodynamic benefits in heart failure patients with a low risk of hypotension (50,51,56,57,122); unfortunately these early studies which prompted enthusiasm for this agent were not blind and not placebo-controlled. Two multicenter, randomized double-blind and placebo-controlled trials of chronic oral amrinone in the management of heart failure have been reported (78,80). These large studies, with contrasting designs, demonstrated unequivocally that chronic oral amrinone lacked efficacy and was associated with unacceptable toxicity in patients with moderately severe heart failure.

The first and largest of these studies was a withdrawal study which enrolled 173 patients with moderately severe heart failure (see Fig. 14 and Table 3). All patients initially received amrinone as a supplement to their other medications for heart failure which were kept constant throughout the trial (89% were concurrently stabilized with digoxin and diuretic, with an additional 62% on one or more vasodilators). After an initial 4-week baseline period, a randomized and placebo-controlled withdrawal was performed in those patients who tolerated amrinone without experiencing limiting side effects and in whom there was a significant increase in exercise capacity during the early introduction of amrinone (see Fig. 14). The patients were evaluated every 2 weeks using the standard clinical tools of symptom diary review, physical examinations, determinations of exercise capacity by a modified Naughton treadmill protocol, systolic time intervals, and echocardiographic indices of left ventricular size and function. The group received a mean dose of

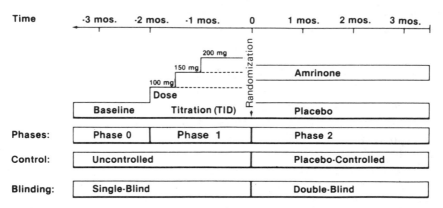

FIGURE 14   Study design of the placebo-controlled withdrawal trial. (From Ref. 79.)

TABLE 3 Patient Sample, Oral Amrinone Withdrawal Study

No. of patients	173 (154 M, 19 F)
Mean age	55 years (range 24-76)
Etiology of heart failure	89 (51%) ischemic heart disease
	79 (45%) history of myocardial infarction
	26 (15%) history of coronary bypass surgery
	64 (37%) idiopathic heart disease
	9 (5%) valvular heart disease
	11 (6%) hypertensive heart disease
NYHA class	2.6 ± 0.5 (67 patients class II; 103 patients class III; 3 patients class IV)
LVEF	25 ± 15%
Medications	89% digoxin
	89% diuretic drug
	62% vasodilator

Note: F = female; LVEF = left ventricular ejection fraction determined by radionuclide multiple gated acquisition scanning; M = male; NYHA class = New York Heart Association functional class.
Source: From Ref. 79.

113 ± 33 mg of oral amrinone three times daily during the initial baseline period. There were no clinically important changes in measures of cardiac performance after treatment with amrinone; although a slight increase in heart rate and exercise time did reach statistical significance (Table 4). From the patient sample, a subgroup of 52 patients was identified, each of whom showed an improved exercise capacity of ≥ 2 minutes after the addition of amrinone. In this group, the double-blind randomized withdrawal of amrinone and 12-week follow-up study failed to reveal a worsening in the symptoms of heart failure, exercise capacity on standardized treadmill protocol, or values on echocardiographic or systolic time interval studies. Exercise capacities fell slightly over the follow-up period to the same extent regardless of treatment with either amrinone (7%) or placebo (10%) (Table 5). Amrinone-treated patients developed increasing and severe heart failure as often as placebo-treated patients did (13% versus 18%, respectively, P = NS). Adverse effects of amrinone treatment were observed during both the initial introduction of amrinone and the double-blind placebo comparison and are presented in Tables 6 and 7 (79).

The second randomized double-blind and placebo-controlled trial of amrinone was of a prospective design; it found the same conclusions as the withdrawal trial (78,80). In this trial, 99 patients were enrolled; each had moderately severe heart failure that was stabilized on digoxin and diuretics (31 also received stable doses of captopril). Patients then randomly received amrinone or placebo, beginning at

TABLE 4 Results of Initial Treatment with Amrinone

	Baseline[a]	Amrinone[a]	P value
No. of patients	173	173	
Symptom score[b]	5.8 ± 1.4	5.3 ± 1.6	NS
NYHA class	2.6 ± 0.5	2.6 ± 0.6	NS
Body weight (kg)	76.8 ± 12	76.4 ± 12	NS
Rest heart rate (beats/min)	85 ± 14	89 ± 17	<0.01
Rest systolic BP (mmHg)	117 ± 18	117 ± 20	NS
Digoxin dosage (mg)	0.23 ± 0.06	0.23 ± 0.07	NS
Furosemide dosage (mg)	99 ± 71	106 ± 90	NS
LV internal size (end-diastole)(cm)	7.0 ± 1.0	6.9 ± 1.1	NS
Shortening fraction (%)	17.2 ± 7.1	17.8 ± 8.7	NS
PEP (seconds)	0.15 ± 0.04	0.14 ± 0.04	NS
LVET (seconds)	0.30 ± 0.07	0.29 ± 0.07	NS
QS2 (seconds)	0.44 ± 0.10	0.43 ± 0.10	NS
Exercise capacity (seconds)	601 ± 141	678 ± 211	<0.001
VO_2 (ml/kg)	15.8 ± 3.7	16.4 ± 4.5	NS

[a]Mean values (±SD) are shown for indicated variables for patients at baseline (left column) and after 4 weeks or more of amrinone (right column).
[b]Symptom score represents an average rating by the patient for symptoms of breathlessness during the day and at night, edema and fatigue. An average rating number is given to symptoms.
Note: BP = blood pressure; LV = left ventricle; LVET = left ventricular ejection time; PEP = pre-ejection period; QS2 = interval from onset of the Q wave to the onset of the second heart sound; VO_2 = maximal oxygen consumption attained with exercise, measured directly; NYHA = New York Heart Association.
Source: From Ref. 79.

1.5 mg/kg three times daily to a maximum dose of 200 mg per dose. After 12 weeks of therapy or prior to discontinuation of treatment, there was no significant difference from baseline between treatments with regard to symptoms, New York Heart Association functional class, left ventricular ejection fraction, cardiothoracic ratio, frequency of ventricular ectopy, or mortality. Both amrinone-treated and placebo-treated groups showed improved exercise capacity (37 ± 10% improvement and 35 ± 11%, respectively; P = NS) (see Figure 15). Adverse reactions were frequent (observed in 83% of the group receiving amrinone) (see Tables 6 and 7). These side effects prompted drug withdrawal in 34% of the amrinone-treated patients and downward adjustment of dose to a significantly lower level compared to placebo (355 mg/day versus 505 mg/day, respectively; P<0.001). The result of these large studies,

TABLE 5 Percent Change in Response Variables Observed in the Withdrawal Phase for Amrinone-Supplemented and Placebo-Substituted Groups Compared with Final Evaluation

	Amrinone	P value	Placebo	P value	A vs. P P value
No. of patients	31		21		
Symptom score	21.4	<0.05	8.4	NS	NS
NYHA class	5.9	NS	7.9	NS	NS
LVEF	-3.3	NS	8.3	NS	NS
Body weight (kg)	0.2	NS	0.7	NS	NS
Rest heart rate (beats/min)	3.6	NS	-6.2	NS	NS
Rest systolic BP (mmHg)	0.5	NS	-3.2	NS	NS
LV internal size (end-diastole) (cm)	3.1	NS	0.7	NS	NS
Shortening fraction (%)	-5.1	NS	14.2	NS	NS
Digoxin dosage (mg)	0.0	NS	5.0	NS	NS
Furosemide dosage (mg)	-4.0	NS	6.0	NS	NS
PEP (seconds)	2.5	NS	-2.6	NS	NS
LVET (seconds)	3.4	NS	0.6	NS	NS
QS2 (seconds)	2.7	NS	3.7	NS	NS
Exercise capacity (seconds)	-6.7	<0.05	-9.8	<0.05	NS
VO$_2$ (ml/kg)	-3.7	NS	-0.6	NS	NS

Note: P values are compared with the values obtained just before withdrawal (that is, at the end of the dose titration phase); A vs. P p value refers to the comparison between the percent change in those taking amrinone and the percent change in those taking placebo. NYHA = New York Heart Association; BP = blood pressure; LV = left ventricular; PEP = pre-ejection period.
Source: From Ref. 79.

along with the development of milrinone, an analog of amrinone with less reported toxicity from early trials, was expressed as the reason for terminating further study of oral amrinone for chronic heart failure (79,80).

That major differences appeared between the early short-term and chronic studies of oral amrinone has prompted much discussion and speculation (74,79-81,131). It is clear that most investigations into the treatment of heart failure, including those concerning pharmacologic agents, have evaluated changes after acute interventions and extrapolated these findings to chronic heart failure. Such extrapolations are not without problems since there may be major differences between

TABLE 6 Adverse Effects Observed During Uncontrolled Addition of Amrinone to Conventional Treatment

	n	%	P value
Gastrointestinal disturbances	69	(39)	
Nausea	46	(27)	
Anorexia	17	(10)	
Abdominal pain	17	(10)	
Diarrhea	22	(13)	
CNS complaints	29	(17)	
Dizziness	3	(2)	
Headache	10	(6)	
Lightheadedness	4	(2)	
Somnolence	5	(3)	
Fatigue	27	(15)	
Increased heart failure	27	(15)	
Upper respiratory infection	22	(13)	
Death	18	(10)	
Thrombocytopenia	17	(10)	
Arrhythmia[a]	16	(9)	
Probable ischemic episode	12	(7)	
Hepatic dysfunction	12	(7)	
Fever	10	(6)	
Virallike illness	7	(4)	
Laboratory abnormalities[b]			
Platelets	(25/172)	-46.3 ± 83.7	<0.001
SGOT	(9/168)	17 ± 24	0.02
SGPT	(10/103)	29 ± 176	NS
LDH	(1/165)	22 ± 75	<0.001
Alk Phos	(0/168)	3 ± 34	NS
Bilirubin	(0/113)	-0.04 ± 0.4	NS
Total	173		

[a]No prospective and systematic survey was made of the prevalence, type, or severity of atrial or ventricular arrhythmia. Only observations considered important by the investigators are recorded.

[b]Absolute change in values from end of phase 1 minus last value measured before amrinone in phase 0 (baseline). Fractions in parentheses represent number of patients with greater than three times the upper limit of normal range divided by number of patients having test performed. In the case of platelets, the numerator represents patients with under 100,000 platelets/mm^3.

Note: Alk Phos = alkaline phosphatase; CNS = central nervous system; LDH = lactic dehydrogenase; SGOT = serum glutamic oxaloacetic transaminase; SGPT = serum glutamic pyruvic transaminase.

Source: From Ref. 79.

TABLE 7 Adverse Effects Observed During Controlled Withdrawal of Amrinone

	Amrinone (n = 55)	Placebo (n = 52)	P value
Gastrointestinal disturbances	15 (27%)	4 (8%)	0.01
Nausea	11	0	
Anorexia	4	1	
Abdominal pain	3	2	
Diarrhea	5	1	
Vomiting	1	0	
CNS complaints	11 (20%)	2 (4%)	0.01
Dizziness	0	1	
Headache	4	1	
Lightheadedness	3	2	
Paresthesia	2	0	
Fatigue	9 (16%)	8 (15%)	NS
Increased heart failure	9 (16%)	17 (33%)	0.05
Upper respiratory infection	12 (22%)	4 (8%)	0.04
Death	1 (2%)	0 (0%)	NS
Thrombocytopenia	2 (4%)	0 (0%)	NS
Arrhythmia	8 (15%)	4 (8%)	NS
Probable ischemic episode	4 (7%)	7 (14%)	NS
Hepatic dysfunction	5 (9%)	2 (4%)	NS
Fever	3 (6%)	2 (4%)	NS
Virallike illness	1 (2%)	0 (0%)	NS
Laboratory abnormalities			
Platelets	(3/52) 215 ± 77	(1/47) 264 ± 100	0.008
SGOT	(2/52) 36 ± 32	(2/48) 49 ± 29	NS
SGPT	(3/27) 45 ± 38	(2/21) 32 ± 22	NS
LDH	(1/52) 222 ± 87	(0/47) 203 ± 78	NS
Alk Phos	(0/52) 48 ± 24	(0/48) 55 ± 33	NS
Bilirubin	(0/32) 0.7 ± 0.3	(0/22) 0.8 ± 0.7	NS

Note: The number of patients includes all patients who were followed up in phase 2 of the study regardless of exercise performance in phase 1. Abbreviations and format as in Table 6.
Source: From Ref. 79.

the acute and chronic response (132-135). Little emphasis has generally been given to the magnitude of observed changes and the extent to which these changes are clinically meaningful in long-term follow-up treatment (132,133). Short-term or acute intervention studies largely neglect the variabilities in both subjective and objective longitudinal patient responses, which must be considered in order to prove long-term effects (134). Acute studies are able to measure small changes

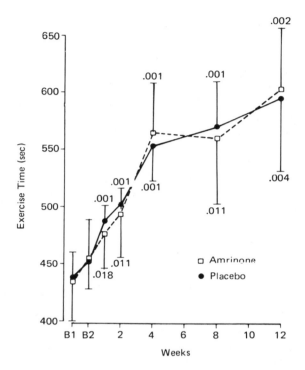

FIGURE 15 Exercise times (mean ± SE) in patients completing the 12-week blind trial. There were 41 placebo patients (solid circles) and 27 amrinone patients (open squares). There is no significant difference between treatments. (From Ref. 80.)

that deviate from closely monitored and stable baselines, thus avoiding confounding training effects, possible drug tolerances, drug interactions, or adverse effects that may appear only after chronic administration. They further avoid the alterations of diet, compliance, and autonomic adjustments that are inherent in patients studied longitudinally. Acute studies are important research tools for registering drug-related changes, but they may not reflect changes found during chronic drug administration. Chronic studies must overcome many more obstacles to demonstrate unequivocal clinical benefit or detriment from a specific treatment. For this reason the benefits of digitalis, hydralazine, prazosin, and nitrates, which have favorable acute drug-related effects, remain controversial during the chronic treatment of CHF (132,134-138) with rare exceptions (139). In the two controlled and blind multicenter studies of oral amrinone, a large patient experience, extensive clinical profiling of subjective and objective variables, prospective study design, and the double-blind testing of amrinone treatments conclusively showed the amrinone did not significantly benefit either the quality of life (that is, symptomatology) or enhance cardiac performance (that is, left ventricular size or function, or exercise tolerance). Although it is argued by some that changes in exercise duration may not correlate with cardiac index or ejection fraction and that this approach can be criticized for its variability with respect to the anaerobic threshold (140,141), it appears necessary to rely on these types of studies for reliable data that more accurately reflect the expected experience for compounds to be placed in general use.

Studies of intravenous milrinone effects in normal subjects, using echocardiography and calibrated carotid pulse tracings, reveal milrinone to produce dose-dependent increases in the end-systolic indices of left ventricular contractility, such as end-systolic pressure dimension, stress shortening, and stress velocity of fiber shortening. This finding suggests that milrinone has a dose-related positive inotropic effect separate from its vasodilator and afterload-reducing actions (142). At concentrations of 81-261 ng/ml (mean 165 ± 49), there was no chronotropic effect; however, the aortic mean and diastolic blood pressures declined, left ventricular diastolic and end-systolic dimensions were reduced, and total vascular resistance fell (-32%) (141).

Milrinone has been studied in preliminary and uncontrolled trials in patients with New York Heart Association class III-IV heart failure (89,143,144). Milrinone was administered both intravenously (143) and orally (89,144). Intravenous milrinone has produced significant increases in left ventricular systolic function as well as concomitant afterload reduction secondary to arteriolar vasodilation in these preliminary studies of patients with heart failure. The administration was well tolerated in a group of 20 patients with severe heart failure (mean cardiac index $1.9 \pm 0.1/m^2$). This early study suggested a favorable acute and chronic response (up to 11 months) though no control group was studied (143). A 27% increase in the resting radionuclide ejection fraction after a dose of 7.5 mg of oral milrinone was shown in 10 patients given milrinone treatment for ≥ 6 months. In a placebo-controlled study of the acute effects of intravenous milrinone ($57 \pm 5\ \mu g/kg$), milrinone was shown to significantly improve exercise duration, peak VO_2, and anaerobic threshold during upright bicycle exercise. At matched submaximal workloads, milrinone produced higher heart rates and blood pressures with lower plasma norepinephrine and lactate levels (144). Milrinone acutely given to patients with heart failure produced favorable effects on left ventricular diastolic function. The peak negative dP/dt increased 18% (P,0.01), the time constant of left ventricular isovolumic contraction decreased 30% (P,0.01), while the heart rate increased slightly by 8% (P<0.01), and aortic pressure fell 11%. These changes were in the opposite direction of those expected for an isolated reduction in arterial pressure; hence, they do not appear to be the result of peripheral vasodilation. Peak left ventricular filling rate was also found to increase (+42%) at a time when the observed driving force for its filling, the left atrial pressure, declined 33%. At present these observations are unexplained. They may be the result of increased levels of cyclic AMP, which may improve relaxation through control of phospholamban, the regulatory protein for sarcoplasmic-reticular-calcium uptake (147). The improved diastolic properties do not appear to result from venodilation, arterial vasodilatation, or peripheral activation of catecholamines, though the latter mechanism is not entirely excluded (148).

The oral administration of milrinone is associated with improved cardiac performance (89,149-151). In 7 patients concurrently on treatment with digitalis and diuretics, milrinone was initiated and titrated to produce an increase in cardiac index of $\geqslant 30\%$ above normal confirmed by hemodynamic monitoring after which patients were given treatment orally every 6 hours and followed as outpatients (89). After 2-9 weeks, patients were withdrawn from milrinone to assess its effects. Oral milrinone at dosages of 2.5-5.0 mg produced prompt improvements in hemodynamics: cardiac index increased from 1.8 to 2.3 liters/m^2; pulmonary capillary wedge pressure decreased from 24 ± 7 to 16 ± 8 mmHg, while systemic arterial resistance and heart rate were not significantly changed. Another study, with similar findings in 11 patients, showed that milrinone could enhance maximal oxygen uptake (145). Interestingly, the acute hemodynamic response in individual patients did not predict the clinical response on follow-up study (89). After approximately 7 weeks of follow-up studies of patients receiving oral milrinone, patients again underwent hemodynamic monitoring before and after milrinone withdrawal. Hemodynamics, which remained improved and stable while patients took milrinone, declined uniformly when milrinone was withdrawn: cardiac index decreased from 2.3 to 1.6 liters/m^2 ($P<0.05$), systemic vascular resistance increased as did the pulmonary capillary wedge pressure (17 to 23 mmHg, $P<0.05$) (89). The stroke volume index after withdrawal was lower than the control level, which prompted questions relating to the reduction in ventricular function. It is unclear whether rapid progression of disease masked by the hemodynamic improvements of milrinone or a drug-related interaction and/or effect of therapy somehow contributed to this observed progressive (and apparent rebound) deterioration upon withdrawal of milrinone. Only controlled studies will be able to adequately address these issues. It is hoped that multicenter, controlled studies currently in progress, which are comparing milrinone to digitalis and placebo, will provide these important answers. It is interesting to note that similar observations were previously made during amrinone treatment; yet, in the controlled trials, no detectable increase in heart failure was produced by amrinone compared to placebo (79,80). An uncontrolled study of the response to oral milrinone suggested both acute and short-term (approximately 1 month) benefits in 37 patients with heart failure (146).

V. ADVERSE REACTIONS

Adverse reactions to intravenous amrinone include cardiovascular effects of hypotension and arrhythmia, gastrointestinal side effects, and laboratory abnormalities such as thrombocytopenia and elevated hepatic enzymes (76,78). These were infrequently noted during early short-term trials and they appear to be infrequent despite increased clinical use, although no postmarketing trials can be cited (121).

The incidence of cardiovascular side effects with intravenous amrinone is low and includes hypotension ($<$2%), which at times is associated with an excessive reduction in diastolic filling pressure; arrhythmia has also been a suggested adverse effect of amrinone ($<$5%). In one uncontrolled early study, the intravenous infusion was accompanied by ventricular tachycardia (130). It is unclear whether intravenous amrinone plays a role with respect to the precipitation of arrhythmia, which can be a spontaneous event observed for the first time during close patient supervision. It is recognized that arrhythmia is common in patients with severe CHF. No placebo-controlled studies of intravenous amrinone are available. The electrophysiological effects of intravenous amrinone were evaluated at dosages between 10 and 20 μg/kg/minute in 15 patients with CHF (see Table 8) (77). Minimal ventricular arrhythmogenesis occurred during amrinone treatment; the frequency of inducible ventricular tachycardia was not changed. The investigators note (without

TABLE 8 Electrophysiological Measurements Before and After Intravenous Amrinone (n = 15)

	Control	Amrinone	P value
SCL	633 ± 106	619 ± 90	NS
PR	169 ± 40	165 ± 40	NS
QRS	107 ± 25	109 ± 23	NS
QTc	410 ± 37	405 ± 42	NS
AH	84 ± 23	81 ± 24	NS
HV	60 ± 13	58 ± 12	NS
Atrial ERP	256 ± 40	240 ± 38	0.015
AV nodal ERP	296 ± 49	280 ± 50	0.077
AV nodal FRP	374 ± 65	356 ± 64	$<$0.05
1:1 max AV	371 ± 46	334 ± 47	0.006
Ventricular ERP	234 ± 23	230 ± 23	NS
MCSNRT	261 ± 72	248 ± 101	NS

Note: All values listed in milliseconds (mean ± standard deviation). AV = atrioventricular; ERP = effective refractory period; FRP = functional refractory period; MCSNRT = maximal corrected sinus node recovery time; NS = not significant; SCL = sinus cycle length.
Source: From Ref. 77.

direct comparison) that these findings are similar to dopamine and dobutamine (77). In this study amrinone did not alter the PR, AH, HV, QRS, or QT intervals (40,77). The maximal corrected sinoatrial nodal recovery time and ventricular effective refractory period were similarly unaffected. Amrinone did, however, reduce the effective refractory period of the atrium and the functional refractory period of the atrioventricular (AV) node while it enhanced AV nodal conduction. These effects may increase the ventricular rate during supraventricular arrhythmia (such as atrial fibrillation or flutter) and may lead to adverse consequences in patients so predisposed. Consideration should be given therefore to pretreatment with digitalis glycoside in order to reduce the maximum ventricular response to this arrhythmia should it occur during amrinone treatment (77).

An arrhythmogenic potential for oral amrinone has been suggested by several investigators (69,75,77), although others have not observed this (80). In 10 patients undergoing 24-48 hr ambulatory electrocardiographic recordings before and after oral amrinone dosages of 75-150 mg three times daily, there was an increased incidence of ventricular couplets (22 ± 34 to 52 ± 55; P<0.05), although the frequency of total premature ventricular beats and runs of ventricular tachycardia were unchanged (80). The most extensive evaluation of oral amrinone's relationship to ventricular arrhythmia was reported in a subgroup of the multicenter experience

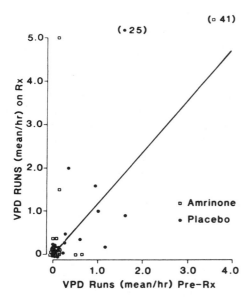

FIGURE 16 Repetitive ventricular premature depolarizations in amrinone- and placebo-treated patients. (From Ref. 80.)

in 41 patients; the findings fail to identify a proarrhythmic effect of oral amrinone (80) (see Figure 16).

Other side effects of intravenous amrinone include gastrointestinal reactions and laboratory abnormalities, most notably thrombocytopenia and elevations of serum liver enzyme levels (67). With short-term intravenous use, gastrointestinal side effects occur with a frequency of <5%; they include nausea (1.7%), vomiting (0.9%), abdominal pain (0.4%), and anorexia (0.4%) (76,78).

The incidence of thrombocytopenia, defined as a platelet count below 100,000/ mm^3 or below the normal laboratory lower limit, occurs with a frequency of <3% with intravenous amrinone use. It is clearly a drug-related, dose-related, and reversible adverse effect, although some controversy persists regarding mechanism (66, 70,113 152) Liver enzyme elevations may appear with intravenous amrinone in low incidence (<1%); they have been predominantly associated with chronic oral amrinone treatment and will be discussed below.

The frequency of adverse reactions is significantly increased with prolonged treatment, as has been demonstrated in studies of chronic oral amrinone administration (68). The first large multicenter study of oral amrinone found a high incidence of side effects during the initial (uncontrolled) addition of amrinone to standard treatment in 173 patients, as shown in Table 7 (79). These adverse reactions are similar to those reported prior to the trial in smaller studies (51,65-70,75-78, 113,152,153). Side effects generally limited treatment to daily dosages of ≤ 350 mg daily. This situation was also found in the most recent multicenter trial, which confirmed the relationship of adverse reactions to amrinone administration with its parallel placebo-treated group (80). The side effects of amrinone in this study occurred with a frequency of 83% in patients treated, and they prompted drug withdrawal in 34% because of increased severity. Despite downward adjustment of the amrinone dosage to a significantly lower level compared to placebo for the management of side effects (355 mg/day versus 505 mg/day, respectively; P<0.001), only 57% of amrinone-treated patients completed the study as opposed to 79% of those taking placebo (P<0.01). Severe episodes of CHF occurred with equal frequency on amrinone and placebo. As in the previous multicenter trial, the most frequent adverse effects were gastrointestinal complaints (usually nausea, vomiting, and diarrhea [49%]). It is clear that the high incidence of gastrointestinal side effects (including hepatitis) are amrinone-related, since these are otherwise uncommon and have been seen with higher frequency than in placebo-treated patients (79,80).

Thrombocytopenia has been observed with both intravenous and oral amrinone treatment (55,64-66,68,70,80). Initially reported to be only associated with patients in severe heart failure associated with oliguria (64,130,154), further study has shown that thrombocytopenia is related to both dose and duration of treatment. There is some controversy, however, regarding the general incidence of this side effect, which ranges from 5% to 50% in different investigations. Wilmshurst et al. (152) found that all of 16 patients had reductions in platelet counts; 9 of 16 had absolute reductions in platelet counts at doses of 300 mg of amrinone daily. The reductions reflected reduced survival of platelets. An increase in peripheral utilization rather than bone marrow suppression appears to be responsible for the reductions in platelet counts attributed to amrinone in other studies as well (69, 152). These observations have not been universally confirmed. Brandt et al. showed no consistent effect on platelet function or survival in a group of 7 patients (153), which suggests that thrombocytopenia may represent an idiosyncratic reaction between drug and a susceptible segment of the population. In most studies, monitoring patients for thrombocytopenia and interrupting therapy for platelet counts below 100,000/mm^3 has precluded bleeding episodes. No bleeding episodes were observed in either of the large multicenter trials (79,80).

Suspected hypersensitivity reactions have been reported in patients receiving amrinone (65,68,69,79). These have included a syndrome of fatigue, malaise, myalgias, and fever. These findings, first reported in uncontrolled trials, have been confirmed by the recent placebo-controlled multicenter study which reported this syndrome in 16% of amrinone-treated patients.

As in the studies of intravenous amrinone, intravenous use of milrinone has been well tolerated (86). Although not yet well studied in the long term, there appears to be a marked difference in the side effect profile and incidence with oral milrinone compared to oral amrinone. Milrinone can cause excessive hypotension associated with reflex tachycardia after oral dosages that usually exceed 15 mg (102). As in the early studies of amrinone in patients with moderate to severe heart failure, an increased incidence of sudden death, arrhythmia, and worsening of heart failure has occurred during milrinone treatment. These reports have been limited to a small group of individuals, often during short-term follow-up studies (143, 145,150). One study testing 10 patients before and after milrinone treatment found no change in the serum hepatic enzyme levels or platelet counts (145). One preliminary report reviewing ambulatory electrocardiograms after milrinone treatment in 15 patients found an increase in the complexity and density of ventricular arrhythmia after treatment (155). Another study confirms that milrinone has some electrophysiological effects—the significance of which is as yet unknown (129).

Some patients may show an increase in myocardial oxygen consumption of greater than 30% (4 of 18 patients in one study [156]). Some have reported increases in angina on long-term use, though this finding is uncontrolled and may be secondary to increased activity or a nonrepresentative sample (143,156). During an uncontrolled follow-up study of 4 patients showing this change in symptomatology, it was found that each patient had severe coronary disease (143).

Withdrawal of milrinone has been associated with prompt reductions in cardiac output and associated elevations of systemic resistance and pulmonary capillary wedge pressure. The observation that the withdrawal level of cardiac performance is less than the level prior to milrinone treatment has engendered speculation that therapy may be the cause for this deterioration of performance. Rapid progression of disease masked by the hemodynamic improvements of milrinone may be an alternate explanation. Controlled studies are necessary to adequately address this question. It is presently only an unproven hypothesis that this observation represents an adverse cardiac effect. Similar observations were previously made during early amrinone treatment which were unconfirmed by controlled trials (79,80). These early, nonblind and uncontrolled trials give only a glimpse of the clinical spectrum of milrinone. The suggestion that milrinone lacks the adverse effects characteristic of amrinone must also await placebo-controlled and double-blind trials of chronic treatment, which are currently in progress. The results of controlled long-term trials should ultimately determine the clinical use of any agent for CHF (154); these results are pending for milrinone.

ACKNOWLEDGMENT

This study was supported in part by the Veterans Administration, Washington, D.C.

REFERENCES

1. A. E. Farah, and A. A. Alousi. New cardiotonic agents: A search for a digitalis substitute. *Life Sci. 22*: 1139-1148 (1978).
2. A. A. Alousi, A. F. Farah, G. Y. Lesher, and C. J. Opalka. Cardiotonic activity of amrinone Win 40680. *Fed. Proc. (abst.) 37*: 914 (1978).
3. A. A. Alousi, A. E. Farah, G. Y. Lesher, and C. J. Opalka, Jr. Cardiotonic activity of amrinone (WIN 40680): 5-amino-3,1-4'1-bipyridin-6 (1H)-one. *Circ. Res. 45*: 666-677 (1979).
4. A. A. Alousi, and A. Helstrosky. Amrinone: A positive inotropic agent with a direct vasodilating activity in the canine isolated perfused hind limb preparation. *Fed. Proc. (abst.) 39* (part 2): 855 (1980).
5. A. A. Alousi, and D. Fort. The inotropic efficacy and safety of amrinone in the presence of other cardiovascular drugs in dogs. *Circulation (abst.) (suppl. 2) 59-60*: II-16 (1979).
6. A. A. Alousi, J. M. Canter, F. Cicero, D. J. Fort, A. Helstosky, G. Y. Lesher, M. J. Montenaro, G. P. Stankus, J. C. Stuart, and L. H. Walton. Pharmacology of milrinone. In *Milrinone—Investigation of a New Inotropic Therapy for Congestive Heart Failure*. E. Braunwald, E. H. Sonnenblick, L. W. Chakrin, and R. P. Schwartz (eds.). Raven Press, New York, 1984, pp. 21-48.
7. M. Endoh, S. Yamashita, and N. Taira. Positive inotropic effect of amrinone in relation to cyclic nucleotide metabolism in the canine ventricular muscle. *J. Pharmacol. Exp. Ther. 221*: 775-783 (1982).
8. P. Honerjager, M. Schafer-Korting, and M. Reiter. Involvement of cyclic AMP in the direct inotropic action of amrinone. *Arch. Pharmacol. 318*: 112-120 (1981).

9. S. D. Levine, M. Jacoby, J. A. Sariano, et al. The effect of amrinone in transport and cyclic AMP metabolism in toad urinary bladder. *J. Pharmacol. Exp. Ther. 216*: 220-224 (1981).
10. M. S. Gaide, S. P. Bakers, A. M. Ezrin, L. T. Potter, H. Golband, and A. L. Bassett. Characterization of the inotropic and biochemical properties of amrinone—a novel cardiotonic agent. *Am. J. Cardiol. (abstr.) 45*: 412 (1980).
11. J. C. Parker, O. R. Robinson, and J. R. Harper, Jr. Effects of amrinone, a cardiotonic drug, on calcium movement in the dog erythrocyte. *J. Clin. Invest. 66*: 254-259 (1980).
12. S. V. Rendig, and E. A. Amsterdam. Positive intropic action of amrinone: Effect of elevated external Ca^{2+}. *J. Cardiovasc. Pharmacol. 6*: 293-299 (1984).
13. R. W. Millard, G. Dube, G. Grupp, I. Grupp, A. Alousi, and A. Schwartz. Direct vasodilator and positive inotropic actions of amrinone. *J. Mol. Cell. Cardiol. 12*: 647-652 (1980).
14. J. S. Hayes, N. Bowling, G. B. Boder, and R. Kauffman. Molecular basis for the cardiotonic activities of amrinone and AR-L57. *J. Pharm. Exp. Ther. 230*: 124-132 (1984).
15. H. R. Adams, J. Rhody, and J. L. Sutko. Amrinone activates K^+-depolarized atrial and ventricular myocardium of guinea pigs. *Circ. Res. 51*: 662-665 (1982).
16. P. K. Siegl, G. Morgan, and C. S. Sweet. Responses to amrinone in isolated cardiac muscles from cat, rabbit and guinea pig. *J. Cardiovasc. Pharmacol. 6*: 281-287 (1984).
17. K. D. Meisheri, R. F. Palmer, and C. Van Breemen. The effects of amrinone on contractility, Ca^{2+} uptake and cyclic AMP in smooth muscle. *Eur. J. Pharmacol. 61*: 159-165 (1980).
18. A. A. Alousi, G. P. Stankus, and J. C. Stuart. The physiologic role of ions in the inotropic response to amrinone. *Circulation 66*: II-309 (1982).
19. S. Mallov. Effect of amrinone on sodium-calcium exchange in cardiac sarcolemmal vesicles. *Res. Commun. Chem. Pathol. Pharmacol. 41*: 197-210 (1983).
20. C. J. Frangakis, K. P. Lasher, and A. A. Alousi. Physiological and biochemical effects of amrinone on cardiac myocytes. *Circulation 66*: II-57 (1982).
21. F. Zannad, Y. Juillere, and R. J. Royer. The effects of amrinone on cardiac function, oxygen consumption and lactate production of an isolated, working guinea-pig heart. *Arch. Int. Pharmacodyn. 263*: 264-271 (1983).
22. J. R. Benotti, W. Grossman, E. Braunwald, D. D. Davalos, and A. A. Alousi. Hemodynamic assessment of amrinone—a new inotropic agent. *N. Engl. J. Med. 299*: 1373-1377 (1978).
23. N. T. de Guzman, O. Munoz, R. F. Palmer, D. Davolos, and A. Alousi. Clinical evaluation of amrinone, a new inotropic agent. *Circulation 58*: II-183 (1978).
24. J. E. Rosenthal, and G. R. Ferrier. Inotropic and electrophysiologic effects of amrinone in untreated and digitalized ventricular tissues. *J. Pharm. Exp. Ther. 22*: 188-196 (1982).
25. R. W. Piwonka, P. C. Canniff, and A. E. Farah. In vitro electrophysiologic properties of amrinone in mammalian cardiac tissue. *J. Cardiovasc. Pharmacol. 5*: 1058-1067 (1983).

26. R. W. Piwonka, J. F. Healey, P. C. Canniff, and A. E. Farah. Electrophysiological actions of amrinone in dogs with cardiac lesions. *J. Cardiovasc. Pharmacol. 5*: 1052-1057 (1983).

27. I. Kodama, N. Kondo, and S. Shibata. Effects of amrinone on the transmembrane action potential of rabbit sinus node pacemaker cells. *Br. J. Pharmacol. 80*: 511-517 (1983).

28. A. Nusrat, D. Tepper, J. Hertzberg, E. H. Sonnenblick, and R. S. Aronson. Effects of amrinone on atrioventricular conduction in the intact canine heart. *J. Clin. Pharmacol. 23*: 257-265 (1983).

29. N. Kondo, S. Shibata, I. Kodama, and K. Yamada. Electrical and mechanical effects of amrinone on isolated guinea pig ventricular muscle. *J. Cardiovasc. Pharmacol. 5*: 903-912 (1983).

30. J. E. Rosenthal, and G. R. Rerrier. Inotropic and electrophysiologic effects of amrinone in untreated and digitalized ventricular tissues. *J. Pharmacol. Exp. Ther. 221*: 188-196 (1982).

31. A. A. Alousi, A. Helstosky, M. J. Montenaro, and F. Cicero. Intravenous and oral cardiotonic activity of WIN 47203, a potent amrinone analog, in dogs. *Fed. Proc. 40*: 663 (1981).

32. A. A. Alousi, J. M. Canter, M. J. Montenaro, D. J. Fort, and R. A. Ferrari. Cardiotonic activity of milrinone, a new and potent cardiac bipyridine, on the normal and failing heart of experimental animals. *J. Cardiovasc. Pharmacol. 5*: 792-803 (1983).

33. R. W. Millard, G. Dube, G. Grupp, I. Grupp, A. A. Alousi, and A. Schwartz. Direct vasodilator and positive inotropic effects of amrinone. *J. Mol. Cell. Biol. 12*: 647-652 (1980).

34. G. Onuaguluchi, and R. D. Tanz. Cardiac effects of amrinone on rabbit papillary muscle and guinea pig Langendorff heart preparation. *J. Cardiovasc. Pharmacol. 3*: 1342-1355 (1981).

35. J. Boncyk, D. Redon, and B. Rusy. Hemodynamic effects of amrinone in dogs anesthetized with helothane: Comparison with isoproterenol and dobutamine. *Res. Commun. Chem. Pathol. Pharmacol. 44*: 347-354 (1984).

36. Y. Ishida, Y. Ohizumi, and S. Shibata. Excitatory and inhibitory actions of amrinone on the guinea pig isolated ileum and vas deferens. *J. Pharm. Pharmacol. 34*: 47-49 (1982).

37. G. Onuaguluchi, and R. D. Tanz. Electromechanical dissociation and possible uncoupling of phosphorylation following tachydysrhythmogenic dose of amrinone in the guinea-pig Langendorff heart preparation. *Arch. Int. Pharmacodyn. Ther. 271*: 81-97 (1984).

38. L. Brown, and E. Erdmann. Non-additive positive inotropic effects of amrinone and ouabain on cat papillary muscles. *Klin. Wochenschr. 62*: 390-393 (1984).

39. K. Satoh, M. Maruyama, and N. Taira. The improvement in cardiac performance by amrinone, a new cardiotonic drug, in experimental failing heart preparation of the dog. *Jpn. Heart J. 23*: 975-980 (1982).

40. J. R. Benotti, W. Grossman, E. Braunwald, and B. A. Carabello. Effects of amrinone on myocardial energy metabolism and hemodynamics in patients

with severe congestive heart failure due to coronary artery disease. *Circulation* 62: 28-34 (1980).

41. J. H. Jentzer, T. H. LeJemtel, E. H. Sonnenblick, and E. S. Kirk. Beneficial effect of amrinone on myocardial oxygen consumption during acute left ventricular failure in dogs. *Am. J. Cardiol.* 48: 75-83 (1981).

42. R. G. Harbison, H. L. Lippton, A. L. Hyman, and P. J. Kadowitz. Pulmonary vascular actions of amrinone and milrinone. *Circulation (abstr.)* 70 (suppl. II): 728 (1984).

43. M. C. Mammel, S. Einzig, T. J. Kulik, T. R. Thompson, and J. E. Lock. Pulmonary vascular effects of amrinone in conscious lambs. *Pediatr. Res.* 17: 720-724 (1983).

44. M. Maruyama, K. Satoh, and N. Taira. Effects of amrinone on the tracheal musculature and vasculature of the dog. *Jpn. J. Pharmacol.* 6: 1095-1097 (1981).

45. R. Osella, G. Piacenza, and R. Borgoglio. Amrinone relaxing effect on the isolated guinea pig trachea and its interaction with aminophylline. *Pharmacol. Res. Commun.* 15: 361-366 (1983).

46. Z. E. Mielens, and D. C. Buck. Relaxant effects of amrinone upon pulmonary smooth muscle. *Pharmacology* 25: 262-271 (1982).

47. S. Einzig, and M. E. Pierpont. Acute effects of amrinone (5-amino-3,4'bipyridin-6[1H]-one) on systemic blood flow distribution. *Am. J. Cardiol. (abstr.)* 47: 491 (1981).

48. P. T. Wilmshurst, D. S. Thompson, B. S. Jenkins, D. J. Calfort, and M. M. Webb-Peploe. The hemodynamic effects of intravenous amrinone in patients with impaired left ventricular function. *Br. Heart J.* 49: 77-82 (1983).

49. T. H. LeJemtel, E. Keung, E. H. Sonnenblick, H. S. Ribner, M. Matsumoto, R. Davis, W. Schwartz, A. A. Alousi, and D. Davolos. Amrinone: A new nonglycosidic, non-adrenergic cardiotonic agent effective in the treatment of intractable myocardial failure in man. *Circulation* 59: 1098-1104 (1979).

50. T. H. LeJemtel, E. Keung, H. S. Ribner, R. Davis, J. Wexler, M. D. Blaufox, and E. H. Sonnenblick. Sustained beneficial effects of oral amrinone on cardiac and renal function in severe congestive heart failure in man. *Am. J. Cardiol.* 45: 123-129 (1980).

51. J. Wynne, R. F. Malacoff, J. R. Benotti, G. D. Curfman, W. Grossman, B. L. Holman, T. W. Smith, and E. Braunwald. Oral amrinone in refractory congestive heart failure. *Am. J. Cardiol.* 45: 1245-1249 (1980).

52. S. J. Siskind, E. H. Sonnenblick, R. Forman, J. Scheuer, and T. H. LeJemtel. Acute substantial benefit of inotropic therapy with amrinone in exercise hemodynamics and metabolism in severe congestive heart failure. *Circulation* 64: 966-973 (1981).

53. P. T. Wilmshurst, et al. Comparison of the effects of amrinone and sodium nitroprusside on hemodynamics, contractility and myocardial metabolism in patients with cardiac failure due to coronary artery disease and dilated cardiomyopathy. *Br. Heart J. 52*: 38-48 (1984).

54. K. T. Weber, V. Andrews, J. S. Janicki, J. R. Wilson, and A. P. Fishman. Amrinone and exercise performance in patients with chronic heart failure. *Am. J. Cardiol.* 48: 164-169

55. C. S. Maskin, R. Forman, N. A. Klein, E. H. Sonnenblick, and T. H. LeJemtel. Long-term amrinone therapy in patients with severe heart failure. Drug-dependent hemodynamic benefits despite progression of the disease. *Am. J. Med. 72*: 113-118 (1982).

56. M. J. Likoff, K. T. Weber, V. Andrews, J. S. Janicki, M. S. T. Sutton, H. Wilson, and M. L. Rocci. Amrinone in the treatment of chronic cardiac failure. *J. Am. Coll. Cardiol. 3*: 1282-1290 (1984).

57. T. H. LeJemtel, E. C. Keung, W. J. Schwartz, C. S. Maskin, M. A. Greenberg, R. S. Davis, R. Formen, H. S. Ribner, and E. H. Sonnenblick. Hemodynamic effects of intravenous and oral administration. *Trans. Assoc. Am. Physicians 42*: 325-333 (1979).

58. N. A. Klein, S. J. Siskind, W. H. Frishman, E. H. Sonnenblick, and T. H. LeJemtel. Hemodynamic comparison of intravenous amrinone and dobutamine in patients with chronic congestive heart failure. *Am. J. Cardiol. 48*: 170-175 (1981).

59. J. Bayliss, M. Norell, R. Canepa-Anson, S. R. Reuben, P. A. Poole-Wilson, and G. C. Sutton. Acute hemodynamic comparison of amrinone and pirbuterol in chronic heart failure—additional effects of isosorbide dinitrate. *Br. Heart J. 49*: 214-221 (1983).

60. B. G. Firth, A. V. Ratner, E. D. Grassman, M. D. Winniford, P. Nicod, and L. D. Hillis. Assessment of the inotropic and vasodilator effects of amrinone versus isoproterenol. *Am. J. Cardiol. 54*: 1331-1336 (1984).

61. J. R. Benotti, J. McCue, D. Love, and J. S. Alpert. Comparative inotropic therapy in heart failure patients. *Circulation (suppl. 3) 68*: 510 (1983).

62. L. A. Siegel, E. Keung, S. J. Siskind, R. Forman, H. Feinberg, J. Strom, D. Efstathakis, E. Sonnenblick, and T. H. LeJemtel. Beneficial effects of amrinonehydralazine combination on resting hemodynamics and exercise capacity in patients with severe heart failure. *Circulation 63*: 838-844 (1981).

63. L. A. Siegel, T. H. LeJemtel, J. Strom, C. Maskin, R. Forman, W. Frishman, J. Wexler, H. Ribner, and E. H. Sonnenblick. Improvement in the exercise capacity despite cardiac deterioration: Noninvasive assessment of long-term therapy with amrinone in severe heart failure. *Am. Heart J. 106*: 1042-1047 (1983).

64. S. A. Rubin, S. Lee, L. O'Conner, A. Hubernette, J. Tober, and H. J. C. Swan. Thrombocytopenia and fever in a patient taking amrinone. (Letter). *N. Engl. J. Med. 301*: 1185 (1979).

65. P. T. Wilmshurst, and M. M. Webb-Peploe. Side effects of amrinone therapy. *Br. Heart J. 49*: 447-451 (1983).

66. E. L. Kinney, J. O. Ballard, B. Carlin, and R. Zelis. Amrinone-mediated thrombocytopenia. *Scand. J. Haematol. 31*: 376-380 (1983).

67. M. E. Gilman, and S. C. Margolis. Amrinone-induced hepatotoxicity. *Clin. Pharm. 3*: 422-424 (1984).

68. W. B. Dunkman, M. M. Wilen, and J. A. Franciosa. Adverse effects of long-term amrinone administration in congestive heart failure. *Am. Heart J. 105*: 861-863 (1983).

69. C. V. Leier, K. Dalpiaz, P. Huss, J. B. Hermiller, R. D. Magorian, T. M. Bashore, and D. V. Unverferth. Amrinone therapy for CHF in outpatients with idiopathic dilated cardiomyopathy. *Am. J. Cardiol. 52*: 304-308 (1983).

70. J. Ansell, et al. Amrinone-induced thrombocytopenia. *Arch. Intern. Med. 144*: 949-952 (1984).

71. A. M. Katz. A new inotropic drug: Its promise and a caution. *N. Engl. J. Med. 299*: 1409-1410 (1978).

72. P. T. Wilmshurst, J. M. Walker, C. H. Fry, et al. Inotropic and vasodilator effects of amrinone on isolated human tissue. *Cardiovasc. Res. 18*: 302-309 (1984).

73. M. Packer. Vasodilator and inotropic therapy for severe chronic heart failure: Passion and skepticism. *J. Am. Coll. Cardiol. 2*: 841-852 (1983).

74. J. A. Franciosa. Intravenous amrinone: An advance or a wrong step? *Ann. Intern. Med. 102*: 399-400 (1985).

75. E. L. Kinney, B. Carlin, J. O. Ballard, J. M. Burks, W. F. Hallahan, and R. Zelis. Clinical experience with amrinone in patients with advanced congestive heart failure. *J. Clin. Pharmacol. 22*: 433-440 (1982).

76. Sterling-Winthrop Research Institute. A summary of laboratory and clinical data on Inocor brand of amrinone, WIN 40680. Jan. 1, 1980. Rensselaer, New York.

77. C. V. Naccarelli, et al. Amrinone: Acute electrophysiologic effects and hemodynamic effects in patients with congestive heart failure. *Am. J. Cardiol. 54*: 600-604 (1984).

78. Winthrop-Breon Laboratories. FDA approved package insert—Inocor lactate injection-brand of amrinone lactate. New York.

79. R. DiBianco, R. Shabetai, B. Silverman, C. Leior, J. R. Benotti, with the Amrinone Multicenter Study Investigators. Oral amrinone for the treatment of chronic congestive heart failure: Results of a multicenter, randomized double-blind and placebo-controlled withdrawal study. *J. Am. Coll. Cardiol. 4*: 855-866 (1984).

80. B. Massie, M. Bourassa, R. DiBianco, M. Hess, M. Konstam, M. Likoff, and M. Packer, for the Amrinone Multicenter Trial Group. Long-term oral administration of amrinone for congestive heart failure: Lack of efficacy in a multicenter controlled trial. *Circulation 71*: 963-971 (1985).

81. M. Packer, N. Medina, and M. Yushak. Failure of low doses of amrinone to produce sustained hemodynamic improvement in patients with severe chronic congestive heart failure. *Am. J. Cardiol. 54*: 1025-1029 (1984).

82. J. R. Evans, K. Pacht, P. Huss, D. V. Unverferth, T. M. Bashore, and C. V. Leier. Chronic oral amrinone therapy in congestive heart failure: A double-blind, placebo-controlled withdrawal study. *Int. J. Clin. Pharmacol. Res. 4*: 9-18 (1984).

83. A. A. Alousi, T. Iwan, J. Edelson, and C. Biddlecome. Correlation of the hemodynamic and pharmacokinetic profile of intravenous milrinone in the anesthetized dog. *Arch. Int. Pharmacodyn. Ther. 267*: 59-66 (1984).

84. G. Pastelin, R. Mendez, E. Kabela, and A. Farah. The search for a digitalis substitute II milrinone (Win 47203): Its action on the heart-lung preparation of the dog. *Life Sci. 33*: 1787-1796 (1983).

85. A. A. Alousi, G. P. Stankus, J. C. Stuart, and L. H. Walton. Characterization of the cardiotonic effects of milrinone, a new and potent bipyridine, on isolated tissues from several species. *J. Cardiovasc. Pharmacol. 5*: 804-811 (1983).

86. Sterling-Winthrop Research Institute. A summary of laboratory and clinical data on Milrinone (Win 47203 cardiotonic). Jan. 13, 1984.

87. R. J. Cody, S. H. Kubo, F. Muller, H. Rutman, and D. Leonard. Vasodilator properties of milrinone: An intra-arterial study. *Circulation (abstr.) 70*: II-11 (1984).

88. R. J. Cody, S. H. Kubo, H. Rutman, and D. Leonard. Inotropic therapy improves abnormal vascular sympathetic responsiveness in chronic heart failure. *Clin. Res. (abstr.) 32*: 156A (1984).

89. L. S. Sinoway, C. S. Maskin, B. Chadwick, R. Forman, E. H. Sonnenblick, and T. H. LeJemtel. Long-term therapy with a new cardiotonic agent, Win 47203: Drug-dependent improvement in cardiac performance and progression of the underlying disease. *J. Am. Coll. Cardiol. 2*: 327-331 (1983).

90. M. P. Kullberg, B. Dorrbecker, J. Lennon, E. Rowe, and J. Edelson. High-performance liquid chromatographic analysis of amrinone and its N-acteyl derivative in plasma: Pharmacokinetics of amrinone in the dog. *J. Chromatog. 187*: 264-270 (1980).

91. M. P. Kullberg, G. B. Freeman, C. Biddlecome, A. A. Alousi, and J. Edelson. Amrinone metabolism. *Clin. Pharm. Ther. 29*: 394-401 (1981).

92. J. F. Baker, B. W. Chalecki, D. P. Benziger, P. E. Omelia, S. D. Clemans, and J. Edelson. Metabolism of amrinone in animals. *Drug. Metab. Dispos. 10*: 168-172 (1982).

93. J. Edelson, T. H. LeJemtel, A. A. Alousi, C. E. Biddlecome, C. S. Maskin, and E. H. Sonnenblick. Relationship between amrinone plasma concentration and cardiac index. *Clin. Pharm. Ther. 29*: 723-728 (1981).

94. J. R. Benotti, L. J. Lesko, and J. E. McCue. Acute pharmacodynamics and pharmacokinetics of oral amrinone. *J. Clin. Pharmacol. 22*: 425-432 (1982).

95. A. A. Alousi, T. Iwan, J. Edelson, and C. Biddlecome. Correlation of the hemodynamic and pharmacokinetic profile of intravenous milrinone in the anesthetized dog. *Arch. Int. Pharmacodyn. Ther. 267*: 59-66 (1984).

96. J. Edelson, R. F. Koss, J. F. Baker, and G. B. Park. High performance liquid chromatographic analysis of Win 47203 in plasma and urine: Intravenous pharmacokinetics in the dog. *J. Chromatogr. 276*: 456-462 (1983).

97. J. F. Baker, and J. Edelson. Metabolism and pharmacokinetics of milrinone in laboratory animals. In *Milrinone—Investigation of a New Inotropic Therapy for Congestive Heart Failure*. E. Braunwald, E. H. Sonnenblick, L. W. Chakrin, and R. P. Schwartz (eds.). Raven Press, New York, 1984, pp. 49-53.

98. R. M. Stroshane, R. F. Koss, C. E. Biddlecome, C. Luczkowec, and J. Edelson. Oral and intravenous pharmacokinetics of milrinone in human volunteers. *J. Pharm. Sci. 73*: 1438-1441 (1984).

99. J. R. Benotti, L. J. Lesko, J. E. McCue, P. Brady, and J. S. Alpert. Pharmacokinetics and pharmacodynamics of intravenous milrinone. *Circulation 70*: II-168 (1984).
100. J. R. Benotti, and W. B. Hood. Dose-ranging study of intravenous milrinone to determine efficacy and pharmacokinetics. In *Milrinone—Investigation of a New Inotropic Therapy for Congestive Heart Failure*. E. Braunwald, E. H. Sonnenblick, L. W. Chakrin, and R. P. Schwartz (eds.). Raven Press, New York, 1984, pp. 95-107.
101. B. E. Jaski, M. A. Fifer, R. F. Wright, E. Braunwald, and W. S. Colucci. Positive inotropic and vasodilator actions of milrinone in patients with severe congestive heart failure. *J. Clin. Invest. 75*: 643-649 (1985).
102. S. H. Kubo, R. J. Cody, K. Chatterjee, C. Simonton, H. Rutman, and D. Leonard. Acute dose range study of milrinone in congestive heart failure. *Am. J. Cardiol. 55*: 726-730 (1985).
103. R. J. Cody, K. Chatterjee, S. H. Kubo, C. Simonton, A. Rutman, and J. Edelson. Pharmacokinetics of milrinone in congestive heart failure. *Clin. Pharmacol. Ther. (abstr.) 35*: 232 (1984).
104. H. Scholz. Pharmacological actions of various inotropic drugs. *Eur. Heart J. 4*: 161-172 (1983).
105. H. Scholtz. Inotropic drugs and their mechanisms of action. *J. Am. Coll. Cardiol. 4*: 389-397 (1984).
106. O. Binah, and M. R. Rosen. Developmental changes in the interactions of amrinone and ouabain in canine ventricular muscle. *Dev. Pharmacol. Ther. 6*: 333-346 (1983).
107. A. Schwartz, I. Grupp, G. Grupp, C. L. Johnson, P. Berner, E. T. Wallick, and K. Imai. Amrinone: A new inotropic agent, studies organelle systems. *Circulation (abstr.) (suppl. 2) 59/60*: II-16 (1979).
108. A. E. Farah, A. A. Alousi, and R. P. Schwartz, Jr. Positive inotropic agents. *Rev. Pharmacol. Toxicol. 24*: 275-328 (1984).
109. N. Toda, M. Nakajima, K. Nishimura, and M. Miyazaki. Responses of isolated dog arteries to amrinone. *Cardiovasc. Res. 18*: 174-182 (1984).
110. R. E. Rude, R. A. Kloner, P. R. Maroko, S. Khuri, S. Karaffa, L. W. V. De-Boer, and E. Braunwald. Effects of amrinone on experimental acute myocardial ischaemic injury. *Cardiovasc. Res. 14*: 419-427 (1980).
111. R. Bossa, I. Gatalulas, G. Savi, R. Supino, and F. Zunino. Reduction in lethal toxicity of doxorubicin by amrinone. *Tumori 68*: 499-504 (1982).
112. R. F. Malacoff, G. D. Curfman, J. Wynne, J. Neill, and E. Braunwald. Inotropic effect of amrinone in severe congestive heart failure: Lack of attenuation with sequential doses. *Am. J. Cardiol. (abstr.) 45*: 433 (1980).
113. G. H. R. Rao, S. Einzig, G. T. Johnson, and J. G. White. Effect of amrinone, a cardio-tonic agent on hemodynamics and platelet function. *Prostaglandins and Medicine 6*: 51-64 (1981).
114. S. Einzig, G. H. R. Rao, M. E. Pierpont, and J. G. White. Acute effects of amrinone on regional myocardial and systemic blood flow distribution in the dog. *Can. J. Physiol. Pharmacol. 60*: 811-8 (1982).

115. A. Timmis, K. Daly, and D. E. Jewitt. Haemodynamic effects of intravenous amrinone in patients with impaired left ventricular function. *Br. Heart J. 50*: 106-108 (1983).

116. A. Ward, R. N. Brogden, R. C. Heel, T. M. Speight, and G. S. Avery. Amrinone—a preliminary review of its pharmacological properties and therapeutic use. *Drugs. 26*: 468-502 (1983).

117. A. M. Katz, D. McCall, F. C. Messineo, A. Pappano, and W. Dobbs. Comments on "Cardiotonic activity of amrinone—Win 40680 [5-amino-3,4'-bipyridin-6(1H)-one]. *Circ. Res. 46*: 887 (1980).

118. A. A. Alousi, and A. E. Farah. Reply to the preceding letter by A. M. Katz et al. Comments on "Cardiotonic acitivity of amrinone—Win 40680 [5-amino-3,4'-bipyridin-6(1H)-one]. *Circ. Res. 46*: 887-888 (1980).

119. T. H. LeJemtel. Side effects of amrinone therapy. *Br. Heart J. 50*: 499-500 (1983).

120. J. H. Chesebro, C. E. Harrison, and S. L. Deets. Intravenous and oral amrinone therapy in refractory heart failure: Hemodynamics, exercise results, and side effects. *Am. J. Cardiol. (abstr.) 47*: 491 (1981).

121. Intravenous amrinone for congestive heart failure. *Med. Lett. Drugs Ther. 26*: 104-105 (1984).

122. D. L. Johnston, P. Mickle, D. Humen, V. Gaphardt, and W. J. Kostuk. Oral amrinone: Lack of early improvement in exercise capacity despite evidence of favorable hemodynamics at rest and during exercise. *Clin. Pharmacol. Ther. 33*: 207 (1983).

123. J. B. Hermiller, M. E. Leithe, R. D. Magorien, D. V. Unverferth, and C. V. Leier. Amrinone in severe congestive heart failure: Another look at an intriguing new cardiactive drug. *J. Pharmacol. Exp. Ther. 228*: 319-326 (1984).

124. J. N. Cohn, and J. A. Franciosa. Vasodilator therapy of heart failure. *N. Engl. J. Med. 297*: 27 (1977).

125. E. Braunwald, and W. S. Colucci. Evaluating the efficacy of new inotropic agents. *J. Am. Coll. Cardiol. 3*: 1570-1574 (1984).

126. K. Chatterjee, and W. W. Parmley. The role of vasodilator therapy in heart failure. *Prog. Cardiovasc. Dis. 19*: 301 (1977).

127. R. M. Grose, J. E. Strain, M. J. Bergman, J. McGinnis, M. A. Greenberg, and T. H. LeJemtel. Milrinone vs dobutamine: A comparative study. *Circulation (abstr.) 7*: II-11 (1984).

128. T. H. LeJemtel, C. S. Maskin, D. Mancini, L. Sinoway, H. Feld, and B. Chadwick. Systemic and regional hemodynamic and metabolic effects of captopril administered alone and concomitantly in patients with heart failure. *Circulation 72*: 364-369 (1985).

129. J. M. Davidenko, and C. Antzelevitch. The effects of milrinone on conduction, reflection, and automaticity in canine Purkinje fibers. *Circulation 69*: 1026-1035 (1984).

130. K. T. Weber, V. Andrews, and J. S. Janicki. Cardiotonic agents in the management of chronic cardiac failure. *Am. Heart J. 103*: 639-649 (1982).

131. M. Packer, N. Medina, and M. Yushak. Hemodynamic and clinical limitations of long-term inotropic therapy with amrinone in patients with severe chronic heart failure. *Circulation 70*: 1038-1047 (1984).

132. R. Engler, R. Ray, C. B. Higgins, C. McNally, W. H. Buxton, V. Bhargava, and R. Shabetai. Clinical assessment and follow-up of functional capacity in patients with chronic congestive cardiomyopathy. *Am. J. Cardiol. 49*: 1832-1837 (1982).

133. B. G. Firth, G. J. Dehner, R. V. Markham, Jr., J. T. Willerson, and L. D. Hillis. Assessment of vasodilator therapy in patients with severe congestive heart failure: Limitations of measurements of left ventricular ejection fraction and volumes. *Am. J. Cardiol. 50*: 954-959 (1982).

134. M. Packer, and T. H. LeJemtel. Physiologic and pharmacologic determinants of vasodilator response: A conceptual framework for rational drug therapy for chronic heart failure. *Prog. Cardiovasc. Dis. 24*: 275 (1982).

135. J. A. Franciosa, K. T. Weber, T. B. Levine, G. T. Kinasewitz, J. S. Janicki, J. West, M. M. J. Benis, and J. N. Cohn. Hydralazine in the long-term treatment of chronic heart failure: Lack of difference from placebo. *Am. Heart J. 104*: 587-594 (1982).

136. D. C. S. Lee, R. A. Johnson, J. B. Bingham, M. Leahy, R. E. Dinsmore, A. H. Goroll, J. B. Newell, H. W. Strauss, and E. Haber. Heart failure in outpatients—a randomized trial of digoxin versus placebo. *N. Engl. J. Med. 206*: 699-705 (1982).

137. M. Gheorghiade, and G. A. Beller. Effects of discontinuing maintenance digoxin therapy in patients with ischemic heart disease and congestive heart failure in sinus rhythm. *Am. J. Cardiol. 51*: 1243-1250 (1983).

138. S. M. Dobbs, W. I. Kenyon, and R. J. Dobbs. Maintenance digoxin after an episode of heart failure: Placebo-controlled trial in outpatients. *Br. Med. J. 1*: 749-752 (1977).

139. C. V. Leier, P. Huss, R. D. Magorien, and D. V. Unverferth. Improved exercise capacity and differing arterial and venous tolerance during chronic isosorbide dinitrate therapy for congestive heart failure. *Circulation 67*: 817-822 (1983).

140. J. A. Patterson, J. Naughton, and Pietras. Treadmill exercise in assessment of the functional capacity of patients with cardiac disease. *Am. J. Cardiol. 30*: 757 (1972).

141. J. A. Franciosa, and J. N. Cohn. Severity of congestive heart failure assessed by exercise and resting hemodynamics. *Clin. Res. 26*: 646A (1978).

142. K. M. Borow, P. C. Come, A. Neumann, D. S. Baim, E. Braunwald, and W. Grossman. Physiologic assessment of the inotropic, vasodilator and afterload reducing effects of milrinone in subjects without cardiac disease. *Am. J. Cardiol. 55*: 1204-1209 (1985).

143. D. S. Baim, A. V. McDowell, J. Cherniles, E. S. Monrad, J. A. Parker, J. Edelson, E. Braunwald, and W. Grossman. Evaluation of a new bipyridine inotropic agent—Milrinone—in patients with severe congestive heart failure. *N. Engl. J. Med. 309*: 748-756 (1983).

144. H. D. White, J. P. Riveiro, L. H. Hartley, and W. S. Colucci. Immediate effects of milrinone on metabolic and sympathetic responses to exercise in severe CHF. *Am. J. Cardiol. 56*: 93-98 (1985).

145. C. S. Maskin, L. Sinoway, B. Chadwick, E. H. Sonnenblick, and T. H. LeJemtel. Sustained hemodynamic and clinical effects of a new cardiotonic

agent, Win 47203, in patients with severe congestive heart failure. *Circulation 67*: 1065-1070 (1983).

146. C. A. Simonton, K. Chatterjee, R. J. Cody, S. H. Cubo, D. Leonard, P. Daly, and H. Rutman. Milrinone in CHF: Acute and chronic hemodynamics and clinical evaluation. *J. Am. Coll. Cardiol. 6*: 453-459 (1985).

147. A. M. Katz, and V. E. Smith. Regulation of myocardial function in the normal and diseased heart: Modification by inotropic drugs. *Eur. Heart J. 3* (suppl. D): 11 (1982).

148. E. S. Monrad, R. G. McKay, D. S. Baim, W. S. Colucci, M. A. Fifer, G. V. Heller, H. D. Royal, and W. Grossman. Improvement in the indices of distolic performance in patients with congestive heart failure with milrinone. *Circulation 70*: 1030-1037 (1984).

149. A. D. Timmis, P. Smyth, M. Monaghan, L. Atkinson, A. A. McLeod, and D. E. Jewitt. Milrinone therapy in heart failure. *Circulation 70*: II-10 (1984).

150. C. Simonton, R. Cody, K. Chatterjee, S. Kudo, H. Rutman, and D. Leonard. Milrinone in chronic heart failure: Hemodynamic and clinical responses during longterm therapy. *Circulation 70*: II-10 (1984).

151. J. P. Ribeiro, H. D. White, J. M. O. Arnold, L. H. Hartley, R. F. Wright, M. A. Fifer, B. E. Jaski, and W. S. Colucci. Chronic milrinone therapy: Differential effects on maximal and submaximal metabolic responses to exercise in heart failure. *Circulation 70*: II-10 (1984).

152. P. T. Wilmshurst, S. F. A. Al-Hasan, M. Semple, A. S. Hamblin, G. F. Savidge, and M. M. Webb-Peploe. The effects of amrinone on platelet count, survival and function in patients with congestive heart failure. *Br. J. Clin. Pharmacol. 17*: 317-324 (1984).

153. J. T. Brandt, et al. Effect of oral amrinone on platelet function and survival. *Clin. Pharmacol. Ther. 36*: 260-264 (1984).

154. P. J. Robinson, R. Lvoff, B. Chong, and P. A. Barrett. Amrinone—a new inotropic agent in chronic resistant congestive heart failure. *Aust. N. Z. J. Med. 11*: 666-668 (1981).

155. J. R. Holmes, S. H. Kubo, R. J. Cody, and P. Kligfield. Milrinone in congestive heart failure: Observations on ambulatory arrhythmias. *Circulation (abstr.) (suppl. 2) 70*: II-11 (1984).

156. E. S. Monrad, D. S. Baim, H. S. Smith, A. Lanque, E. Braunwald, and W. Grossman. Effects of milrinone on coronary hemodynamics and myocardial energetics in patients with congestive heart failure. *Circulation 71*: 972-979 (1985).

157. R. E. Rude, W. Grossman, W. S. Colucci, J. R. Benotti, B. A. Carabello, J. Wynne, R. Malacoff, and E. Braunwald. Problems in assessment of new pharmacologic agents for the heart failure patient. *Am. Heart J. 102*: 584-590 (1981).

8

Endogenous Inotropes

DONALD V. UNVERFERTH
Ohio State University College of Medicine, Columbus, Ohio

I. INTRODUCTION

Living organisms contain a wealth of substances that act to increase or to regulate the force of myocardial contraction. In most cases, the cardiac effect is not part of the primary role but a secondary effect that may enhance the substance's role. In some cases, the hormone or vasoactive substance has a direct effect on the heart, but in others, it may indirectly influence cardiovascular function. This chapter discusses each of these substances and attempts to determine the mechanism of the inotropy. For many compounds the available data are incomplete; I will summarize available information.

II. ENDOGENOUS SUBSTANCES WITH POTENTIAL POSITIVE INOTROPIC ACTIVITY

A. Gastrointestinal Peptides

In 1902, Bayliss and Starling described secretin, a substance from the gut which stimulated juice secretion from the pancreas (1). This discovery not only challenged Pavlov's concept that the gut was controlled entirely by neural reflexes but also described the first hormone (2). In 1905, Edkins described the action of another gut hormone, gastrin, which stimulated gastric acid secretion (3). Research moved slowly until the 1960s when Jorpes and Mutt described the structure of both gastrin and secretin (4). Since then, however, an additional 20 to 30 gastrointestinal peptides with "hormone-like" and "neurotransmitter-like" effects have been discovered. These peptides constitute a diverse group of extremely potent substances with characteristic individual distribution and complex mutual interactions. Some

TABLE 1 Amino Acid Sequences of Some Gastrointestinal Hormones

Hormone	Amino Acid Sequence
Glucagon	His-Ser-Gln-Gly-Thr-Phe-Thr-Ser-Asp-Tyl-Ser-Lys-Tyr-Leu-Asp-Ser-Arg-Arg-Ala-Gln-Asp-Phe-Val-Gln-Trp-Leu-Met-Asp-Thr
VIP	His-Ser-Asp-Ala-Val-Phe-Thr-Asp-Asn-Tyr-Thr-Arg-Leu-Arg-Lys-Gln-Met-Ala-Val-Lys-Lys-Tyr-Leu-Asn-Ser-Ile-Leu-Asn-NH$_2$
Secretin	His-Ser-Asp-Gly-Thr-Phe-Thr-Ser-Glu-Leu-Ser-Arg-Leu-Arg-Asp-Ser-Ala-Arg-Leu-Gln-Arg-Leu-Leu-Gln-Gly-Leu-Val-NH$_2$
Substance P	Arg-Pro-Lys-Pro-Gln-Gln-Phe-Phe-Gly-Leu-Met-NH$_2$
PHI	His-Ala-Asp-Gly-Val-Phe-Thr-Ser-Asp-Phe-Ser-Arg-Leu-Leu-Gly-Gln-Leu-Ser-Ala-Lys-Lys-Tyr-Leu-Glu-Ser-Leu-Ile

Note: VIP = vasoactive intestinal polypeptide; PHI = peptide histidine isoleucine.

of them were first isolated from the brain and, conversely, most of the other gastrointestinal peptides were subsequently found in the brain.

Although some of the gastrointestinal peptides clearly function as hormones (such as secretin), others function as neurotransmitters (such as vasoactive intestinal polypeptide, VIP) and still others function as paracrine regulators of cellular function (such as somatostatin) (5). In addition to their location in the gastrointestinal tract, some of these gastrointestinal peptides have been found in nerve endings in the heart (VIP, neurotensin, and substance P) (6). These three compounds occur in separate multitarget nerve fibers, although they may also be codistributed about some vessels (6). The distribution of VIP, neurotensin, and substance P in cardiac nerves suggest multiple and complex peptide-peptide and peptide-transmitter interactions that may contribute to the regulation of various cardiac functions (6).

Myocyte membrane receptors also show an interaction between some of the gut peptides. Membrane adenylate cyclase from rat heart is activated by glucagon, secretin, VIP, and catecholamines (7). Beta-blockade inhibits only the catecholamine stimulation (8). Secretin and VIP act on the same binding sites which differ from the glucagon binding sites (7). Gastric inhibitory polypeptide does not stimulate any of these receptors (7).

The amino acid sequences of these polypeptides are quite closely related (Table 1). A change of one or two amino acids may drastically alter the physiological properties. For example, removal of the amino acids 1 through 6 of the 27 amino acid sequence of secretin, results in a secretin antagonist (7). There is a remarkable sequence homology of the newly discovered polypeptide, peptide histidine isoleucine (PHI), which also has 27 amino acids (Table 1), to VIP, secretin, glucagon, and gastrointestinal polypeptide (GIP) (8). A change of only two amino acids between VIP and gastrointestinal polypeptide results in a change from cardiac inotropy (VIP) to none (GIP). Another characteristic of the gastrointestinal peptide is that it can exist in multiple forms. Gastrin can exist in six different molecular forms including three different sizes (5). Thus, the polypeptides can be altered to produce various effects. None of these compounds has the property of a perfect inotrope, that is, a peptide that improves contractility without chronotropy and without any other hormonal effects. However, the manipulation of these compounds may yet yield a better inotrope than presently available.

The following sections discuss the characteristics of several of the gut peptides. Too little is known about some of the newer compounds to treat them in full. However, much has been learned about glucagon and VIP and they will be discussed in depth.

B. Glucagon

Glucagon is a polypeptide hormone produced in the alpha cells of the pancreatic islets of Langerhans. Glucagon is also found in the fundus of the stomach and a closely related compound, enteroglucagon, is found in the intestine. Pancreatic glucagon and insulin direct the storage of exogenous fuels and serve to maintain euglycemia (9). In pharmacologic doses, glucagon has cardiovascular, gastrointestinal, and genitourinary effects. Enteroglucagon differs from the pancreatic variety in its physicochemical and biological properties and in its mode of release (10). The roles of glucagon from the gastric fundus and enteroglucagon from small intestine are not clear (10).

Some of the earliest observations on the effects of commercial "insulin" on the heart were made in 1927 by Visscher and Muller (11). They observed an increase in heart rate and improved contractility of the dog heart-lung preparation with some amorphous insulin preparations, while others were inactive (11). However, Farah determined that some insulin preparations contained a contaminant that had epinephrine-like properties (12). Pure crystalline insulin had no positive chronotropic or inotropic properties. Later this contaminant in amorphous insulin was found to be glucagon (13).

The cardiovascular effects of glucagon include positive inotropy, positive chronotropy, and peripheral vascular dilatation. In addition to these primary effects, some secondary effects occur due to the glucagon-induced release of epinephrine from the adrenal gland (14). Glucagon reduces the epinephrine content of the adrenal medulla (15). The effects of glucagon on renal function were first recorded by Staub et al. (16). Glucagon apparently acts as a natriuretic factor (17) and increased glucagon and decreased insulin have been recorded in the fasting state to account for the natriuresis (17-19). The mechanism of the glucagon-induced natriuresis and diuresis is probably that of renal artery dilatation (20) as well as a direct effect on the kidney tubules to increase sodium, potassium, chloride, and water excretion (21,22). This effect is inhibited by indomethacin, a prostaglandin synthetase inhibitor (23). A higher dose of glucagon (1 μg/min), when infused into the renal artery, also increased glomerular filtration rate (21).

The vascular effects of glucagon are generally those of dilatation. Glucagon increases aortic, superior mesenteric, and renal blood flow, while splenic and femoral blood flow does not increase significantly (24-27). Blood flow through skeletal muscle of dog and humans during intravenous infusions of glucagon increases only slightly (28). Thus, the major effect of glucagon on blood flow is to redistribute flow to the splanchnic area to the detriment of blood flow through the limbs (29). Glucagon also lowers pulmonary artery pressure and decreases pulmonary vascular resistance in the abnormal pulmonary circulation (30,31) and in congestive heart failure (28).

No evidence exists that glucagon dilates coronary arteries. The increase of coronary blood flow during an infusion of glucagon is secondary to increased myocardial oxygen consumption (32). The reduction of coronary resistance produced by glucagon is due to the chronotropic and inotropic effects of this hormone (33). In nonbeating hearts, glucagon does not increase coronary blood flow (34,35).

Glucagon has a positive chronotropic effect on the heart. It accelerates the rate of spontaneously beating myocardial fibers (36), and increases conduction velocity and membrane responsiveness in Purkinje fibers (37). In fact, glucagon can reverse the propranolol-induced decrease of atrioventricular conduction velocity (38). The spontaneous discharge rate of a Purkinje fiber (39,40) or an idioventricular focus (41) can be increased by glucagon.

Glucagon has a positive inotropic effect on the myocardium. Many studies have reported the positive effects of glucagon on contractility (42-47). Even in cultured heart cells, glucagon increases rate and contractility (48). Glucagon increases the maximum positive dP/dt both in dog heart (44) and rat heart (49) and the time to peak tension is decreased (49-51). In addition, diastolic function is improved with a decreased relaxation time (51). In humans, glucagon elicits a dose-related effect on heart rate, ejection fraction, and end-systolic volume (52-54). However, the doses required to elicit positive inotropy result in greater plasma levels than those seen in the normal physiological situation (54). In addition, the response of the severely failing human heart (New York Heart Association functional class III or IV) is less dramatic than that of the normal or mildly failing heart (52,55,56). However, in a comparison of glucagon, epinephrine, and ouabain, Gruhzit and Farah (57) found that the inotropic response in severe heart failure to all three was significantly less than in mild heart failure. Thus, glucagon has a positive inotropic effect on most intact and isolated heart preparations, but large nonphysiological doses are needed and the inotropic effect is dissipated in a failing heart.

Glucagon elicits its positive chronotropic and inotropic effects by the stimulation of cyclic AMP (48). The effects of glucagon on cardiac contractility and on cyclic AMP production are not blocked by beta-blockers (51). In addition, the response of cyclic AMP production and the force of contraction is less when glucagon is placed in the tissue bath with muscle from a failing heart (56,58,59). Glucagon and cyclic AMP have similar effects on the heart but cyclic AMP may not be the sole messenger for glucagon's action. Glucagon may activate sarcolemmal calcium channels independent of cyclic AMP (51). Further study on the mechanism of action of glucagon is still in progress.

C. Vasoactive Intestinal Polypeptide

Said and Mutt isolated vasoactive intestinal polypeptide from the porcine intestine and reported their work in 1972 (60). VIP is a member of the secretin family of hormones that includes secretin, glucagon, gastric inhibitory polypeptide, and more recently PHI. This family shares the anatomical localization of the upper small intestine and pancreas. However, VIP has distinguished itself by its additional distribution in the central and peripheral nervous system (61) as well as in the heart in the region of the sinus node (62). The distribution of VIP in mammalian heart has been intensively studied by immunohistochemistry (6). The VIP nerve fibers predominate in the atria and conduction system and are less common in the ventricles (6). The large vessels of the heart and periarterial cardiac glomeruli also are rich in VIP fibers. A recent study from our laboratory has also found by radioimmunoassay, that VIP is present in normal human and canine ventricular tissue, but that the levels are only about 1% of the level of catecholamines (63). In addition, the tissue levels are significantly decreased in heart failure (63).

The noncardiovascular effects of VIP are diverse and include a stimulation of electrolyte and water secretion by the pancreas and stimulation of small intestinal secretion in dogs (64). VIP raises levels of cyclic AMP in rabbit ileal mucosa by stimulation of adenylate cyclase (65). Often, VIP-secreting tumors of the pancreas induce watery diarrhea (syndrome of Verner-Morrison) (66). There are numerous other activities of VIP, including bronchodilation and pulmonary artery dilation (67). It also inhibits gastric acid secretion and relaxes gastric muscle (68). In addition, VIP stimulates lipolysis and glycogenolysis (69-71) and stimulates the release of prolactin.

One of the first observations about VIP was its potent vasodilatation of peripheral and splanchnic vascular beds (69). In later studies it was also found to be a coronary vasodilator (70,71). Our laboratory has extended these observations by an intravenous infusion of VIP into normal and cardiomyopathic dogs to determine the relative change of blood flow in the vascular system. Brain blood flow markedly decreased while cardiac and pancreatic blood flow doubled and tripled, respectively (72). A study in anesthetized humans has demonstrated that intravenous VIP lowers blood pressure and increases blood flow to the splanchnic bed (73).

It is known that VIP induces an increase in tension of isolated isometrically contracting cat papillary muscle; it also increases left ventricular dP/dt in intact anesthetized dogs when the heart rate, preload, and afterload are kept constant (74). Our laboratory has made similar observations in anesthetized dogs; however, blood pressure fell significantly as cardiac output, heart rate, and dP/dt_{max} rose (72). Isolated hearts from monkeys have also been studied; VIP increased the rate of beating of the atria and increased contractility as well (75). Increased contractility was also noted in a monkey papillary muscle preparation and the efficiency was equivalent to isoproterenol (75).

The mechanism of the vascular effect of VIP has been studied in brain vessels (76). In that study, direct topical applications of VIP onto exposed pial arterioles resulted in vasodilatation. Beta-blockers did not prevent the arteriolar vasodilation but indomethacin did (76). The authors hypothesized that the peripheral vascular effect of VIP was mediated by prostaglandins (76). Human cerebral arteries have also been studied and have been found to dilate with VIP in the tissue bath (77).

The mechanism of the positive chronotropy and inotropy of VIP is probably mediated by specific heart cell membrane receptors (78,79) and subsequent stimulation of adenylate cyclase (78,79). Some VIP receptors have been found in rat myocardial cell membranes (80). The VIP-stimulated adenylate cyclase activity in cardiac membranes was significantly decreased (35%) in a hypertensive strain of rats and this alteration actually took place before the onset of the hypertension (80). Some VIP receptors have also been found in human atrial and ventricular tissues (79). Thus, VIP release from local myocardial stores may stimulate VIP receptors and activate adenylate cyclase, with a resultant increase of cyclic AMP (81).

It is not known what stimuli cause a release of VIP. Perhaps the increased left ventricular ejection fraction found after a meal (82) is due to VIP release. However, the role of VIP in the cardiovascular system remains a mystery.

D. Secretin

Hydrochloric acid in the duodenum stimulates the release of secretin which acts on the pancreas to produce a watery secretion low in enzyme activity but high in bicarbonate. Secretin also acts in a feedback mechanism to inhibit gastrin-stimulated acid production and gastric motility.

Secretin belongs to the same peptide family as glucagon and VIP and seems to share many activities with them. In anesthetized cats, a rapid injection of secretin increases cardiac output and heart rate (83). In perfused dog atria, a positive inotropic and chronotropic effect has been recorded (84). In rat papillary muscles, secretin stimulated an increase in tension that was comparable to that found with isoproterenol, and the stimulation of adenylate cyclase by secretin in a heart membrane preparation was also equivalent to that of isoproterenol (85).

The receptors for secretin and VIP appear to be the same (80). Depending on the species, however, these receptors seem to prefer one peptide over the other. For example, the rat heart secretin/VIP receptor prefers secretin (79). The secretin/VIP receptor on cardiac membrane in humans, monkeys, and dogs prefers VIP (79). Beta-blockers do not inhibit the secretin-induced stimulation of adenylate cyclase (86).

Some factors do depress the physiological response to secretin. Obese rats have a 70% reduction in inotropic response and adenylate cyclase activity compared to lean rats (85). Depressed responses have also been recorded in cases of hypertension (80), hypothyroidism, and diabetes (79). Thus, it appears that secretin plays some role in the modulation of cardiac activity and data suggests that the effect is mediated by the activation of adenylate cyclase and the production of cyclic AMP (86).

E. Peptide Histidine Isoleucine

Peptide histidine isoleucine is also a member of the secretin family of intestinal polypeptides. The PHI consists of 27 amino acid residues and shows a remarkable amino acid sequence homology to other members of the glucagon-secretin family

(8). (See Table 1.) It has been shown that PHI stimulates cyclic AMP production
in rat liver and intestinal membranes, stimulates the release of insulin and glucagon
from isolated rat pancreas, and stimulates rat pancreatic secretion, while it relaxes
tracheal smooth muscle and relaxes the gallbladder (87).

Due to the recent development of a specific radioimmunoassay to measure PHI,
the peptide has been found in high concentrations not only in intestine but also in
brain, respiratory tract, urogenital tract, and other peripheral tissues. Its distribution is similar to that of VIP and there is a significant correlation between the concentration of these two peptides (87). The parallel distribution and release is due
to the cosynthesis of VIP and PHI from the same prohormone peptide.

F. Thyroid Hormone

The earliest clinical descriptions of the signs and symptoms of thyrotoxicosis were
made by Parry (88) and Groves (89) when they observed the hyperdynamic circulatory state. The increased atrial rate with hyperthyroidism and the decreased rate
with hypothyroidism was documented in 1918 (90). Although the cardiac output
was increased by as much as 100% in thyrotoxicosis, there was no difference of
arteriovenous oxygen gradient from normal (91). Some of these effects were
thought to be due to peripheral vascular dilatation (92) and the hypermetabolic
state (93), which returned to normal after the patients were rendered euthyroid
(93,94). Cardiac catheterization studies confirmed these findings, as well as an increased stroke volume and borderline elevated right-sided pressures in hyperthyroidism (94,95). The inotropic effect of thyroid hormone was also demonstrated
by noninvasive tests that showed an increase of the velocity of circumferential fiber
shortening and a decrease of the pre-ejection period (96,97). Despite this hypermetabolic state of the ventricle and the higher oxygen consumption, the coronary
blood flow is adequate in most patients at rest to satisfy oxygen requirements and
the percentage of oxygen extraction from the coronary blood is normal (98).

Exercise studies in thyrotoxic human subjects have suggested some abnormalities. Although heart rate, cardiac output, and total body oxygen consumption rise
with exercise, there is also an inappropriate rise of right ventricular pressures (95).
In addition, the left ventricular ejection fraction demonstrated by radionuclide
ventriculography was high at rest but fell during exercise (99). When these same
patients were returned to a euthyroid state, their ejection fraction returned to
normal at rest and rose appropriately with exercise (99). This effect was independent of beta-receptor blockade. Both normal and hyperthyroid subjects experienced
a fall of the ejection fraction at rest after propranolol administration, but only the
thyrotoxic group fell even further with exercise (99). This may indicate either a
mild reversible cardiomyopathy or it may indicate that the muscle metabolism
outstrips coronary blood supply with exercise and thyrotoxicosis.

In order to isolate the primary myocardial effects from the peripheral vasculature
effects of thyroid hormone, animal hearts have been studied. Thyroid hormone

markedly increases heart size (100). In the isolated rat heart, L-triiodothyronine (T_3) or L-thyroxine (T_4) increases the maximum positive dP/dt and shortens the contraction and relaxation times (101). In isolated papillary muscles, T_3 increases the velocity of muscle shortening (102), and the tension and the rate of tension development (103). However, if the tissue is made ischemic, it loses its properties of increased contractility (103) which may pertain to the exercising thyrotoxic human heart.

The time course of the thyrotoxic effect has also been studied. One day after initiation of T_3 treatment, the developed tension and maximal rate of rise of tension are significantly greater than normal in guinea pigs (104). The maximum functional effect is observed on day 8 (104), but hypertrophy continues to develop until at least day 16 (100).

Thyroid hormone also affects the electrophysiological properties of cardiac muscle. Exogenous thyroid hormone administration increases diastolic depolarization to raise heart rate (105). In addition, it decreases action potential duration (105), lowers the threshhold for tachycardia, and shortens the effective refractory period (106). These effects are returned to normal in the euthyroid state (107). Excessive thyroid hormone administration has been reported to cause atrioventricular block (108).

The mechanism by which T_3 and T_4 induce the cardiac effects has been extensively studied. Thyroid hormone affects target organs by reversible binding to high-affinity nuclear receptors which alter the transcription of specific genes (109-111). Nuclear receptor site activation stimulates RNA synthesis, which in turn increases protein production (111). One important change after T_3 stimulation is the increase in myosin ATPase activity (112,113). The myosin isoenzyme V1 (with high ATPase activity) becomes the predominant form, while V3 (low ATPase activity) recedes (114-117). The change is noted at 1 to 2 days and is maximum by 7 days (117) but can be reversed by a return to the euthyroid state (116). This shift of ventricular isoenzymes is not the pattern seen with other hypertrophic states such as pressure afterload (115), nor are these changes seen in atrial muscle (118). Other changes found in the cell may also be mediated via nuclear stimulation or they may be extranuclear effects of the hormone (111). The T_3 treatments increase cation movements by increasing the activity of sodium-potassium ATPase, potassium ATPase (119-121), and calcium ATPase (122). The T_3 increases phosphorylase-A activity (101) but does not seem to affect the rate of oxidative phosphorylation (123) or excitation-contraction coupling (124).

The interaction of T_3 with the sympathetic nervous system and their combined effect on the heart has been debated for decades. Some of the early studies suggested that the hyperdynamic state of thyrotoxicosis was due to increased catecholamines (125) or that there was a close relationship of thyroid hormone and the sympathetic nervous system (126). However, other investigators found that catecholamine depletion or beta-receptor blockade had no effect on cardiac function (127,128) and others found no need to interdict an intermediary substance to obtain the thyrotoxic heart (129,130). However, the thyrotoxic heart is more sensitive to beta-adrenergic stimulation (131-134). Radiolabeled alprenolol studies have determined that T_3 increases myocyte cell membrane beta-receptor number but not affinity (135-140). This effect is specific to the heart and is not seen in other tissues such as lymphocytes (139). This effect increases the sensitivity of myocytes to isoproterenol stimulation and decreases the number of alpha-adrenergic receptors and diminishes cyclic GMP and cyclic GMP protein kinase activity (140).

Thus, thyroid hormone is a powerful inotrope that has unique and multiple actions on the heart. The T_3 stimulates nuclear receptors and raises protein production, increases the activity of several enzymes, and raises beta-receptor number to enhance beta-adrenergic sensitivity.

G. Thyrotropin Releasing Hormone

Thyrotropin releasing hormone (TRH) is a tripeptide that has been found throughout the brain as well as in the spinal cord, retina, pancreas, gastrointestinal tract, placenta, and adrenal gland (141). It is a modulator and neurotransmitter that also resides in the adenohypophysis and releases thyrotropin (TSH) and prolactin. In addition, it may release vasopressin, growth hormone, corticotropin, and somatostatin (141). The hormone TRH is of interest because it has been increasingly used for testing in human subjects.

Infusion of TRH increases heart rate, and raises systolic blood pressures by 21 ± 2 mmHg and diastolic pressure by 14 ± 1.0 mmHg (142). Individuals experienced increases in pressure by as much as 56 mmHg (142) and some patients have noted chest pain and premature ventricular contractions (141). The mechanism of action is not known but it is probably due to the local release of catecholamines (142).

H. Parathyroid Hormone

Parathyroid hormone (PTH) is initially synthesized as a prohormone which contains about 106 amino acids (143). This prohormone is rapidly converted to a storage or glandular form which consists of 84 amino acids. After appropriate stimuli, PTH is secreted into the circulation where metabolism of the hormone generates one or more immunoreactive peptide fragments (144). The intact 84 amino acid polypeptide is not required for biological activity. In humans, the first 34 amino terminal residues of PTH have been identified (145); studies of this fragment from human sera suggest that it contains biological activity (146). High plasma concentrations of calcium inhibit and low concentrations stimulate the parathyroids (147). Low concentrations of magnesium can also acutely stimulate PTH secretion (147). Hyperphosphatemia may indirectly stimulate PTH secretion by depressing plasma calcium concentration (148). Once in the circulation, the half-life of PTH is about 30 minutes.

The actions of PTH are mediated via adenylate cyclase and cyclic AMP in the osteocytes (149). Under PTH stimulation the cells increase in size, cause absorption of bone, and release calcium in the plasma (146,150). In addition, PTH increases renal cortical, tubular cyclic AMP (151) and induces the rapid renal excretion of phosphate, sodium, potassium, and bicarbonate and promotes the reabsorption of calcium, hydrogen ion, magnesium, and ammonia (146). In addition, PTH may cause an increase in gastrointestinal calcium absorption (152).

It has been shown that PTH infusions produce dose-related arterial hypotension in dogs and rats (153). Only the first 34 amino acids of the PTH polypeptide are necessary to exert this action (154). In perfused rat hind limbs and in dog renal, hepatic, pancreatic, and coronary vascular beds, PTH exerts a direct vasodilator action; it also relaxes isolated strips of rabbit aorta (153) and rat tail artery (154).

Hypercalcemia (155) and intravenous administration of calcium (156) cause an increase of blood pressure. Renal failure is often characterized by hypercalcemia as well as hyperparathyroidism. The opposite effects of calcium (to raise pressure) and PTH (to lower pressure) often result in normal or mildly elevated blood pressure (157).

When PTH has been placed with rat heart cells grown in culture, PTH stimulated cyclic AMP production with a dose-related rise of heart rate (158). The total 84 amino acid moiety of PTH was more potent than the 1-34 amino acid fragment (158). In addition, the PTH increased the influx of calcium into the myocytes (158). Bullfrog atria also respond with positive chronotropy and inotropy to PTH (159,160), as does the isolated papillary muscle of the rat (161).

The mechanism of action of PTH on cardiac tissue may be at least partially due to the release of myocardial stores of catecholamines and the subsequent stimulation of beta-receptors and rise of cyclic AMP (161). However, most studies have found the effects to be independent of beta-receptors (that is, not blocked by propranolol) and catecholamine stores (158-160). Apparently PTH has a separate receptor that stimulates adenylate cyclase and induces a rise of cyclic AMP with a remarkable influx of calcium (158). This influx of calcium can be blocked by verapamil (158).

The PTH-induced rise of myocardial calcium results in increased inotropy (158-160). However, high doses of PTH cause a remarkable and toxic rise of myocardial calcium that is synergistic with catecholamines (158). This observation is clinically pertinent in chronic renal failure in which high plasma calcium levels induce PTH secretion and a subsequent rise of myocardial calcium. The myocyte calcium concentration rises past the inotropic state to the toxic state and results in the early death of cells (158). This pathway may be important in the cardiomyopathy of chronic renal failure.

The dystrophic hamster model of cardiomyopathy has been studied. Parathyroid ablation with a subsequent decrease of PTH and a fall of myocyte calcium accumulation decreases the severity of the cardiomyopathy (162). On the other hand, chronic hypoparathyroidism and subsequent hypocalcemia and hypomagnesemia result in cardiomyopathy and congestive heart failure (163). The congestive heart failure resolves with PTH replacement (163). Treatment directed only at normalizing plasma calcium and magnesium may also reverse the heart failure of hypoparathyroidism. Apparently both hyper- and hypoparathyroidism can result in adverse myocardial effects. It appears that the adverse effects are linked to calcium and magnesium metabolism and may be independent of catecholamines.

I. Sex Hormones

Uterine activity is under the control of the ovaries. After ovariectomy, the contractile actomyosin system of the uterus and the ATPase activity decrease. With subsequent administration of estrogen to ovariectomized rats, the excised uterus exhibits rhythmic contractility. Also, the estrogen initiates a recovery toward the situation existing in estrus by causing an increase in the actomyosin concentration and an increase in ATPase activity (164).

Estrogens have a similar effect on myocardial muscle. There is a reduction of myocardial contractility and actomyosin content in ovariectomized albino rats without any alterations in excitability or refractoriness (165). Treatment with alpha-estradiol (0.1 μg/day) returns tension production and actomyosin concentration to normal (165). Androgens influence the myocardial muscle in a similar manner. There is a reduction in heart weight and work capacity in castrated male rats. These changes are prevented by administration of androgens (166).

An intravenous infusion of estrogens produces generalized vasodilatation which is most pronounced in the pelvic organs, skin, brain, and coronaries (167). Injection of estradiol into human subjects results in an increase of skin temperature in the extremities for 2-3 hr as well as a drop of blood pressure. X-ray studies have demonstrated that estrogens dilate the uterine artery and increase uterine blood flow by 25-90% (167). The acute intravenous infusions raise heart rate, cardiac output, stroke volume, and force of contraction. Of the estrogen compounds, the order of potency was Premarin > estradiol > estriol (167). Chronic administration of estrogens causes an expansion of blood volume by 15% or more (167).

Early studies suggested that estrogens had a "glycoside-like" effect. Acute infusions result in T-wave changes (168) and bigeminy (169). Estrogens augment the effect of digitalis on the heart and appear to have a direct glycosidic effect (167). This action has been explained on the basis of the similarity of structure between the glycoside digitalis and the sex steroids.

Studies of the rabbit heart in vitro have demonstrated the positive inotropic effect of estradiol, the negative inotropic effect of progesterone, and the absence of effect of testosterone (170). In a Langendorff preparation, estradiol-17-beta enhances the rate of pressure development and decreases the time to reach peak pressure. Progesterone decreases both the rate of pressure development and the time to reach peak pressure (170).

The mechanism of action of estradiol-17-beta to increase inotropy is thought to be by receptor binding (170). The presence of estrogen receptors in the atrium of the rat have been reported (171). In addition, a recent study has demonstrated that estrogens increase the number of atrial histamine receptors so that the chronotropic response to histamine from estradiol-treated rabbits was significantly greater compared to those from control rabbits (172). However, estrogens appear to have no effect on myocardial alpha-receptors (173).

The sarcolemmal membrane is thought to be the site of the estrogen receptors, although receptor sites within the cytosol cannot be excluded (171,174). The sarcolemmal site is favored because of the very short time delay needed for the observed inotropic effects after the introduction of the hormone (170). The ultimate effect of estradiol on the myocardial cell appears to be on the slow inward calcium current (170). The influx of calcium is increased and thus the calcium available for the actin-myosin interaction is enhanced (170).

Progesterone shows the opposite effects. There is a decreased calcium influx (175) which is consistent with the observed decline of pressure development (170). Progesterone also counteracts the digitalis effect (176). The decrease in calcium flux can also explain the changes in the crest of the action potential as reported by deBeer et al. (177). An inbalance of sex hormones with an overabundance of progesterone has been hypothesized to be a potential etiology of peripartum cardiomyopathy (175,178).

Thus, although the precise role of sex hormones in the cardiovascular system is not well understood, it is thought that testosterone and the estrogens promote normal growth of the myocyte as well as the production of actomyosin. Estradiol may have acute inotropic capabilities mediated by specific receptors that allow an increased influx of calcium. Progesterone counterbalances that effect. The role of these hormones in the pathological states such as peripartum cardiomyopathy is speculative at this time.

J. Adrenal Glucocorticosteroids

Several centers within the central nervous system control the elaboration and secretion of corticotropin releasing factor (CRF) by the hypothalamus. The CRF is carried in the hypothalamic hypophyseal portal system to the anterior pituitary where it directly stimulates the release of adrenocorticotropic hormone (ACTH). A polypeptide with 39 amino acids, ACTH has its major physiological effect in stimulating cortisol secretion and release by the adrenal cortex. Cortisol is synthesized from cholesterol and after release is bound to transcortin. Cortisol enters target organs by diffusion and combines with a specific high-affinity cytoplasmic receptor protein. The receptor-cortisol complex is transferred to specific acceptor sites on nuclear chromatin where it produces an increase in RNA and protein synthesis (179).

Almost any significant stress will lead to increased release of CRF, ACTH, and cortisol. In addition, there is a normal diurnal variation with peak secretion around 8 A.M. and a nadir at midnight (180). Cortisol exerts widespread effects on the metabolism of most tissue. Fat and protein catabolism is enhanced while glucose is formed. Lipolysis adds glycerol for further gluconeogenesis and the released free fatty acids provide an energy source which allows for glucose sparing. Within the liver, cortisol stimulates both gluconeogenesis and glycogen formation (181). The rise of blood glucose levels is counteracted by hyperinsulinism.

Other important effects of cortisol include lysis of lymphoid tissue, decrease in circulating lymphocytes, suppression of eosinophils and basophils, osteoporosis, increased gastric secretion, and altered central nervous system activity including mood changes. In physiological amounts, cortisol improves muscle strength, while deficiency results in weakness. Adrenal corticosteroids also have anti-inflammatory properties and they have a major effect on the distribution and excretion of body water (179).

An acute infusion of cortisol produces diverse effects on the cardiovascular system. Most of these effects can be ascribed to enhanced sensitivity to catecholamine stimulation (182). It also appears that cortisol increases the response to epinephrine more than to norepinephrine (183). Specifically, adrenocorticosteroids enhance the positive inotropic response of heart muscle (184), enhance vascular response (185,186), and enhance hepatic glucose production (187). Catecholamine exposure from endogenous or exogenous sources leads to diminished physiological responsiveness to further catecholamine stimulation (188). The desensitization of beta-receptors is attenuated by adrenocorticosteroid administration (182). It may also be that the enhanced response to catecholamine stimulation from cortisol is due to the inhibition of catechol-O-methyl transferase, the primary enzyme for the metabolism of catecholamines (183).

A chronic loss of adrenal corticosteroids (Addison's syndrome) is characterized by increased capillary permeability, inadequate vasomotor response of the small vessels, chronic hypotension, and reduction in cardiac size and output. Chronic cortisol excess (Cushing's syndrome) is characterized by hypertension due to retention of salt and water, enhanced peripheral vascular sensitivity to catecholamine stimulation (183,189), and increases in renin substrate or angiotensin II (190). Accelerated atherosclerosis is also seen in Cushing's syndrome (179). The cause for the accelerated atherosclerosis is not clear but it may be due to the hypertension and hyperlipidemia (191).

K. Corticotropin Releasing Factor and Adrenocorticotropic Hormone

Corticotropin releasing factor is located in the hypothalamus and is secreted in response to stress to stimulate the release of ACTH. In addition, CRF is anatomically distributed in brain regions outside of the hypothalamus (192) and acts to modify the activity of the sympathetic and parasympathetic nervous systems, cardiovascular function, endocrine-pancreatic function, and carbohydrate metabolism (193). The CRF induces the release of vasopressin as well as angiotensin II. It also causes the release of epinephrine and norepinephrine from the adrenal medulla (193). Thus, CRF may be physiologically involved in integrating the neuroendocrine, autonomic, cardiovascular, and metabolic responses to stressful stimuli (193).

The ACTH receptors in the adrenal cortex are responsible for the release of cortisol. However, peripheral sympathetic nerves also have presynaptic ACTH receptors. Stimulation of these ACTH receptors increases the norepinephrine release (194). Stressful stimuli cause both ACTH release and activation of the sympathetic nervous system. Thus, the ACTH receptors may play a physiological role in the regulation of norepinephrine release (195). It is not known, however, whether ACTH also stimulates the release of norepinephrine from myocardial stores.

L. Insulin

Insulin is an anabolic hormone affecting all metabolic substrates including carbohydrates, fats, and protein. In general, the actions of insulin are to stimulate transport of metabolites and ions through cell membranes, biosynthesis of various molecules and macromolecules, and cell growth (196). Insulin reacts with a specific receptor on the cell membrane (197,198) to initiate its metabolic effect. In the fed state, insulin levels are high and the myocardial uptake of glucose and amino acids as well as protein synthesis are increased (199). In the patients with diabetes, there is a delay in the uptake and the disposal of fuels into their respective depots, which leads to abnormal circulating levels of these substrates.

The determination of the precise actions of insulin on the cardiovascular system is complicated by accompanying metabolic effects such as hyper- or hypoglycemia, or hypothyroidism, as well as by differing responses in different species. One consistent and important effect of insulin is that it is an anabolic hormone and allows for the normal growth and maturation of myocytes (200) and even promotes the viability of cardiac tissue in vitro (201,202). This factor alone may account for the cardiomyopathy reported in the absence of insulin, that is, in diabetes (203-207).

Several investigators have shown in animal studies and in isolated preparations that insulin increases cardiac muscle contractility, an effect that is not dependent on glucose or catecholamines (208-210). In addition, insulin increases heart rate (211,212), an effect not inhibited by autonomic nervous system blockade (212). The mechanism of the insulin-induced inotropy and chronotropy is not known (213). One study (214) has suggested that the direct positive inotropic effect of insulin is minimal but this study was done in the isolated septic rat heart.

Some of the effects of insulin on inotropy are undoubtedly due to the release of norepinephrine. Intravenous insulin increases plasma norepinephrine in subjects with a normal autonomic nervous system (215-217). The rise in plasma norepineph-

rine is also observed when blood glucose concentration is kept constant (217).
Plasma epinephrine does not change with insulin (216). The release of norepinephrine occurs from peripheral sympathetic fibers but is probably due to the stimulation of the central nervous system (213,217). This release of catecholamines con-
bributes to the increased inotropy of insulin administration in intact organisms
(213).

Insulin is a general anabolic hormone. Some specific proteins important to myocardial contractility have been studied and found to be depressed in diabetes. Calcium ATPase activity and actomyosin ATPase activities are depressed in strepto-
zoticin-induced diabetic rats (218). In addition, the myosin isoenzyme V1 is converted to the slower V3 (219). Graded therapy with insulin (too little to correct
hyperglycemia, polydipsia, or body or heart weight) normalizes cardiac contractile
function (219,220). Calcium ATPase, magnesium ATPase, and the myosin isoenzyme pattern is also returned to normal (219). No evidence exists at present, however, to suggest that abnormal myocardial enzyme function in nondiabetic heart
failure can be corrected by insulin.

In the Framingham study, the risk of developing heart failure for diabetics was
substantially increased (221). Even when patients with prior coronary or rheumatic
heart disease are excluded, diabetics have a four- to fivefold increased risk of congestive heart failure. This risk persists after age, blood pressure, weight, and cholesterol levels are taken into account (221). Thus, this excessive risk of heart failure
is caused by factors other than accelerated atherosclerosis and coronary heart disease. One suggested possibility is diabetic cardiomyopathy. This cardiomyopathy
consists of more than the previously described enzyme abnormalities (218-220)
and abnormalities of calcium handling (222). Pathology studies have described
heavy interstitial collagen deposition (204,206,207) as well as a PAS-positive gly-
coprotein material (204,207). In addition, the basement membrane may be markedly thickened. The thickened basement membrane of diabetes can be reduced in
size by compulsive insulin therapy with precise blood sugar control (223).

M. Growth Hormone

Growth hormone is a single-chain polypeptide with 190 amino acid residues. The
hormone is present in the anterior pituitary throughout life. Unlike many hormones
it does not exert its effect by increasing the activity of adenyl cyclase. Growth hormone appears to increase RNA synthesis, amino acid transport, and protein synthesis in a variety of tissues (224,225), resulting in nitrogen retention. The anabolic
effect of growth hormone on the heart has been clearly demonstrated (226). The
anabolic effect of growth hormone on the heart is further demonstrated by the
production of cardiac enlargement with acromegaly (chronic secretion of excessive growth hormone). Cardiomegaly usually occurs in acromegaly before there
are any other signs of cardiac disease.

An animal model of acromegaly has been created in the rat (227). Several weeks after implantation of a growth-hormone-secreting tumor, the serum level is nearly 100 times normal. At that time, the cardiac index, max + dP/dt, and aortic flow are markedly increased, while systemic vascular resistance is decreased (227). It is not clear whether the improved cardiac function is a primary event or secondary to the depressed peripheral vascular resistance.

Despite this rat model of acromegaly, human acromegaly is often characterized not only by cardiomegaly but congestive heart failure as well. An echocardiographic study reported thick hypertrophic ventricular walls (228); about 20% of patients have an asymmetrically thickened septum (229). Hypertension is common in acromegaly (230) and is associated with higher growth hormone levels and thicker ventricular walls (231). Some patients without hypertension or atherosclerosis develop significant congestive heart failure (232,233). Focal cardiac interstitial fibrosis and a myocarditis with lymphocyte infiltration have been reported in some of these cases (232,233). The increased collagen formation may be a direct effect of the growth hormone (234).

In summary, growth hormone has an anabolic effect on the heart and increased levels may have an inotropic effect during short exposure (1-2 weeks). However, chronic excessive growth hormone levels are probably detrimental to cardiac function.

N. Prolactin

It has become apparent that prolactin has many effects and that lactation is only one aspect of its function (235). In both sexes, there is an increase in secretion at night and there are bursts of secretion in response to stress, especially exercise, surgery, and myocardial infarction (236-238). Prolactin has striking renal actions causing sodium, potassium, and water retention and it also modulates the effects of aldosterone and antidiuretic hormone (239,240).

Prolactin also has effects on the cardiovascular system. Modest doses of prolactin potentiate the effects of angiotensin and norepinephrine on vascular smooth muscle (241). However, very high doses of prolactin depress the vasoconstrictor response (241). The effect on the isolated rat heart is similar. At lower prolactin levels (50 ng/ml) the heart rate rises 40% above control but at higher levels (200 ng/ml) heart rate falls to 25% below control (242). The cardiac response varies according to sex and time of year. Only male rat hearts studied in the winter respond to prolactin with an increased amplitude and rate of contraction (243). Prepubertal males and female rats do not respond at any time of year (243).

The mechanism of inotropic action of prolactin has been well studied by Karmazyn et al. (244). They studied the isolated rat heart and found that these animals increase inotropic force by 60% with 50 ng/ml of prolactin. The addition of beta-blockers to the bath prevents the response as does the pretreatment of the rats with reserpine. The investigators suggest that the inotropic influence of prolactin is mediated by endogenous catecholamine release (244).

The role of prolactin in normal physiology and in stressful situations is not clear. The diverse conditions necessary and the variable responses of the myocardium to prolactin have made this a difficult hormone to study. At present there are more questions than answers about this fascinating hormone.

O. Angiotensin

Decreased renal artery pressure leads to the renal release of renin, an enzyme that initiates the conversion of angiotensinogen to angiotensin I. Angiotensin I is a decapeptide that is converted to the octapeptide, angiotensin II, by converting enzyme. Angiotensin II and angiotensin III, a heptapeptide formed by hydrolysis, are the pharmacologically active forms (245,246). Further cleavage yields peptides with little activity.

The most familiar and best-studied effects of angiotensin II are vasoconstriction and stimulation of the synthesis and secretion of aldosterone by the adrenal cortex. However, this peptide has numerous other effects, including the stimulation of thirst and increased secretion of antidiuretic hormone, both of which compliment the effects of aldosterone and contribute to the retention of sodium and water. Angiotensin II directly stimulates the central nervous system in a way that causes a rise of systemic blood pressure by enhancement of sympathetic outflow. In addition, angiotensin stimulates sympathetic ganglion cells and facilitates transmission. Increased output of norepinephrine from the sympathetic nerve terminals is due to increased biosynthesis of norepinephrine, decreased re-uptake of the transmitter, and increased output of norepinephrine per impulse (247).

Angiotensin is by far the most potent pressor agent known; on a molar basis, it is about 40 times more potent than norepinephrine. Vasoconstriction involves precapillary arterioles and postcapillary venules (248). The peptide has a direct action on vascular smooth muscle and indirectly stimulates contraction by means of the sympathetic nervous system. The vasoconstrictor effect of intravenous angiotensin II is strongest in the vessels of the skin, splanchnic region, and kidney (248).

The positive inotropic effect of angiotensin II has been described in the dog, cat, and rabbit (249-253). The mechanism of increased contractility is probably due to two mechanisms: (1) the release of myocardial catecholamines, and (2) a direct stimulation of a cell membrane receptor and subsequent increased influx of calcium into the myocyte. In isolated rat heart and rabbit heart, angiotensin II facilitates adrenergic transmission by enhancing the release of norepinephrine (254, 255). Angiotensin II facilitates cardiac norepinephrine synthesis (256), inhibits neuronal uptake of norepinephrine (247,257), and increases responsiveness of the adrenergic effector sites (258). In isolated hearts, angiotensin II potentiates the inotropic (259) and chronotropic (260) response to sympathetic nerve stimulation;

this effect appears to be due to facilitation of norepinephrine release from the adrenergic nerve terminals in the heart (261). Prostaglandins at least partially interfere with the release of norepinephrine; inhibition of cyclo-oxygenase with indomethacin further increases angiotensin II-mediated norepinephrine release and contractility (262).

Angiotensin also directly stimulates the myocardial cell membrane (263). Pretreatment with reserpine (249,251,253,264), acetylcholine (265), beta-adrenergic antagonists (252), or extrinsic cardiac denervation (250) does not eliminate the inotropic response to angiotensin II. Thus, the hormone exerts a direct myocardial effect that is independent of the beta-adrenergic system. In addition, basal adenylate cyclase activity and cyclic AMP need not be affected by angiotensin II to develop increased contractility (265). The contractile response is blocked by verapamil, suggesting that the inotropic response is related to the slow inward current of calcium (265). Baker et al. (263) have used radiolabeled angiotensin II to demonstrate a specific cell membrane receptor which mediates the inotropic effects. The angiotensin II binding sites have high affinity, and are saturable, reversible, specific, and modulated by divalent cations and guanine nucleotides. The data from their study suggest that these binding sites represent the receptors that mediate the positive inotropic effects (263).

Thus, angiotensin II has profound effects on the cardiovascular system and these include positive inotropy. The positive inotropy is mediated by at least two mechanisms, including release of norepinephrine and direct stimulation of myocyte membrane receptors.

P. Histamine

Histamine, 2-(4-imidazolyl) ethylamine, is found throughout the body and is involved in diverse physiological processes. It is now clear that two distinct subclasses of histamine receptors exist, H_1 (266) and H_2 (267). These receptors show different structural requirements for both binding and activation; structure-activity relationships have been described (268,269).

Histamine contracts many smooth muscles, such as those of the bronchi and gut, but powerfully relaxes others, including those of blood vessels. It is a very potent stimulus to gastric acid production and elicits various other exocrine secretions (270). Stimulation of H_1 receptors induces bronchoconstriction and contraction of the gut (266). Stimulation of H_2 receptors induces gastric acid secretion (267), while vasodilatation is mediated by both H_1 and H_2 receptor types (271). Capillary dilatation is also mediated by both H_1 and H_2 receptor types, while increased capillary permeability and edema formation is primarily an H_1 function (272).

Histamine has a well-established positive inotropic effect on the heart (273, 274). This effect is quantitatively similar to that produced by the beta-adrenergic catecholamines and is also related to stimulation of adenylate cyclase and an increased cyclic AMP level (275). The positive inotropic effects of histamine are not mediated by beta-adrenoceptors and are not impaired by beta-blockers (275). The response appears to be mediated by H_2 receptors since it is mimicked by selective H_2 agonists and antagonized by H_2 blockers (271,276-278).

Histamine also has a positive chronotropic effect mediated by H_2 receptors. It is of interest that the increased inotropy occurs temporally before the increased heart rate (279). The H_2 stimulation increases the automaticity of the sinus node (267,280). Despite fears that H_2 receptor antagonism with cimetidine would cause bradycardia and worsen the sick sinus syndrome, a clinical study determined that cimetidine did not affect heart rate, sinus node recovery time, or sinoatrial conduction time (281). The H_1 receptor stimulation decreases heart rate and slows conduction through the atrial ventricular node (279) and may even cause various arrhythmias (270).

Although cardiac H_2 receptor stimulation results in increased inotropy, H_1 receptor stimulation decreases contractility (279,282). Thus, H_2 receptor blockade can unmask the histamine H_1 receptor and result in mild negative inotropy (282). Catecholamine and histamine stimulation of myocardial function seems to lead to the breakdown of ATP and the generation of adenosine. Adenosine also functions to block histamine H_2 receptor and the beta-adrenergic receptors so that H_1 stimulation may moderate the positive inotropy (282). Further modulation of the response to sympathetic stimulation has been demonstrated by Gross et al. (283). Cardiac histamine is released together with norepinephrine upon stimulation of the sympathetic nerves (283). A histamine-stimulated heart will release less norepinephrine, thereby conserving stores. In addition, the presence of histamine reduces the duration of the inotropic effect of norepinephrine (283). Thus, both H_1 and H_2 receptors modulate the effect of sympathetic nerve stimulation of the heart.

Q. Serotonin

Serotonin (5-hydroxytryptamine, 5-HT) is found throughout the plant and animal kingdoms and occurs in many venoms. Related compounds can be found in hallucinogenic mushrooms and the psychotomimetic drug, LSD (270). It is known that 5-HT stimulates or inhibits a variety of smooth muscles and nerves with a resultant wide spectrum of responses (270). The responses are variable between species, and tachyphylaxis occurs rapidly (284).

Most (90%) 5-HT is found in the gastrointestinal tract in enterochromaffin cells. Of the remaining 5-HT, most is in platelets and the central nervous system (270) although some is found in the myocardium (285). Most 5-HT is synthesized by the individual cells. Platelets, however, take up 5-HT from the environment and release it on destruction. Metabolism occurs rapidly in the liver and lung (270).

An intravenous injection of 5-HT increases respiratory minute volume but also induces pulmonary artery constriction (286) and bronchoconstriction (270). It has been demonstrated that 5-HT plays some role in the pulmonary hypertension of chronic hypoxia in rats (286). As early as 1953, Comroe and co-workers (287) suggested that 5-HT might be the responsible agent for the reflex embolism (287). Serotonin is found in abundance in platelets and may be released after embolization (288).

Motility of the small intestine is also stimulated by 5-HT; diarrhea is one of the manifestations of the carcinoid syndrome produced by a 5-HT secreting tumor (289). In some species but not in humans, 5-HT stimulates uterine contraction (270). Intravenous infusions in dogs and humans reduce the volume, acidity, and pepsin of gastric juice, while increasing the production of mucus. One of the most important physiological roles of 5-HT is in the central nervous system as a neurotransmitter (290).

Serotonin (or 5-HT) has a powerful vasoconstrictor effect on human (291) and animal (288,292-294) vascular systems. The arteries of hypertensive subjects seem to be more sensitive to 5-HT (291). A model of hypertension in the rat has revealed that platelets in some animals may release their 5-HT at a certain stage and this release is associated with vascular injury (288). 5-HT also appears to have a vasoconstricting effect on coronary arteries (295-297) although not all investigators agree (298). Sympathetic nerves in the myocardium can accumulate 5-HT and then release the transmitter with sympathetic stimulation (297). The general effects of 5-HT on vascular tissue is due to a direct stimulation of 5-HT receptors (299) but it is also due to a stimulated release of catecholamines (300). Thus, the sympathetic nervous system and 5-HT have a complex interaction to stimulate vascular constriction in apparently healthy states as well as in disease.

The interaction of catecholamines and 5-HT in the myocardium is equally complex. The 5-HT stores in the myocardium are at about 30% of those of norepinephrine, are extraneural, and are not due to platelet contamination (285). Myocardial 5-HT content and synthesis are markedly decreased in the failing Syrian hamster cardiomyopathy (285). Serotonin has also been found in human papillary muscles (285). Administration of 5-HT to ventricular muscle results in increased contractility (301-307), heart rate (306,307), and dysrhythmias (307). Large or prolonged doses of 5-HT result in rapid tachyphylaxis and a subsequent decline of the force of contraction to baseline levels (284,302,304). The mechanism of the positive inotropy and chronotropy is due to two actions: (1) direct stimulation of 5-HT receptors, activation of adenylate cyclase, and a rise of cyclic AMP (302,303,305), and (2) release of catecholamines at high doses (302).

The effects of 5-HT in the atria contrast with the ventricular effects. Within 6 seconds after injection of 5-HT into the left atrium, the left ventricular dP/dt doubles, and peripheral vascular resistance increases by 75% but atrial force declines by 82% (306). The atrial effect is partially due to a vagally mediated reflex (307) but 5-HT directly depresses atrial function as well (308). Isolated frog atrial tissue responds to 5-HT by a depressed isometric contraction; the depression is atropine resistant (308). Amplitude and duration of the atrial action potential are reduced by 5-HT (308). In addition, some investigators have found greater quantities of 5-HT in atrial than in ventricular muscle of rabbits and rats; the 5-HT localized to the atrial-specific granules (309). These investigators hypothesized that atrial granules may function in the storage and retention of 5-HT and may accumulate other amines as well (309).

In summary, 5-HT is a ubiquitous compound with diverse effects. Its role in normal physiology is not well understood but it probably functions as a neurotransmitter in the central nervous system. The presence of 5-HT in atrial and ventricular tissue implies some ill-defined supportive role. In pathology, it may have a role in systemic and pulmonary hypertension, migraine (vascular) headaches, and pulmonary embolism. Tumors of enterochromaffin or related cells (carcinoid tumor) release large quantities of 5-HT and other compounds. Many of the pathological effects of this tumor, including pulmonary hypertension and diarrhea, are due to 5-HT. Better understanding of this compound may lead to more effective cardiotonic and/or antiarrhythmic therapy.

R. Prostaglandins

The primary prostaglandins (PGE_2, $PGF_{2\alpha}$) were isolated and characterized in the early 1960s. However, the most active compounds thromboxane A_2 (TXA_2, and its degradation product TXB_2) and prostacyclin (PGI_2) were not found until 1975 and 1965 (310-312). The prostaglandins with a subscript 2 are derivatives of arachidonic acid metabolism and fall into several main classes designated by letters and distinguished by substitutions on a cyclopentane ring. In humans, arachidonic acid is either derived from dietary linoleic acid or is ingested as a constituent of meat. It is then esterified as a component of the phospholipids of cell membranes or is found in ester linkage in other complex lipids (313).

The primary prostaglandins (PGE_2, $PGF_{2\alpha}$) are synthesized by cyclo-oxygenase and then oxygenated to PGG_2 and PGH_2. These endoperoxides are unstable; PGH_2 is metabolized to TXA_2 and PGI_2. Tissues are able to synthesize the intermediate prostaglandin endoperoxides from arachidonic acid but further metabolism varies according to the tissue (313). Platelets primarily synthesize TXA_2, while blood vessel walls primarily produce PGI_2 (313).

The prostaglandins are not stored in the tissue. Therefore, release reflects de novo biosynthesis (314-316). They are synthesized by virtually every tissue in the body and their release can be stimulated by hormones (such as bradykinin and angiotensin II), nerve stimulation, exogenous neurotransmitters, mechanical damage, and decreased oxygen tension (316). Little prostaglandin is detected in arterial blood largely because of efficient pulmonary destruction (317). Thus, prostaglandins should be considered local hormones that are synthesized at or near their site of action (316).

The pharmacologic properties of prostaglandins include inhibition of platelet aggregation by PGE_2, PGD_2, and most powerfully by PGI_2; TXA_2 induces aggregation. Moreover, PGF_2 and TXA_2 contract bronchial and tracheal muscle, while PGE and PGI_2 (weakly) dilate these muscles (313). Gastric acid secretion is inhibited by PGE, PGA, and PGI_2, while mucus secretion is enhanced. Prostaglandin PGF causes a contraction of intestinal smooth muscle. When infused into the renal artery, PGE, PGA, and PGI_2 increase renal blood flow and provoke diuresis, natriuresis, and kaliuresis (313). The prostaglandins have variable effects in the central nervous system; various prostaglandins cause release of ACTH, growth hormone, prolactin, gonadotropin, and thyrotropin in the endocrine system. The signs and symptoms of the inflammatory process are largely due to prostaglandins. Prostaglandins may control the immunological response, and PGE and PGI_2 enhance the pain-producing activity and edema-inducing activity of bradykinin (313).

The cardiovascular effects of the prostaglandins are equally varied. An intra-arterial or intravenous infusion of prostacyclin (PGI_2) in humans induces a fall of peripheral and pulmonary vascular resistance (317). This is accompanied by a fall of blood pressure and an acceleration of heart rate (317). Further, PGI_2, PGD_2, and PGE_2 dilate the systemic circulation of dogs with a resultant fall of blood pressure (318,319). In addition, PGI_2 will directly relax arterial strips when isolated in the bath (311). It has been shown that PGE_2 relaxes the pulmonary circulation and has been used for the treatment of pulmonary hypertension (320). An intravenous infusion in patients with pulmonary hypertension results in a significant decline of pulmonary artery pressure and total pulmonary resistance without increasing myocardial inotropy (320). Systemic pressure and left ventricular end diastolic pressure fall while cardiac output increases (320).

The prostaglandins play an important role in the coronary circulation. Myocytes contain no prostaglandin biosynthetic capability while the coronary microvessels (<100 μm in diameter) contain very little (321). We know that PGI_2 is primarily synthesized in larger coronary arteries, while PGE is synthesized in the veins (321). The prostaglandin PGI_2 is a powerful coronary vasodilator (322-324) as well as an antiplatelet aggregatory agent (325). By an undefined mechanism PGI_2 also helps to preserve ischemic myocardial cells (326). Thus, PGI_2 has been used for the treatment of coronary vasospasm (with variable success) (323,327) as well as atherosclerotic coronary disease (325,328).

In the pathogenesis of coronary artery disease TXA_2 may be an important agent. Part of the mechanism by which hyperlipidemia, diabetes mellitus, smoking, hypertension, sex hormones, age, heredity, emotional stress, and diet contribute to the development and progression of atherosclerosis may be through an imbalance between TXA_2 and PGI_2 (328). The prostaglandin TXA constricts coronary arteries (329,330), induces platelet aggregation, and increases thrombus formation (325);

TXA$_2$ also appears to play a role in acute coronary occlusion. With acute occlusion, TXA$_2$ and catecholamines are released with a resultant coronary vasoconstruction that inhibits reactive hyperemia (329). These compounds may be responsible for the coronary circulatory failure during reperfusion of irreversibly damaged myocardium (329).

Several of the prostaglandins have a positive myocardial inotropic effect but the effect varies with the preparation and the species. The addition of PGE$_1$ to the perfusion medium increases the contractile force of isolated frog, rat, and guinea pig hearts but not rabbit heart (331). In newborn rabbits PGE$_1$ and PGD$_2$ increase maximum systolic dP/dt to a greater degree than in adults (332). However, PGE$_1$ is a positive inotrope in adult dogs (318,319,333) without any inotropy recorded in human subjects (320). The prostaglandin PGI$_2$ has no apparent inotropic action in isolated muscle strips (334) in dogs (318) or in humans (323). In some preparations, PGI$_2$ even has a negative inotropic effect (334). In isolated muscle strips (334), rabbit hearts (335), and human subjects TXA$_2$ consistently depresses myocardial contractility (336). An increased production of TXA$_2$ has even been recorded in sepsis and shock and may be an important factor in the myocardial depression in that clinical state (337).

The mechanism of action of the prostaglandins is not totally understood. However, specific receptors for PGE$_1$ and PGE$_2$ have been identified; most of the prostaglandins do stimulate adenyl cyclase and cyclic AMP production (313). The specific prostaglandin receptors and subsequent stimulation of adenyl cyclase are not inhibited by beta-blockers (319,332). The coronary artery dilatation properties of PGI$_2$ are also due to activation of adenyl cyclase and production of cyclic AMP (324,338). The cardiac effects of PGE$_1$ and the coronary effects of PGI$_2$ are mediated by calcium fluxes that may or may not be related to cyclic AMP (322,334). Nevertheless, these calcium exchanges can be inhibited by verapamil, which also inhibits the cardiac and vascular effects (322,334). Another study has suggested that the stimulation of rat heart sarcolemmal ATPases results in the increased inotropy in that model (339).

Improved knowledge of the prostaglandins and their metabolism and effects has already been applied to the treatment of ischemic coronary disease (323,325, 327,328), peripheral vascular disease (336), and congestive heart failure (340), in addition to their manipulation for the treatment of fever, inflammation, and asthma. The prospects for the effective prevention of atherosclerosis hold promise. Prostaglandins probably play less of a role as a positive myocardial inotrope but they may be important in some situations.

III. SUMMARY

In summary, the body contains numerous endogenous inotropes that interact in a complex manner to support myocardial function. The mechanism by which each

TABLE 2 Mechanism of Action of Endogenous Inotropes

Endogenous inotrope	Circulating or local hormone	Specific myocyte receptor	Relationship with catecholamines	Other mechanisms of action
Glucagon	Circulates	Sarcolemmal receptor, stimulation activates adenyl cyclase, ↑ cAMP	Releases epinephrine from adrenal gland	May activate sarcolemmal Ca^{2+}
VIP	Local	Sarcolemmal receptor, activates adenyl cyclase, ↑ cAMP	None known	May release prostacyclin in blood vessels
Secretin	Circulates	Common receptor with VIP and perhaps PHI	None known	None known
PHI	Local	No specific receptor	Releases catecholamines?	Releases glucagon and insulin
Thyroid	Circulates	Stimulates receptor on nuclear membrane, alters transcription of specific genes, and increases protein production	Increases beta-receptor number but not affinity	Changes V3 to V1 myosin isoenzyme
TRH	Local	None known	Local release of catecholamines	Local modulator and neuro-transmitter
PTH	Circulates	Sarcolemmal receptor, activates adenyl cyclase, ↑ cAMP	May release myocardial catecholamines	No
Estradiol	Circulates	Sarcolemmal receptor, increases cAMP which ↑ Ca^{2+} flux	None known	Promotes normal myocyte growth ↑ histamine receptors
Cortisol	Circulates	Intracellular receptor to increase protein synthesis	↑ Sensitivity to epinephrine, → beta-receptor tachyphylaxis or desensitization; May → catechol-O-methyl transferase	No

(Table 2 continues)

267

TABLE 2 (continued)

Endogenous inotrope	Circulating or local hormone	Specific myocyte receptor	Relationship with catecholamines	Other mechanisms of action
CRF	Local	None known	Releases epinephrine and norepinephrine from adrenals (other sites too?)	Integrates autonomic nervous system
ACTH	Circulates	None known	Releases catecholamines from periphery and adrenal gland	Releases cortisol
Insulin	Circulates	Sarcolemmal receptor primarily to facilitate glucose transport, also facilitates ion transport	Releases norepinephrine	Facilitates cell growth
Growth hormone	Circulates	Receptor stimulation leads to ↑ RNA synthesis and ↑ amino acid transport	None known	Chronically elevated levels promote cardiomyopathy
Prolactin	Circulates	Unknown	Releases myocardial catecholamines	No
Angiotensin	Circulates	Sarcolemmal receptor activation leads to ↑ Ca^{2+} influx	↑ Releases catecholamines ↑ Synthesis of norepinephrine Inhibits neuronal uptake of norepinephrine ↑ Responsiveness of adrenergic effector sites	No
Histamine	Circulates	Sarcolemmal receptor, activates adenyl cyclase, ↑ cAMP	Modulates response to catecholamines	No
Serotonin	Circulates	Sarcolemmal receptor, activates adenyl cyclase, ↑ cAMP	Releases norepinephrine	Sympathetic stimulation also releases serotonin
Prostaglandins PGE$_1$, PGD$_2$?	Local	Sarcolemmal receptor, activates adenyl cyclase, ↑ cAMP	None known	↑ Ca^{2+} flux

Note: cAMP - cyclic -3'5'-adenosine monophosphate; VIP = vasoactive intestinal polypeptide; PHI = peptide histidine isoleucine; TRH - thyrotropin releasing hormone; PTH = parathyroid hormone; CRF = corticotropin releasing factor; ACTH = adrenocorticotrophic hormone.

exerts its myocardial effect may be simply through the stimulation of a specific membrane receptor with subsequent activation of adenyl cyclase, increase of cyclic AMP, and stimulation of protein kinases, or they may release catecholamines (see Table 2). Of great interest are the compounds that have intracellular effects to accelerate protein production or increase ion exchange. Perhaps one or a group of these mechanisms can be effectively mimicked to improve our pharmacopeia of agents for the treatment of heart failure.

ACKNOWLEDGMENTS

The author would like to thank Tom O'Dorisio for review and Tami Smith for preparation of the manuscript.

REFERENCES

1. W. M. Bayliss, and E. H. Starling. The mechanism of pancreatic secretion. *J. Physiol. 28*: 325-353 (1902).
2. T. E. Adrian, and S. R. Bloom. Physiology of the porcine gastrointestinal regulatory peptides. In *Nutrition in Health and Disease and International Development: Symposia from the XII International Congress of Nutrition*. Alan R. Liss, New York, pp. 873-882.
3. J. S. Edkins. The chemical mechanism of gastrin release. *J. Physiol. 34*: 133-144 (1906).
4. J. E. Jorpes, and E. Mutt. Secretin, cholecystokinin (CCK). In *Secretin, Cholecystokinin, Pancreozymin and Gastrin*. J. E. Jorpes (ed.). Springer-Verlag, Berlin, 1973, pp. 1-144.
5. J. D. Gardner, and R. T. Jensen. Gastrointestinal peptides: The basis of action at the cellular level. *Recent Prog. Horm. Res. 39*: 211-243 (1983).
6. E. Weihe, M. Reinecke, and W. G. Forssmann. Distribution of vasoactive intestinal polypeptide-like immunoreactivity in the mammalian heart: Interrelation with neurotensin- and substance P-like immunoreactive nerves. *Cell Tissue Res. 236*: 527-540 (1984).
7. P. Chatelain, P. Robberecht, P. De Neef, M. Deschodt-Lanckman, W. Konig, and J. Christophe. Secretin and VIP-stimulated adenylate cyclase from rat heart. I. General properties and structural requirements for enzyme activation. *Pflugers Arch. 389*: 21-27 (1980).
8. K. Tatemoto, and V. Mutt. Isolation and characterization of the intestinal peptide porcine PHI (PHI-27), a new member of the glucagon-secretin family. *Proc. Natl. Acad. Sci. USA 78*: 6603-6607 (1981).
9. R. H. Unger, and L. Orci. Physiology and pathophysiology of glucagon. *Physiol. Rev. 56*: 778-826 (1976).
10. A. G. E. Pearse, J. M. Polak, and S. R. Bloom. Progress in gastroenterology. The newer gut hormones. Cellular sources, physiology, pathology, and clinical aspects. *Gastroenterology 72*: 746-761 (1977).

11. M. B. Visscher, and E. A. Muller. The influence of insulin upon the mammalian heart. *J. Physiol.* *62*: 341-348 (1927).
12. A. Farah. Beitrag zur wirking des insulins und isolierte abschnitte des dunndarmes. *Arch. Exp. Pathol. Pharmakol.* *188*: 548-553 (1938).
13. A. Farah, and R. Tuttle. Studies on the pharmacology of glucagon. *J. Pharmacol. Exp. Ther.* *129*: 49-55 (1960).
14. L. F. Scian, C. D. Westermann, A. S. Verdesca, and J. G. Hilton. Adrenocortical and medullary effects of glucoagon. *Am. J. Physiol.* *199*: 867-870 (1960).
15. P. Lefebvre, and A. Dresse. Influence de glucagon sur le taux des catecholamines surreniennes chez le rat. *C. R. Soc. Biol.* *155*: 412-414 (1961).
16. A. Staub, V. Springs, F. Stoll, and H. Elrick. A renal action of glucagon. *Proc. Soc. Exp. Biol. Med.* *94*: 57-60 (1957).
17. R. H. Unger, A. M. Eisentraut, and L. L. Medison. The effects of total starvation upon the levels of circulating glucagon and insulin in man. *J. Clin. Invest.* *42*: 1031-1039 (1963).
18. F. G. Benedict. A study of prolonged fasting. Carnegie Institute, Washington. Publ. No. 203 (1915). Quoted in E. Veverbrants, and R. A. Arky. Effects of fasting and refeeding. I. Studies on sodium, potassium and water excretion on a constant electrolyte and fluid intake. *J. Clin. Endocrinol. Metab.* *29*: 55-62 (1969).
19. W. L. Bloom. Inhibition of salt excretion by carbohydrate. *Arch. Intern. Med.* *109*: 26-32 (1962).
20. G. Gagnon, D. Regoli, and F. Rioux. Studies on the mechanism of action of glucagon in strips of rabbit renal artery. *Br. J. Pharmacol.* *69*: 389-396 (1980).
21. M. A. Kirschenbaum, and E. T. Zawada. The role of prostaglandins in glucagon-induced natriuresis. *Clin. Sci.* *58*: 393-401 (1980).
22. T. N. Pullman, A. R. Lavender, and I. Aho. Direct effects of glucagon on renal hemodynamics and excretion of inorganic ions. *Metabolism* *16*: 358-373 (1967).
23. U. B. Olsen. Prostaglandin mediated natriuresis during glucagon infusion in dogs. *Acta Endocrinol.* *84*: 429-438 (1977).
24. P. F. Hulstaert, H. J. M. Beijer, F. A. S. Brouwer, A. J. Teunissen, and G. A. Charbon. Glucagon: Hemodynamic action related to the effect of K^+ and Na^+ metabolism. *J. Appl. Physiol.* *37*: 556-561 (1974).
25. S. Tibblin, N. G. Kock, and W. T. Schenk, Jr. Splanchnic hemodynamic responses to glucagon. *Arch. Surg.* *100*: 84-89 (1970).
26. N. G. Kock, S. Tibblin, and W. G. Schenk, Jr. Hemodynamic responses to glucagon: An experimental study of central, visceral and peripheral effects. *Ann. Surg.* *171*: 147-149 (1970).
27. J. J. Madden, Jr., R. M. Ludewig, and S. L. Wagensteen. Effects of glucagon on the splanchnic and the systemic circulation. *Am. J. Surg.* *122*: 85-90 (1971).
28. J. G. Murtagh, P. F. Binnion, S. Lal, K. J. Hutchison, and E. Fletcher. Haemodynamic effects of glucagon. *Br. Heart J.* *32*: 307-315 (1970).
29. A. Kazmers, W. M. Whitehouse, Jr., S. M. Lindenauer, and J. C. Stanley. Dissociation of glucagon's central and peripheral hemodynamic effects: Mechanism

of reduction and redistribution of canine hindlimb blood flow. *J. Surg. Res. 30*: 384-390 (1981).

30. M. M. Kirsh, D. R. Kahn, B. Lucchesi, O. Gago, J. H. Dufek, R. W. S. Lee, D. Stutz, and H. Sloan. Effect of glucagon on pulmonary vascular resistance. *Surgery 70*: 439-442 (1971).

31. G. E. Gisgard, and J. A. Will. Glucagon and aminophylline as pulmonary vasodilators in the calf with hypoxic pulmonary hypertension. *Chest 71*: 263-265 (1977).

32. V. J. Tarnow, J. W. Gethmann, D. Patschke, A. Weymar, and H. J. Eberlein. Hamodynamik, koronardurchblutung und sauerstoffverbrauch des herzens unter glukagon. *Arzneim. Forsch. 25*: 1906-1910 (1975).

33. T. W. Moir, and W. G. Nayler. Coronary vascular effects of glucagon in the isolated dog heart. *Circ. Res. 26*: 29-34 (1970).

34. R. Gmeiner, and N. Brachfeld. Wirkungen von glukagon auf des kohlenhydratstoffwechsel des isolierten rattenherzens. *Arch. Kreislaufforsch. 65*: 151-161 (1971).

35. R. Gmeiner, and N. Brachfeld. Wirkungen auf den sauerstoffverbrauch und aus die hamodynamik des isolierten rattenherzens. *Z. Kreislaufforsch. 49*: 999-1006 (1970).

36. J. K. Pruett, E. F. Woods, and H. B. Daniell. Glucagon enhanced automaticity in spontaneously beating Purkinje fibres of canine false tendons. *Cardiovasc. Res. 5*: 436-439 (1971).

37. K. Prasad. Electrophysiologic effects of glucagon on human cardiac muscle. *Clin. Pharmacol. Ther. 18*: 22-30 (1975).

38. L. S. Whitsitt, and B. R. Lucchesi. Effects of beta-receptor blockade and glucagon on the atrio-ventricular transmission system in the dog. *Circ. Res. 23*: 585-595 (1968).

39. J. W. Stewart, R. J. Myerburg, and B. F. Hoffman. The effect of glucagon on quinidine-induced changes in Purkinje fibers. *Circulation 40*: 196 (1969).

40. K. Prasad, and P. Weckworth. Glucagon in procainamide-induced cardiac toxicity. *Toxicol. Appl. Pharmacol. 46*: 517-528 (1978).

41. R. D. Wilkerson, J. K. Pruett, and E. F. Woods. Glucagon-enhanced ventricular automaticity in dogs: Its concealment by positive chrontropism. *Circ. Res. 29*: 616-625 (1971).

42. B. R. Lucchesi. Cardiac actions of glucagon. *Circ. Res. 22*: 777-787 (1968).

43. G. G. Boder, and I. S. Johnson. Comparative effects of some cardioactive agents on the automaticity of cultured heart cells. *J. Mol. Cell. Cardiol. 4*: 453-463 (1972).

44. G. Glick, W. W. Parmley, A. S. Wechsler, and E. H. Sonnenblick. Glucagon: Its enhancement of cardiac performance in the cat and dog and persistence of its inotropic action in spite of beta-receptor blockade and propranolol. *Circ. Res. 22*: 789-799 (1968).

45. Y. Matsuura, M. Tamura, E, Kato, S. Uehara, and T. Mochizuki. Experimental studies on the effects of glucagon on the denervated transplanted heart. *Hiroshima J. Med. Sci. 20*: 207-213 (1971).

46. T. J. Regan, P. H. Lehan, D. H. Henneman, A. Behar, and H. K. Hellemi. Myocardial, metabolic and contractile response to glucagon and epinephrine. *J. Lab. Clin. Med. 63*: 638-647 (1964)'

47. F. W. Whitehouse, and I. N. James. Chronotropic action of glucagon on the sinus node. *Proc. Soc. Exp. Biol. Med. 122*:

48. A. M. Moura, and H. Simpkins. Cyclic AMP levels in cultured myocardial cells under the influence of chronotropic and inotropic agents. *J. Mol. Cell. Cardiol. 7*: 71-77 (1975).

49. K. M. MacLeod, R. L. Rodgers, and J. H. McNeill. Characterization of glucagon-induced changes in rate, contractility and cyclic AMP levels in isolated cardiac preparations of the rat and guinea pig. *J. Pharmacol. Exp. Ther. 217*: 798-804 (1981).

50. K. Greeff. Einfluss von pharmaka suf die kontraktilitat des herzens. *Verh. Dtsch. Ges. Kreislaufforsch. 42*: 80-92 (1976).

51. A. E. Farah. Glucagon and the circulation. *Pharmacol. Rev. 35*: 181-217 (1983).

52. R. J. Kones, and J. H. Phillips. Glucagon: Present status in cardiovascular disease. *Clin. Pharmacol. Ther. 12*: 427-444 (1971).

53. H. Lydtin, L. Leidl, S. T. Schewe, W. Daniel, W. Schieri, and G. Lohmoller. Kreislaufwirkungen verschiedener applikationsformen von glucagon. *Verh. Dtsch. Ges. Inn. Med. 78*: 1551-1554 (1972).

54. T. Smitherman, R. C. Osborn, and J. M. Atkins. Cardiac dose response relationship for intravenously infused glucagon in normal intact dogs and men. *Am. Heart J. 96*: 363-371 (1978).

55. P. W. Armstrong, H. B. Gold, W. M. Daggett, W. G. Austen, and C. A. Sanders. Hemodynamic evaluation of glucagon in symptomatic heart disease. *Circulation 44*: 67-73 (1971).

56. L. Westlie, A. Andersen, J. Jervell, K. Rassmussen, and O. Storstein. Cardiovascular effects of glucagon. *Acta Med. Scand. 189*: 179-184 (1971).

57. C. C. Gruhzit, and A. Farah. Determination of the therapeutic range of gitalin in the heart-lung preparation of the dog. *J. Pharmacol. Exp. Ther. 108*: 112-116 (1953).

58. R. E. Goldstein, C. L. Skelton, G. S. Levey, D. L. Glancy, G. D. Beiser, and S. E. Epstein. Effects of chronic heart failure on the capacity of glucagon to enhance contractility and adenyl cyclase activity of human papillary muscles. *Circulation 44*: 638-648 (1971).

59. W. W. Parmley, L. Chuck, and J. Matloff. Diminished responsiveness of the failing human myocardium to glucagon. *Cardiology 55*: 211-217 (1970).

60. S. I. Said, and V. Mutt. Isolation from porcine intestinal wall of a vasoactive octocosa peptide related to secretin and glucagon. *Eur. J. Biochem. 28*: 199-204 (1972).

61. M. G. Bryant, J. M. Polak, I. Modlin, S. R. Bloom, R. H. Albuquerque, and A. G. E. Pearse. Possible dual role for vasoactive intestinal peptide as gastrointestinal hormone and neurotransmitter substance. *Lancet*: 991-993 (1976).

62. E. Weihe, and M. Reinecke. Peptidergic innervation of the mammalian sinus nodes: Vasoactive intestinal polypeptide, neurotensin, substance P. *Neurosci. Letter 26*: 283-288 (1981).

63. M. M. Miller, T. O. O'Dorisio, R. Hunsaker, C. V. Leier, D. V. Unverferth. The decline of vasoactive intestinal polypeptide (VIP) in canine myocardium during the induction of cobalt cardiomyopathy. *Circulation (abstr.) 62*: III-302 (1980).

64. G. O. Barbezat, and M. I. Grossman. Intestinal secretion: Stimulation by peptides. *Science 174*: 422-424 (1971).

65. C. J. Schwartz, D. V. Kimberg, H. E. Sherrin, M. Field, and S. I. Said. Vasoactive intestinal peptide stimulation of adenylate cyclase and active electrolyte secretion in intestinal mucosa. *J. Clin. Invest. 54*: 536-544 (1974).

66. S. R. Bloom, J. M. Polak, and A. G. E. Pearse. Vasoactive intestinal peptide and watery-diarrhea syndrome. *Lancet 2*: 14-16 (1973).

67. S. I. Said, and G. M. Makhlouf. Vasoactive intestinal polypeptide: Spectrum of biologic activity. In *Endocrinology of the Gut.* W. Y. Chey, and F. P. Brooks (eds.). Charles B. Slack, Thorofare, N.J., 1974, pp. 83-87.

68. G. M. Makhlouf, and S. I. Said. The effect of vasoactive intestinal peptide (VIP) on digestive and hormonal function. In *Gastrointestinal Hormones.* J. C. Thompson (ed.). University of Texas Press, Austin, 1975, pp. 599-610.

69. B. Desbuquois, M. H. Laudat, and P. Laudat. Vasoactive intestinal polypeptide and glucagon: Stimulation of adenylate cyclase activity via distinct receptors in liver and fat cell membranes. *Biochem. Biophys. Res. Commun. 53*: 1187-1194 (1973).

70. E. K. Frandsen, and A. J. Moody. Lipolytic action of a newly isolated vasoactive intestinal polypeptide. *Horm. Metab. Res. 5*: 196-199 (1973).

71. C. Kerins, and S. I. Said. Hyperglycemic and glycogenolytic effects of vasoactive intestinal polypeptide. *Proc. Soc. Exp. Biol. Med. 142*: 1014-1017 (1973).

72. D. V. Unverferth, M. M. Miller, R. L. Hamlin, C. V. Leier, and T. M. O'Dorisio. The role of vasoactive intestinal polypeptide in the cardiovascular system. *J. Am. Coll. Cardiol. (abstr.) 1*: 696 (1983).

73. L. Thulin, B. Nyberg, G. Tyden, and T. Sonnenfeld. Circulatory effects of VIP in anesthetized man. *Peptides 5*: 319-323 (1984).

74. S. I. Said, L. P. Bosher, J. A. Spath, and H. A. Kontos. Positive inotropic action of newly isolated vasoactive intestinal polypeptide (VIP). *Clin. Res. (abstr.) 20*: 29 (1972).

75. P. DeNeef, P. Robberecht, P. Chatelain, M. Waelbroeck, and J. Christophe. The in vitro chronotropic and inotropic effects of vasoactive intestinal peptide (VIP) on the atria and ventricular papillary muscle from cynomolgus monkey heart. *Regul. Pept. 8*: 237-244 (1984).

76. E. P. Wei, H. A. Kontos, and S. I. Said. Mechanism of action of vasoactive intestinal polypeptide on cerebral arterioles. *Am. J. Physiol. 239*: H765-H768 (1980).

77. Y. Suzuki, D. McMaster, K. Lederis, and O. P. Rorstad. Characterization of the relaxant effects of vasoactive intestinal peptide (VIP) and PHI on isolated brain arteries. *Brain Res. 322*: 9-16 (1984).

78. P. Chatelain, P. Robberecht, M. Waelbroeck, P. DeNeef, J. C. Camus, A. N. Huu, J. Roba, and J. Christophe. Topographical distribution of the secretin-

and VIP-stimulated adenylate cyclase system in the heart of five animal species. *Pflugers Arch. 397*: 100-105 (1983).

79. J. Christophe, M. Waelbroeck, P. Chatelain, and P. Robberecht. Heart receptors for VIP, PHI and secretin are able to activate adenylate cyclase and to mediate inotropic and chronotropic effects: Species variations and physiopathology. *Peptides 5*: 341-353 (1984).

80. P. Robberecht, L. Gillet, P. Chatelain, P. DeNeef, J. C. Camus, M. Vincent, J. Sassard, and J. Christophe. Specific decrease of secretin/VIP-stimulated adenylate cyclase in the heart from the lyon strain of hypertensive rats. *Peptides 5*: 355-358 (1984).

81. G. Taton, P. Ghatelain, M. Delhaye, J. C. Camus, P. DeNeef, M. Waelbroeck, K. Tatemoto, P. Robberecht, and J. Christophe. Vasoactive intestinal peptide (VIP) and peptide having N-terminal histidine and C-terminal isoleucine amide (PHI) stimulate adenylate cyclase activity in human heart membranes. *Peptides 3*: 897-900 (1982).

82. J. M. Brown, C. J. White, S. M. Sobol, and R. J. Lull. Increased left ventricular ejection fraction after a meal: Potential source of error in performance of radionuclide angiography. *Am. J. Cardiol. 51*: 1709-1711 (1983).

83. G. Ross. Cardiovascular effects of secretin. *Am. J. Physiol. 218*: 1166-1170 (1970).

84. S. Chiba. Effect of secretin on pacemaker activity and contractility in the isolated blood perfused atrium of the dog. *Clin. Exp. Pharmacol. Physiol. 3*: 167-172 (1976).

85. P. Robberecht, P. DeNeef, J. C. Camus, M. Waelbroeck, J. Fontaine, and J. Christophe. The cardiac inotropic response to secretin is lower in genetically obese (fa/fa) than in lean (fa/?) Zucker rats. *Pflugers Arch. 398*: 217-220 (1983).

86. P. Robberecht, P. DeNeef, M. Waelbroeck, J. C. Camus, J. Fontaine, J. Christophe. Secretin-induced changes in rate, contractility and adenylate cyclase activity in rat heart atria. *Pflugers Arch. 401*: 1-5 (1984).

87. N. D. Christofides, J. M. Polak, and S. R. Bloom. Studies on the distribution of PHI in mammals. *Peptides 5*: 261-266 (1984).

88. C. H. Parry. Collections from the unpublished papers of the late Caleb Hilliel Parry. *Diseases of the Heart 2*: 111-165 (1825).

89. R. J. Graves. Newly observed affection of the thyroid gland in females. *London Med. Surg. J. 7*: 516-517 (1835).

90. J. C. Aub, and N. S. Stern. The influence of large doses of thyroid extract on the total metabolism and heart in a case of heart-block. *Arch. Intern. Med.* 130-138 (1918).

91. C. S. Burwell, W. C. Smith, and D. Neighbors. The output of the heart in thyrotoxicosis, with the report of a case of thyrotoxicosis combined with primary pernicious anemia. *Am. J. Med. 178*: 157-168 (1929).

92. H. M. Thomas, Jr. Effect of thyroid hormone on circulation. *JAMA 163*: 337-341 (1957).

93. S. Humerfelt, O. Muller, and O. Storstein. The circulation in hyperthyroidism: A cardiac catheterization study before and after treatment. *Am. Heart J. 56*: 87-94 (1958).

94. A. M. Abrahamsen, J. Haarstad, and C. Oulie. Haemodynamic studies in thyrotoxicosis. Before and after treatment. *Acta Med. Scand. 174*: 463-467 (1963).

95. J. M. Bishop, K. W. Donald, and O. L. Wade. Circulatory dynamics at rest and on exercise in the hyperkinetic states. *Clin. Sci. 14*: 329-360 (1955).

96. J. J. Leonard, and W. J. deGroot. The thyroid state and the cardiovascular system. *Mod. Concepts Cardiovasc. Dis. 38*: 23-27 (1969).

97. M. V. Cohen, I. C. Schulman, A. Spenillo, and M. I. Surks. Effects of thyroid hormone on left ventricular function in patients treated for thyrotoxicosis. *Am. J. Cardiol. 48*: 33-38 (1981).

98. L. Leight, V. DeFazio, F. N. Talmers, T. J. Regan, and H. K. Hellems. Coronary blood flow, myocardial oxygen consumption, and myocardial metabolism in normal and hyperthyroid human subjects. *Circulation 14*: 90-99 (1956).

99. J. C. Forfar, A. L. Muir, S. A. Sawers, and A. D. Toft. Abnormal left ventricular function in hyperthyroidism: Evidence for a possible reversible cardiomyopathy. *N. Engl. J. Med. 307*: 1165-1170 (1982).

100. K. Talafih, K. L. Briden, and H. R. Weiss. Thyroxine-induced hypertrophy of the rabbit heart: Effect on regional oxygen extraction, flow and oxygen consumption. *Circ. Res. 52*: 272-279 (1983).

101. M. L. Marriott, and J. H. McNeill. Effect of thyroid hormone treatment on responses of the isolated working rat heart. *Can. J. Physiol. Pharmacol. 61*: 1382-1390 (1983).

102. R. A. Buccino, J. F. Spann, Jr., P. E. Pool, E. H. Sonnenblick, and E. Braunwald. Influence of the thyroid state on the intrinsic contractile properties and energy stores of the myocardium. *J. Clin. Invest. 46*: 1669-1682 (1967).

103. R. R. Taylor. Contractile properties of cardiac muscle in hyperthyroidism. *Circ. Res. 27*: 539-549 (1970).

104. M. J. Goodkind, G. E. Dambach, P. T. Thyrum, and R. J. Luchi. Effect of throxine on ventricular myocardial contractility and ATPase activity in guinea pigs. *Am. J. Physiol. 226*: 66-72 (1974).

105. P. N. Johnson, A. S. Freedberg, and J. M. Marshall. Action of thyroid hormone on the transmembrane potentials from sino-atrial node cells and atrial muscle cells in isolated atria of rabbits. *Cardiology 58*: 273-289 (1973).

106. M. F. Arnsdorf, and R. W. Childers. Atrial electrophysiology in experimental hyperthyroidism in rabbits. *Circ. Res. 26*: 575-581 (1970).

107. M. Amidi, D. F. Leon, W. J. DeGroot, F. W. Kroetz, and J. J. Leonard. Effect of the thyroid state on myocardial contractility and ventricular ejection rate in man. *Circulation 38*: 229-239 (1968).

108. R. H. Miller, F. H. Corcoran, and W. P. Baker. Second and third degree atrioventricular block with Graves' disease: A case report and review of the literature. *PACE 3*: 702-711 (1980).

109. I. Klein, and G. S. Levey. New perspectives on thyroid hormone, catecholamines, and the heart. *Am. J. Med. 76*: 167-172 (1984).

110. E. Morkin, I. L. Flink, and S. Goldman. Biochemical and physiologic effects of thyroid hormone on cardiac performance. *Prog. Cardiovasc. Dis 25*: 435-464 (1983).

111. J. H. Oppenheimer, H. L. Schwartz, M. I. Surks, D. Koerner, and W. H. Dillmann. Nuclear receptors and the initiation of thyroid hormone action. In *Recent Progress in Hormone Research*. R. O. Greep (eds.). Academic Press, New York, 1976, pp. 529-565.

112. M. J. Rovetto, A. C. Hjalmarson, H. E. Morgan, M. J. Barrett, and R. A. Goldstein. Hormonal control of cardiac myosin adenosine triphosphatase in the rat. *Circ. Res. 31*: 397-409 (1972).

113. R. Z. Litten, III, B. J. Martin, E. R. Howe, N. R. Alpert, and R. J. Solaro. Phosphorylation and adenosine triphosphatase activity of myofibrils from thyrotoxic rabbit hearts. *Circ. Res. 48*: 498-501 (1981).

114. R. A. Chizzonite, A. W. Everett, W. A. Clar, S. Jakovcic, M. Rabinowitz, and R. Zak. Isolation and characterization of two molecular variants of myosin heavy chain from rabbit ventricle. *J. Biol. Chem. 257*: 2056-2065 (1982).

115. R. Z. Litten, III, B. J. Martin, R. B. Low, and N. R. Alpert. Altered myosin isozyme patterns from pressure-overloaded and thyrotoxic hypertrophied rabbit hearts. *Circ. Res. 50*: 856-864 (1982).

116. E. Morkin, I. L. Flink, and S. Goldman. Biochemical and physiologic effects of thyroid hormone on cardiac performance. *Prog. Cardiovasc. Dis. 25*: 435-464 (1983).

117. A. F. Martin, E. D. Pagani, and R. J. Solaro. Thyroxine-induced redistribution of isoenzymes of rabbit ventricular myosin. *Circ. Res. 50*: 117-124 (1982).

118. S. K. Banerjee. Comparative studies of atrial and ventricular myosin from normal, thyrotoxic, and thyroidectomized rabbits. *Circ. Res. 52*: 131-136 (1983).

119. J. H. Oppenheimer. Thyroid hormone action at the cellular level. *Science 203*: 971-979 (1979).

120. G. D. Curfman, T. J. Crowley, and T. W. Smith. Thyroid-induced alterations in myocardial sodium- and potassium-activated adenosine triphosphatase, monovalent cation active transport, and cardiac glycoside binding. *J. Clin. Invest. 59*: 586-590 (1977).

121. K. D. Philipson, and I. S. Edelman. Thyroid hormone control of Na^+-K^+-ATPase and K^+-dependent phosphatase in rat heart. *Am. J. Physiol. 232*: C196-C201 (1977).

122. J. Suko. The calcium pump of cardiac sarcoplasmic reticulum. Functional alterations at different levels of thyroid state in rabbits. *J. Physiol. 228*: 563-582 (1973).

123. W. W. Stocker, F. J. Samaha, and L. J. DeGroot. Coupled oxidative phosphorylation in muscle of thyrotoxic patients. *Am. J. Med. 44*: 900-909 (1968).

124. J. Y. Su, H. G. Lahrtz, and P. E. Pool. Effects of hyperthyroidism on glycerol-extracted cardiac muscle. *Circulation (abstr.) 41/42*: III-202 (1970).

125. R. T. Knight. The use of spinal anesthesia to control sympathetic overactivity in hyperthyroidism. *Anesthesiology 6*: 225-230 (1945).

126. W. R. Brewster, Jr., J. P. Isaacs, P. F. Osgood, and T. L. King. The hemodynamic and metabolic interrelationships in the activity of epinephrine, norepinephrine and the thyroid hormones. *Circulation 13*: 1-20 (1956).

127. S. Goldstein, and T. Killip, III. Catecholamine depletion in thyrotoxicosis. Effect of guanethidine on cardiovascular dynamics. *Circulation 31*: 219-227 (1965).

128. W. Grossman, N. I. Robin, L. W. Johnson, H. L. Brooks, H. A. Selenkow, and L. Dexter. The enhanced myocardial contractility of thyrotoxicosis. *Ann. Intern. Med. 74*: 869-874 (1971).

129. C. Markowtiz, and W. M. Yater. Response of explanted cardiac muscle to thyroxine. *Am. J. Physiol. 100*: 162-166 (1932).

130. J. B. Van Der Schoot, and N. C. Moran. An experimental evaluation of the reputed influence of thyroxine on the cardiovascular effects of catecholamines. *J. Pharmacol. Exp. Ther. 149*: 336-345 (1965).

131. K. Wildenthal. Studies of fetal mouse hearts in organ cultures: Influence of prolonged exposure to triiodothyronine on cardiac responsiveness to isoproterenol, glucagon, theophylline, acetylcholine and dibutyryl cyclic 3',5'-adenosine monophosphate. *J. Pharmacol. Exp. Ther. 190*: 272-279 (1974).

132. K. Wildenthal, and J. R. Wakeland. Studies of isolated fetal hearts in organ culture. Evidence for a direct effect of triiodothyronine in enhancing cardiac responsiveness to norepinephrine. *J. Clin. Invest. 51*: 2702-2709 (1972).

133. J. D. Rutherford, S. F. Vatner, and E. Braunwald. Adrenergic control of myocardial contractility in conscious hyperthyroid dogs. *Am. J. Physiol. 237*: H590-H596 (1979).

134. G. S. Levey. Catecholamine sensitivity, thyroid hormone and the heart. *Am. J. Med. 50*: 413-420 (1971).

135. L. R. Williams, R. J. Lefkowitz, A. M. Watannabe, D. R. Hathaway, and H. R. Besch, Jr. Thyroid hormone regulation of β-adrenergic receptor number. *J. Biol. Chem. 252*: 2787-2789 (1977).

136. W. Krawietz, K. Werdan, and E. Erdmann. Effect of thyroid status on β-adrenergic receptor, adenylate cyclase activity and guanine nucleotide regulatory unit in rat cardiac and erythrocyte membranes. *Biochem. Pharmacol. 31*: 2463-2469 (1982).

137. J. A. Whitsett, J. Pollinger, and S. Matz. β-adrenergic receptors and catecholamine sensitive adenylate cyclase in developing rat ventricular myocardium: Effect of thyroid status. *Pediatr. Res. 16*: 463-469 (1982).

138. L. T. Williams, R. J. Lefkowitz, A. M. Watanabe, D. R. Hathaway, and H. R. Besch, Jr. Thyroid hormone regulation of β-adrenergic receptor number. *J. Biol. Chem. 252*: 2787-2789 (1977).

139. P. J. Scarpace, and I. B. Abrass. Thyroid hormone regulation of rat heart, lymphocyte, and lung β-adrenergic receptors. *Endocrinology 108*: 1007-1011 (1981).

140. J. Tse, R. W. Wrenn, and J. F. Kuo. Thyroxine-induced changes in characteristics and activities of β-adrenergic receptors and adenosine 3',5'-monophosphate and guanosine 3',5'-monophosphate systems in the heart may be related to reputed catecholamine supersensitivity in hyperthyroidism. *Endocrinology 107*: 6-16 (1980).

141. Extrathyroidal actions of TRH. *Lancet 2*: 560-561 (1984).

142. G. D. Borowski, C. D. Garofano, L. I. Rose, and R. A. Levy. Blood pressure response to thyrotropin-releasing hormone in euthyroid subjects. *J. Clin. Endocrinol. Metab. 58*: 197-200 (1984).

143. D. V. Cohn, R. R. MacGregor, and L. I. Chiu. Calcemic fraction A: Biosynthesis peptide precursor of parathyroid hormone. *Proc. Natl. Acad. Sci. USA 69*: 1521 (1972).

144. J. F. Habener, D. Powell, and T. M. Murray. Parathyroid hormone: Secretion and metabolism in vivo. *Proc. Natl. Acad. Sci. USA 68*: 2986 (1971).

145. J. M. Carterbury, G. S. Levey, and E. Reiss. Activation of renal cortical adenylate cyclase by circulating immunoreactive parathyroid hormone fragments. *J. Clin. Invest. 52*: 524-531 (1977).

146. C. D. Arnaud, and A. Tenenhouse. Parathyroid hormone. In *International Encyclopedia of Pharmacology and Therapeutics*, Vol. 1, section 51: Parathyroid hormone thyroidictonin and related drugs. H. Rasmussen (ed.). Pergamon Press, Oxford, 1970, p. 197.

147. L. M. Sherwood, W. B. Lundberg, and J. H. Tarqovnik. Synthesis and secretion of PTH in vitro. *Am. J. Med. 50*: 568-570 (1971).

148. E. Reiss, J. M. Canterbury, M. A. Bercovitz, and E. L. Kaplan. Role of phosphate in secretion of parathyroid hormone in man. *J. Clin. Invest. 49*: 2146-2153 (1970).

149. G. D. Aurbach, and L. R. Chase. Cyclic 3'5'-adenylic acid in bone and the mechanism of action of PTH. *Fed. Proc. 29*: 1179 (1970).

150. H. Rasmuss. Ionic and hormonal control of calcium homeostasis. *Am. J. Med. 50*: 567-575 (1971).

151. G. L. Nelson, L. R. Chase, and G. D. Aurbach. Parathyroid hormone sensitive adenyl cyclase in isolated renal tubules. *Endocrinology 86*: 511-520 (1970).

152. M. R. Wills, J. Wortzman, C. Y. C. Pak, and F. C. Bartter. The role of PTH in the gastrointestinal absorption of calcium. *Clin. Sci. 39*: 89-95 (1970).

153. G. A. Charbon. A rapid and selective vasodilator effect of parathyroid hormone. *Eur. J. Pharmacol. 3*: 275-278 (1968).

154. P. K. T. Pang, M. C. M. Yang, R. Shew, and T. E. Tenner, Jr. The vasorelaxant action of parathyroid hormone fragments on isolated rat tail artery. *Blood Vessels 22*: 57-64 (1985).

155. P. Weidmann, S. G. Massry, J. W. Coburn, M. H. Maxwell, J. Atleson, and C. R. Kleeman. Blood pressure effects of acute hypercalcemia. Studies in patients with chronic renal failure. *Ann. Intern. Med. 76*: 741-745 (1972).

156. S. Sialer, D. H. McKenna, R. J. Corliss, and G. R. Rowe. Systemic and coronary hemodynamic effects of intravenous administration of calcium chloride. *Arch. Int. Pharmacodyn. Ther. 169*: 177-184 (1967).

157. I. Christensson, K. Hellstrom, and B. Wengle. Blood pressure in subjects with hypercalcaemia and primary hyperparathyroidism detected in a health screening programme. *Eur. J. Clin. Invest. 7*: 109-113 (1977).

158. E. Bogin, S. G. Massry, and I. Harary. Effect of parathyroid hormone on rat heart cells. *J. Clin. Invest. 67*: 1215-1227 (1981).

159. P. B. Furspan, J. S. K. Sham, R. L. Shew, G. Peng, and P. K. T. Pang. Cardiac action of bovine parathyroid hormone fragment (1-34) in some lower vertebrates. *Gen. Comp. Endocrinol. 56*: 246-251 (1984).

160. J. S. K. Sham, A. D. Kenny, and P. K. T. Pang. Cardiac actions and structural-activity relationship of parathyroid hormone on isolated frog atrium. *Gen. Comp. Endocrinol. 55*: 373-377 (1984).

161. Y. Katoh, K. L. Klein, R. A. Kaplan, W. G. Sanborn, and K. Kurokawa. Parathyroid hormone has a positive inotropic action in the rat. *Endocrinology 109*: 2252-2254 (1981).

162. G. M. A. Palmieri, D. F. Nutting, S. K. Bhattacharya, T. E. Bertorini, and J. C. Williams. Parathyroid ablation in dystrophic hamsters: Effects on a Ca content and histology of heart, diaphragm, and rectus femoris. *J. Clin. Invest. 68*: 646-654 (1981).

163. T. D. Giles, B. J. Iteld, and K. L. Rives. The cardiomyopathy of hypoparathyroidism: Another reversible form of heart muscle disease. *Chest 79*: 225-229 (1981).

164. A. Csapo. Actomyosin formation by estrogen action. *Am. J. Physiol. 162*: 406-410 (1950).

165. T. M. King, W. V. Whitehorn, B. Reeves, and R. Kubota. Effects of estrogen on composition and function of cardiac muscle. *Am. J. Physiol. 196*: 1282-1285 (1959).

166. K. Hall, R. C. Burbank, and J. Cohen. Hepatotrophic and cardiotrophic properties of sex hormones. *Br. Med. J. 1*: 396-399 (1941).

167. K. Ueland, and J. T. Parer. Effects of estrogens on the cardiovascular system of the ewe. *Am. J. Obstet. Gynecol. 96*: 400-406 (1966).

168. M. Gulzow, and G. Brusch. Elektrokardiogrammveranderungen durch einen follikelhormonstofs. *Med. Klin. 42*: 140 (1947).

169. H. F. H. Hamilton. The cardiac output in normal pregnancy: As determined by the Cournand right heart catheterization technique. *J. Obstet. Gynaecol. Br. Emp. 56*: 548-552 (1949).

170. E. L. DeBeer, H. A. Keizer, and P. Schiereck. The effect of some sex hormones on the isovolumetric pressure curve of the rabbit's left ventricle. *Steroids 41*: 67-77 (1983).

171. W. E. Stumpf, M. Sar, and G. Aumuller. The heart: A target organ for estradiol. *Science 196*: 319-321 (1977).

172. S. N. Baksi, and M. J. Hughes. Modulation by estradiol of rabbit atrial chronotropic response to histamine. *Basic Res. Cardiol. 78*: 505-509 (1983).

173. W. S. Colucci, M. A. Gimbrone, Jr., and R. W. Alexander. Regulation of myocardial and vascular α-adrenergic receptor affinity: Effects of guanine nucleotides, cations, estrogen, and catecholamine depletion. *Circ. Res. 55*: 78-88 (1984).

174. H. C. McGill, Jr., V. C. Anselmo, J. M. Buchanan, and P. J. Sheridan. The heart is a target organ for androgen. *Science 207*: 775-777 (1980).

175. J. Mendoza, and W. C. DeMello. Influence of progesterone on membrane potential and peak tension of myocardial fibres. *Cardiovasc. Res. 8*: 352-361 (1974).

176. F. S. LaBella, I. Bihler, and R. S. Kim. Progesterone derivatives that bind to the digitalis receptor: Effects on ^{86}Rb uptake and contractility in the isolated guinea pig heart. *Can. J. Physiol. Pharmacol. 62*: 1057-1064 (1984).

177. E. L. DeBeer, H. A. Keizer, P. Schiereck, and C. Van Amerongen. In *Cardiovascular System Dynamics: Models and Measurements*. T. Kenner, R. Busse, and H. Hinghofer-Szalkay (eds.). Planum Press, New York, 1982, pp. 613-620.

178. D. C. Homans. Peripartum cardiomyopathy. *N. Engl. J. Med. 312*: 1432-1436 (1985).

179. G. H. Williams, and E. Braunwald. Endocrine and nutritional disorders and heart disease. In *Heart Disease, a Textbook of Cardiovascular Medicine*. E. Braunwald (ed.). Saunders, Philadelphia, 1984, pp. 1722-1747.

180. D. N. Orth, D. P. Island, and G. W. Liddle. Experimental alteration of the circadian rhythm in plasma cortisol concentration in man. *J. Clin. Endocrinol. Metab. 27*: 549-558 (1967).

181. G. F. Cahill, Jr. Action of adrenal cortical steroids on carbohydrate metabolism. In *The Human Adrenal Cortex*. N. P. Christy (ed.). Harper & Row, New York, 1971, p. 205.

182. A. O. Davies, and R. J. Lefkowitz. In vitro desensitization of beta adrenergic receptors in human neutrophils. *J. Clin. Invest. 71*: 565-571 (1983).

183. S. Kalsner. Mechanism of hydrocortisone potentiation of responses to epinephrine and norepinephrine in rabbit aorta. *Circ. Res. 24*: 383-395 (1969).

184. A. J. Kauman. Potentiation of the effects of isoproterenol and noradrenalin by hydrocortisone in cat heart muscle. *Naunyn-Schmiedebergs Arch. Pharmacol. 273*: 134-153 (1972).

185. J. C. Besse, and A. D. Bass. Potentiation by hydrocortisone of responses to catecholamines in vascular smooth muscle. *J. Pharmacol. Exp. Ther. 154*: 224-238 (1966).

186. S. Kalsner. Steroid potentiation of responses to sympathomimetic amines in aortic strips. *Br. J. Pharmacol. 36*: 582-593 (1969).

187. J. H. Exton, E. H. Friedman, A. Wong, J. D. Brineaux, J. D. Corbin, and C. R. Park. Interaction of glucocorticoids with glucagon and epinephrine in the control of gluconeogenesis and glycolysis in liver and of lipolysis in adipose tissue. *J. Biol. Chem. 247*: 3579-3588 (1972).

188. S. T. Holgate, C. J. Baldwin, and A. E. Tattersfield. Beta adrenergic agonist resistance in normal human airways. *Lancet 2*: 375-377 (1977).

189. G. W. Liddle. Pathogenesis of glucocorticoid disorders. *Am. J. Med. 53*: 638-649 (1972).

190. L. Krakoff, G. Nicolis, and B. Amsel. Pathogenesis of hypertension in Cushing's syndrome. *Am. J. Med. 58*: 216-220 (1975).

191. L. J. Soffer, A. Iannaecone, and J. L. Gabrilove. Cushing's syndrome (study of 50 patients). *Am. J. Med. 45*: 116-124 (1961).

192. L. W. Swanson, P. E. Sawchenko, J. Rivier, and W. W. Vale. Organization of ovine corticotropin releasing factor (CRF)—immunoreactive cells and fibers in the rat brain: An immunohistochemical study. *Neuroendocrinology 36*: 165-186 (1983).

193. M. R. Brown, and L. A. Fisher. Corticotropin-releasing factor: Effects on the autonomic nervous system and visceral systems. *Fed. Proc. 44*: 243-248 (1985).

194. M. Gothert. ACTH increases stimulation-evoked norepinephrine release from sympathetic fibers by acting on presynaptic ACTH receptors. *Eur. J. Pharmacol. 76*: 295-296 (1981).

195. M. Gothert. Facilitatory effect of adrenocorticotropic hormone and related peptides on Ca^+-dependent noradrenaline release from sympathetic nerves. *Neuroscience 11*: 1001-1009 (1984).

196. A. Hershko, P. Mamont, R. Shields, and G. M. Tomkins. Pleiotypic response. *Nature 232*: 206-211 (1971).

197. P. Cuatrecasas. Insulin receptor of liver and fat cell membranes. *Fed. Proc. 32*: 1838-1846 (1973).

198. S. Jacobs, Y. Schecter, K. Bissell, and P. Cuatrecasas. Purification and properties of insulin receptors from rat liver membranes. *Biochem. Biophys. Res. Commun. 77*: 981-988 (1977).

199. G. F. Cahill, Jr. Physiology of insulin in man. *Diabetes 20*: 785-802 (1971).

200. P. Libby. Long-term culture of contractile mammalian heart cells in a defined serum-free medium that limits non-muscle cell proliferation. *J. Mol. Cell. Cardiol. 16*: 803-811 (1984).

201. J. S. Ingwall, and K. Wildenthal. Fetal mouse hearts in organ culture studies in cardiac metabolism. *Recent Adv. Stud. Cardiac Struct. Metab. 12*: 621-633 (1978).

202. P. Libby, and K. V. O'Brien. Culture of quiescent arterial smooth muscle cells in a defined serum free medium. *J. Cell. Physiol. 115*: 217-223 (1983).

203. S. S. Ahmed, G. A. Jaferi, R. M. Narang, and T. J. Regan. Preclinical abnormality of left ventricular function in diabetes mellitus. *Am. Heart J. 89*: 153-158 (1975).

204. T. J. Regan, M. M. Lyons, S. S. Ahmed, G. E. Levinson, H. A. Oldewurtel, M. R. Ahmad, and B. Haider. Evidence for cardiomyopathy in familial diabetes mellitus. *J. Clin. Invest. 60*: 885-899 (1977).

205. J. A. D'Elia, L. A. Weinrauch, R. W. Healy, J. A. Libertino, R. F. Bradley, and O. S. Leland, Jr. Myocardial dysfunction without coronary artery disease in diabetic renal failure. *Am. J. Cardiol. 43*: 193-199 (1979).

206. S. M. Factor, T. Minase, and E. H. Sonnenblick. Clinical and morphological features of human hypertensive-diabetic cardiomyopathy. *Am. Heart J. 99*: 446-458 (1980).

207. L. M. Shapiro, A. P. Howat, and M. M. Calter. Left ventricular function in diabetes mellitus. I. Methodology, and prevalence and spectrum of abnormalities. *Br. Heart J. 45*: 122-128 (1981).

208. B. R. Lucchesi, M. Medina, and F. J. Kniflen. The positive inotropic action of insulin on the canine heart. *Eur. J. Pharmacol. 18*: 107-115 (1972).

209. J. C. Lee, and S. E. Downing. Effects of insulin on cardiac muscle contraction and responsiveness to norepinephrine. *Am. J. Physiol. 230*: 1360-1365 (1976).

210. B. Bhagat, W. J. Burke, and W. S. Dhalla. Insulin induced enhancement of uptake of noradrenaline in atrial strips. *Br. J. Pharmacol. 74*: 325-332 (1981).

211. M. M. B. Page, R. B. W. Smith, and P. J. Watkins. Cardiovascular effects of insulin. *Br. Med. J. 1*: 430-432 (1976).

212. F. Jacobsen, and N. J. Christensen. Stimulation of heart rate by insulin: Uninfluenced by beta adrenergic blockade in rabbits. *Scand. J. Clin. Lab. Invest. 39*: 253-256 (1979).

213. N. J. Christensen. Acute effects of insulin on cardiovascular function and noradrenaline uptake and release. *Diabetologia 25*: 377-381 (1983).

214. L. J. Markovitz, and H. R. Freund. Insulin and glucagon have significant inotropic properties in the normal and septic isolated rat heart. *Curr. Probl. Surg. 41*: 274-277 (1984).

215. J. Christensen, H. J. G. Gunderson, L. Hegedus, F. Jacobsen, C. E. Mogensen, R. Osterby, and E. Vittinghus. Acute effects of insulin on plasma norepinephrine and the cardiovascular system. *Metabolism 29*: 1138-1145 (1980).

216. N. J. Christensen. Plasma epinephrine and norepinephrine in untreated diabetics during fasting and after insulin administration. *Diabetes 23*: 1-8 (1974).

217. J. W. Roew, J. B. Young, K. L. Minaker, A. L. Stevens, J. Pallotta, and L. Landsberg. Effect of insulin and glucose infusions on sympathetic nervous system activity in normal man. *Diabetes 30*: 219-225 (1981).

218. A. Malhotra, S. Penpargkul, F. S. Fein, E. H. Sonnenblick, and J. Scheuer. The effect of streptozotocin-induced diabetes in rats on cardiac contractile proteins. *Circ. Res. 49*: 1243-1250 (1981).

219. M. Rubinstein, T. F. Schaible, A. Malhotra, and J. Scheuer. Effects of graded insulin therapy on cardiac function in diabetic rats. *Am. J. Physiol. 246*: H453-H458 (1984).

220. T. J. Regan, C. F. Wu, C. K. Yeh, H. A. Oldewurtel, and B. Haider. Myocardial composition and function in diabetes. The effects of chronic insulin use. *Circ. Res. 49*: 1268-1277 (1981).

221. W. B. Kannel, M. Hjortland, and W. P. Castelli. The role of diabetes in congestive heart failure: The Framingham study. *Am. J. Cardiol. 34*: 29-36 (1974).

222. F. S. Fein, R. S. Aronson, C. Nordin, B. Miller-Green, and E. H. Sonnenblick. Altered myocardial response to ouabain in diabetic rats: Mechanics and electrophysiology. *J. Mol. Cell. Cardiol. 15*: 769-784 (1983).

223. P. Rakin, A. O. Pietri, R. Unger, and W. A. Shannon, Jr. The effect of diabetic control on the width of skeletal-muscle capillary basement membrane in patients with type I diabetes mellitus. *N. Engl. J. Med. 309*: 1546-1550 (1983).

224. J. L. Kostyo. Rapid effects of growth hormone on amino acid transport and protein synthesis. *Ann. NY Acad. Sci. 148*: 389-396 (1968).

225. A. Karner. Anabolic action of growth hormone. *Ann. NY Acad. Sci. 148*: 408-418 (1968).

226. C. Frelin. The regulation of protein turnover in newborn rat heart cell cultures. *J. Biol. Chem. 255*: 11149-11155 (1980).

227. D. G. Penney, J. C. Dunbar, Jr., and M. S. Baylerian. Cardiomegaly and haemodynamics in rats with a transplantable growth hormone-secreting tumour. *Cardiovasc. Res. 19*: 270-277 (1985).

228. M. Csanady, L. Gaspar, M. Hogye, and N. Gruber. The heart in acromegaly: An echocardiographic study. *Int. J. Cardiol. 2*: 349-357 (1983).

229. R. C. Smallridge, S. Rajfer, J. Davia, and M. Schaaf. Acromegaly and the heart. An echocardiographic study. *Am. J. Med. 66*: 22-27 (1979).

230. J. V. Souadjian. Hypertension in acromegaly. *Am. J. Med. Sci.* November: 629-633 (1967).

231. W. L. McGuffin, Jr., B. M. Sherman, J. Roth, P. Gorden, R. Kahn, W. C. Roberts, and P. L. Frommer. Acromegaly and cardiovascular disorders. A prospective study. *Ann. Intern. Med, 81*: 11-18 (1974).

232. J. T. Lie, and S. J. Grossman. Pathology of the heart in acromegaly: Anatomic findings in 27 autopsied patients. *Am. Heart J. 100*: 41-53 (1980).

233. L. Rossi, G. Thiene, L. Caregoro, R. Giordano, and S. Lauro. Dysrhythmias and sudden death in acromegalic heart disease. A clinicopathologic study. *Chest 72*: 495-504 (1977).

234. J. A. Kellgron, J. Ball, and G. K. Tutton. The articular and other limb changes in acromegaly. *Q. J. Med. 21*: 405-412 (1952).

235. D. F. Horrobin. In *Prolactin: Physiology and Clinical Significance*. Medical and Technical Publishing, Lancaster, 1973.

236. A. G. Frantz, D. L. Kleinberg, and G. L. Noel. *Recent Prog. Horm. Res. 28*: 527-534 (1972).

237. H. Friesen, C. Belanger, H. Guyda, and P. Hwang. In *Lactogenic Hormones*. G. E. W. Woldstenholme, and J. Knight (eds.). Churchill-Livingston, London, 1972.

238. J. F. Sassin, A. G. Frantz, E. D. Weitzman, and S. Kapen. Human prolactin: 24-hour pattern with increased release during sleep. *Science 177*: 1205-1207 (1972).

239. D. F. Horrobin, P. G. Burstyn, I. J. Lloyd, N. Durkin, A. Lipton, and K. L. Muiruri. Actions of prolactin on human renal function. *Lancet 2*: 352-355 (1971).

240. P. G. Burstyn, D. F. Horrobin, and M. S. J. Mankin. *Endocrinology 55*: 369-377 (1972).

241. M. S. Manku, B. A. Nassar, and D. F. Horrobin. Effects of prolactin on the responses of rat aortic and arteriolar smooth-msucle preparations to noradrenaline and angiotensin. *Lancet 2*: 991-994 (1973).

242. B. A. Nassar, M. S. Manku, J. D. Reed, M. Tynan, and D. F. Horrobin. Actions of prolactin and frusemide on heart rate and rhythm. *Br. Heart J. 2*: 27-29 (1974).

243. B. A. Nassar, D. F. Horrobin, M. Tynan, M. S. Manku, and P. A. Davies. *Endocrinology 97*: 1008-1013 (1975).

244. M. Karmazyn, M. J. Daly, M. P. Moffat, and N. S. Dhalla. A possible mechanism of inotropic action of prolactin on rat heart. *Am. J. Physiol. 243*: E458-E463 (1982).

245. I. H. Page and F. M. Bumpus. In *Angiotensin, Handbuch der Experimentellen Pharmakologies*. I. H. Page, and F. M. Bumpus (eds.). Springer-Verlag, Berlin, 1974.

246. J. R. Blair-West, J. P. Coghlan, D. A. Denton, J. W. Funder, B. A. Scoggins, and R. D. Wright. The effect of the heptapeptide and hexapeptide fragments of angiotensin II on aldosterone secretion. *J. Clin. Endocrinol. Metab. 32*: 575-578 (1971).

247. B. G. Zimmerman. Actions of angiotensin on adrenergic nerve endings. *Fed. Proc. 37*: 199-202 (1978).

248. W. W. Douglas. Polypeptides-angiotensin, plasma kinins and others. In *The Pharmacological Basis of Therapeutics*. A. G. Gilman, L. S. Goodman, and A. Gilman (eds.). Macmillan, New York, 1980, pp. 647-667.

249. N. O. Fowler, and J. C. Holmes. Coronary and myocardial actions of angiotensin. *Circ. Res. 14*: 191-201 (1964).

250. P. Dempsey, Z. McCallum, K. Kent, and T. Cooper. Direct myocardial effects of antiotensin II. *Am. J. Physiol. 220*: 477-481 (1971).

251. J. Koch-Weser. Nature of the inotropic action of angiotensin on ventricular myocardium. *Circ. Res. 16*: 230-237 (1965).

252. J. Koch-Weser. Myocardial actions of angiotensin. *Circ. Res. 14*: 337-344 (1964).

253. A. Ilanes, J. Perex-Olea, Q. Quevedo, A. Ortiz, and M. Lazo. Influence of angiotensin on the effects of tyramine upon the contractile force of isolated rabbit atria. *J. Pharmacol. Exp. Ther. 158*: 487-493 (1967).

254. K. Starke. Action of angiotensin on uptake, release, and metabolism of 14C-noradrenalin by isolated rabbit hearts. *Eur. J. Pharmacol. 14*: 112-123 (1971).

255. S. M. Lanier, and K. U. Malik. Attenuation by prostaglandins of the facilitory effect of angiotensin II at adrenergic prejunctional sites in the isolated rat heart. *Circ. Res. 51*: 594-601 (1982).

256. R. H. Roth. Action of angiotensin on adrenergic nerve endings: Enhancement of norepinephrine biosynthesis. *Fed. Proc. 31*: 1358-1363 (1972).

257. M. J. Peach, F. M. Bumpus, and P. A. Khairallah. Inhibition of norepinephrine uptake in hearts by angiotensin II and analogs. *J. Pharmacol. Exp. Ther. 169*: 291-300 (1969).

258. B. G. Zimmerman. Effect of acute sympathectomy on responses to angiotensin and norepinephrine. *Circ. Res. 11*: 780-791 (1962).

259. H. Iven, R. Pursche, and G. Zetler. Field stimulation responses of guinea pig atria as influenced by the peptides angiotensin, bradykinin and substance P. *Naunyn. Schmiedebergs Arch. Pharmacol. 312*: 63-69 (1980).

260. J. L. Thompson. Effect of angiotensin on the cardio-accelerator response to sympathetic nerve stimulation in isolated rabbit hearts. *Proc. Soc. Exp. Biol. Med. 135*: 825-831 (1970).

261. Y. Furukawa, P. Scipione, and M. N. Levy. Effects of angiotensin II on the cardiac responses to sympathetic nerve stimulation in dogs. *Hypertension 5*: 26-33 (1983).

262. S. M. Lanier, and K. U. Malik. Facilitation of adrenergic transmission in the canine heart by intracoronary infusion of angiotensin II: Effect of prostaglandin synthesis inhibition. *J. Pharmacol. Exp. Ther. 227*: 676-682 (1983).

263. K. M. Baker, C. P. Campanile, G. J. Trachte, and M. J. Peach. Identification and characterization of the rabbit angiotensin II myocardial receptor. *Circ. Res. 54*: 286-293 (1984).

264. A. M. Lefer. Influence of mineralocorticoids and cations on the inotropic effect of angiotensin and norepinephrine in isolated cardiac muscle. *Am. Heart J. 73*: 674-680 (1967).

265. M. J. Peach. Molecular actions of angiotensin. *Biochem. Pharmacol. 30*: 2745-2751 (1981).

266. A. S. F. Ash, and H. O. Schild. Receptors mediating some actions of histamine. *Br. J. Pharmacol. 27*: 427-439 (1966).

267. J. W. Black, W. A. M. Duncan, C. J. Durant, C. R. Ganellin, and E. M. Parsons. Definition and antagonism of histamine H_1 receptors. *Nature 236*: 385-390 (1972).

268. G. J. Durant, C. R. Ganellin, and M. E. Parsons. Chemical differentiation of histamine H_1 and H_2 receptor antagonists. *J. Med. Chem. 18*: 905-909 (1975).

269. G. J. Durant, C. R. Ganellin, and M. E. Parsons. Dimaprit, a highly specific histamine H_1 receptor agonist. Part 2 structure-activity considerations. *Agents Actions 7*: 39-43 (1977).

270. W. W. Douglas. Histamine and 5 hydroxytryptamine (serotonin) and their antagonists. In *The Pharmacological Basis of Therapeutics*. A. G. Gilman, L. S. Goodman, and A. Gilman (eds.). Macmillan, New York, 1980, pp. 609-646.

271. D. A. A. Owen. Histamine receptors in the cardiovascular system. *Gen. Pharmacol. 8*: 141-156 (1977).

272. G. Majno, S. M. Shea, and M. Leventhal. Endothelial contraction induced by histamine-type mediators. An electron microscopic study. *J. Cell. Biol. 42*: 647-672 (1969).

273. D. Reinhardt. Hirzwirkungen von histamin. *Anaesthesist 28*: 67-77 (1979).

274. R. Levi. Effects of exogenous and immunologically released histamine on the isolated heart: A quantitative comparison. *J. Pharmacol. Exp. Ther. 182*: 227-238 (1972).

275. H. Scholz. Inotropic drugs and their mechanisms of action. *JACC 4*: 389-397 (1984).

276. J. H. McNeill, and S. C. Verma. Blockade by burinamide of the effects of histamine and histamine analogs on cardiac contractility, phosphorylase activation and cyclic adenosine monophosphate. *J. Pharmacol. Exp. Ther. 188*: 180-188 (1974).

277. R. Levi, N. Capurno, and C. H. Lee. Pharmacologic characterization of cardiac histamine receptors: Sensitivity to H_1 and H_2 receptor agonists and antagonists. *Eur. J. Pharmacol. 30*: 328-335 (1975).

278. R. Levi, G. Allan, and J. H. Zavecz. Cardiac histamine receptors. *Fed. Proc. 35*: 1942-1947 (1976).

279. J. H. Zavecz, and L. Roberto. Histamine-induced negative inotropism: Mediation by H_1-receptors. *J. Pharmacol. Exp. Ther. 206*: 274-280 (1978).

280. R. Levi, A. Hordof, and R. Edie. Histamine effects on human atria. *Circulation 57/58*: II-105 (1978).

281. T. R. Engel, and J. C. Luck. Histamine$_2$ receptor antagonism by cimetidine and sinus-node functions. *N. Engl. J. Med. 301*: 591-592 (1979).

282. Y. Hattori, and R. Levi. Adenosine selectively attenuates H_2- and beta-mediated cardiac responses to histamine and norepinephrine: An unmasking of H_1- and alpha-mediated responses. *J. Pharmacol. Exp. Ther. 231*: 215-223 (1984).

283. S. S. Gross, Z. G. Guo, R. Levi, W. H. Bailey, and A. A. Chenouda. Release of histamine by sympathetic nerve stimulation in the guinea pig heart and modulation of adrenergic responses: A physiologic role for cardiac histamine? *Circ. Res. 54*: 516-526 (1984).

284. W. J. Higgins. 5-Hydroxytryptamine-induced tachyphylaxis of the molluscan heart and concomitant desensitization of adenylate cyclase. *J. Cycl. Nucl. Res. 3*: 293-302 (1977).

285. M. J. Sole, A. Shum, and G. R. VanLoon. Serotonin metabolism in the normal and failing hamster heart. *Circ. Res. 45*: 629-634 (1979).

286. J. M. Kay, P. M. Keane, and K. L. Suyama. Pulmonary hypertension induced in rats by monocrotaline and chronic hypoxia is reduced by p-chloraphenylalanine. *Respiration 47*: 48-56 (1985).

287. J. Comroe, B. VanLingen, B. Stroud, and A. Roncoroni. Reflex and direct cardiopulmonary effects of 5HT (serotonin). *Am. J. Physiol. 173*: 379-385 (1953).

288. T. Tomita, K. Umegaki, and E. Hayashi. The appearance of exhausted platelets due to a duration of hypertension in stroke-prone spontaneously hypertensive rats. *Thromb. Res. 37*: 195-200 (1985).

289. D. G. Grahame-Smith. The cardinoid syndrome. In *Metabolic Control and Disease*. P. K. Boudy, and L. E. Rosenberg (eds.). Saunders, Philadelphia, 1980. p. 1703.

290. G. K. Aghajanion, and R. Y. Wang. Physiology and pharmacology of central serotonergic neurons. In *Psychopharmacology: A Generation of Progress*. M. A. Lipton, A. DiMascio, and K. F. Killam (eds.). Raven Press, New York, 1978, pp. 171-183.

291. D. G. Wyse. Relationship of blood pressure to the responsiveness of an isolated human artery to selected agonists and to electrical stimulation. *J. Cardiovasc. Pharmacol. 6*: 1083-1091 (1984).

292. C. Su, and T. Uruno. Excitatory and inhibitory effects of 5-hydroxytrypamine in mesenteric arteries of spontaneously hypertensive rats. *Eur. J. Pharmacol. 106*: 283-290 (1984).

293. P. L. McLennan. Antagonism by ketanserin of 5-HT-induced vasodilation. *Pharmacology 104*: 313-318 (1984).

294. T. E. Mecca, and R. C. Webb. Vascular responses to serotonin in steroid hypertensive rats. *Hypertension 6*: 887-892 (1984).

295. T. Godfraind, M. Finet, J. S. Lima, and R. C. Miller. Contractile activity of human coronary arteries and human myocardium in vitro and their sensitivity to calcium entry blockade by nifedipine. *J. Pharmacol. Exp. Ther. 230*: 514-518 (1984).

296. E. Bassenge. Tonus of epicardial main arteries and dynamic dynamic stenosis. *Z. Kardiol. 73*: 55-61 (1984).

297. R. A. Cohen. Platelet-induced neurogenic coronary contractions due to accumulation of the false neurotransmitter, 5-hydroxytryptamine. *J. Clin. Invest. 75*: 286-292 (1985).

298. M. A. Mena, and H. Vidrio. On the mechanism of the coronary dilator effect of serotonin in the dog. *Eur. J. Pharmacol. 36*: 1-5 (1976).

299. M. L. Cohen, R. W. Fuller, and K. S. Wiley. Evidence for 5-HT$_2$ receptors mediating contraction in vascular smooth muscle. *J. Pharmacol. Exp. Ther. 218*: 421-425 (1981).

300. J. R. Fozard, and A. T. M. Mobarok Ali. Receptors for 5-hydroxytryptamine on the sympathetic nerves of the rabbit heart. *Naunyn-Schmiedebergs Arch. Pharmacol. 301*: 223-235 (1978).

301. V. Kecskemieti, K. Kelemen, R. Marko, and J. Knoll. Drugs affecting the calcium-dependent slow depolarization mechanism of the cardiac cell membrane. *Adv. Myocardiol. 3*: 205-214 (1982).

302. T. J. C. Higgins, D. Allsopp, and P. J. Bailey. Mechanisms of stimulation of rat cardiac muscle by 5-hydroxytryptamine. *J. Pharmacol. 30*: 2703-2707 (1981).

303. K. Sakai, and M. Akima. An analysis of the stimulant effects of 5-hydroxytryptamine on isolated, blood-perfused rat heart. *Eur. J. Pharmacol. 55*: 421-424 (1979).

304. J. R. Fozard, and A. T. Mobarok Ali. Dual mechanism of the stimulant action of N.N-dimethyl-5-hydroxy-tryptamine (bufotenine) on cardiac sympathetic nerves. *Eur. J. Pharmacol. 49*: 25-30 (1978).

305. W. J. Higgins, D. A. Price, and M. J. Greenberg. FMRFamide increases the adenylate cyclase activity and cyclic AMP level of molluscan heart. *Eur. J. Pharmacol. 48*: 425-430 (1978).

306. F. Urthaler, G. R. Haoeman, and T. N. James. Hemodynamic components of a cardiogenic hypertensive chemoreflex in dogs. *Circ. Res. 42*: 135-142 (1978).

307. J. A. Ojewole, and K. I. Akinwanda. Effects of cholinomimetic drugs on reptilian atrial muscles. *Methods Find. Exp. Clin. Pharmacol. 6*: 378-387 (1984).

308. T. Tokimasa. The effect of 5-hydroxytryptamine on the slow inward current of bullfrog atrium. *Jpn. Heart J. 22*: 227-237 (1981).

309. J. J. Theron, R. Biagio, A. C. Meyer, S. Boekkooi, and J. C. Seegers. The effect of a serotonin inhibitor on the serotonin content and ultrastructure of rat atria and ventricles with special reference to atrial granules. *Life Sci. 23*: 111-120 (1978).

310. M. Hamberg, J. Svensson, and B. Samuelsson. Thromboxane: A new group of biologically active compounds derived from prostaglandin endoperoxides. *Proc. Natl. Acad. Sci. USA 72*: 2994-2998 (1975).

311. S. Moncada, R. Gryglewski, S. Buting, and J. R. Vane. An enzyme isolated from arteries transforms prostaglandin endoperoxides to an unstable substance that inhibits platelet aggregation. *Nature 263*: 663-665 (1976).

312. A. J. Marcus. The role of lipids in platelet function with particular reference to the arachidonic acid pathway. *J. Lipid Res. 19*: 793-826 (1978).

313. S. Moncada, R. J. Flower, and J. R. Vane. Prostaglandins, prostacycline and thromboxane A2. In *The Pharmacological Basis of Therapeutics*. A. G. Gilman, L. S. Goodman, and A. Gilman (eds.). Macmillan, New York, 1980, pp. 668-681.

314. P. Needleman. The synthesis and function of prostaglandins in the heart. *Fed. Proc. 35*: 2376-2381 (1976).

315. M. Sivakoff, E. Pure, W. Hsueh, and P. Needleman. Prostaglandins and the heart. *Fed. Proc. 38*: 78-82 (1979).

316. P. Needleman, and G. Kaley. Cardiac and coronary prostaglandin synthesis and function. *N. Engl. J. Med. 298*: 1122-1128 (1978).

317. J. Szczeklik, A. Szczeklik, and R. Nizankowski. Haemodynamic changes induced by prostacyclin in man. *Br. Heart J. 44*: 254-258 (1980).

318. T. M. Fitzpatrick, I. Alter, E. J. Corey, P. W. Ramwell, J. C. Rose, and P. A. Kot. Cardiovascular responses to PGI_2 (prostacyclin) in the dog. *Circ. Res. 42*: 192-194 (1978).

319. J. Nakano, and J. R. McCurdy. Cardiovascular effects of prostaglandin E_1. *J. Pharmacol. Exp. Ther. 156*: 538-547 (1967).

320. J. Szczeklik, J. S. Dubiel, M. Mysik, Z. Pyzik, R. Krol, and T. Horzela. Effects of prostaglandin E_1 on pulmonary circulation in patients with pulmonary hypertension. *Br. Heart J. 40*: 1397-1401 (1978).

321. M. E. Gerritsen, and M. P. Printz. Sites of prostaglandin synthesis in the bovine heart and isolated bovine coronary microvessels. *Circ. Res. 49*: 1152-1163 (1981).

322. P. Mentz, and K. E. Pawelski. The dependence of cardiac eicosanoid effects of changes of calcium concentration. *Biomed. Biochim. Acta. 43*: S167-S170 (1984).

323. S. Chierchia, C. Patrono, F. Crea, G. Ciabattoni, R. De Caterina, G. A. Cinotti, A. Distante, and A. Maseri. Effects of intravenous prostacyclin in variant angina. *Circulation 65*: 470-477 (1982).

324. M. Karmazyn, and N. S. Dhalla. Physiological and pathophysiological aspects of cardiac prostaglandins. *Can. J. Physiol. Pharmacol. 61*: 1207-1225 (1983).

325. B. Pitt, M. J. Shea, J. L. Romson, and B. R. Lucchesi. Prostaglandins and prostaglandin inhibitors in ischemic heart disease. *Ann. Intern. Med. 99*: 83-92 (1983).

326. W. G. Nayler, M. Purchase, and G. J. Dusting. Effect of prostacyclin infusion during low-flow ischaemia in the isolated perfused rat heart. *Basic Res. Cardiol. 79*: 125-134 (1984).

327. P. Ganz, J. Gaspar, W. S. Golucci, W. H. Barry, G. H. Mudge, and R. W. Alexander. Effects of prostacyclin on coronary hemodynamics at rest and in response to cold pressor testing in patients with angina pectoris. *Am. J. Cardiol. 53*: 1500-1504 (1984).

328. P. D. Hirsh, W. B. Campbell, J. T. Willerson, and L. D. Hillis. Prostaglandins and ischemic heart disease. *Am. J. Med. 71*: 1009-1026 (1981).

329. M. Tanabe, Z. I. Terashita, S. Fujiwara, N. Shimamoto, N. Goto, K. Nishikawa, and M. Hirata. Coronary circulatory failure and thromboxane A_2

release during coronary occlusion and reperfusion in anaesthetised dogs. *Cardiovasc. Res. 16*: 99-106 (1982).

330. T. Godfraind, M. Finet, J. S. Lima, and R. C. Miller. Contractile activity of human coronary arteries and human myocardium in vitro and their sensitivity to calcium entry blockade by nifedipine. *J. Pharmacol. Exp. Ther. 230*: 514-518 (1984).

331. F. Berti, M. Lentati, and M. Usardi. The species specificity of prostaglandin E_1 effects on isolated hearts. *Med. Pharmacol. Exp. 13*: 233-240 (1965).

332. S. Uemura, T. Nakanishi, S. Matsuoka, W. F. Friedman, and J. M. Jarmakani. Inotropic effects of prostaglandin D_2 and E_1 on the newborn rabbit heart. *Pediatr. Res. 18*: 1277-1281 (1984).

333. S. Roux, J. G. Latour, P. Theroux, J. P. Clozel, and M. G. Bourassa. Prostaglandin E_1 increases myocardial contractility in the conscious dog. *Can. J. Physiol. Pharmacol. 62*: 1505-1510 (1984).

334. U. N. Das, A. M. Lee, and G. J. Barritt. Prostanoids can modify response to electrical stimulus and $^{45}Ca^{2+}$ exchange in isolated myocardial muscle cells. *Prostaglandins Leukotrienes Med. 12*: 305-314 (1983).

335. P. Mentz, K. E. Pawelski, and C. H. Giessler. Drug induced inhibition of the cardiac effects of U 46619 as a thromboxane A_2-like agonist. *Biomed. Biochim. Acta 43*: S163-S166 (1984).

336. W. V. Huval, S. Lelcuk, P. D. Allen, J. A. Mannick, D. Shepro, and H. B. Hechtman. Determinants of cardiovascular stability during abdominal aortic aneurysmectomy (AAA). *Ann. Surg. 199*: 216-222 (1984).

337. R. H. Carmona, T. C. Tsao, and D. D. Trunkey. The role of prostacyclin and thromboxane in sepsis and septic shock. *Arch. Surg. 119*: 189-192 (1984).

338. W. R. Kukovetz, S. Holzmann, A. Wurm, and G. Poch. Prostacyclin increases cAMP in coronary arteries. *J. Cycl. Nucl. Res. 5*: 469-475 (1979).

339. M. Karmazyn, B. S. Tuana, and N. S. Dhalla. Effect of prostaglandins on rat heart sarcolemmal ATPases. *Can. J. Physiol. Pharmacol. 59*: 1122-1130 (1981).

340. Y. Yui, H. Nakajima, C. Kawai, and T. Murakami. Prostacyclin therapy in patients with congestive heart failure. *Am. J. Cardiol. 50*: 320-324 (1982).

Index